Midwifery Skills
at a Glance

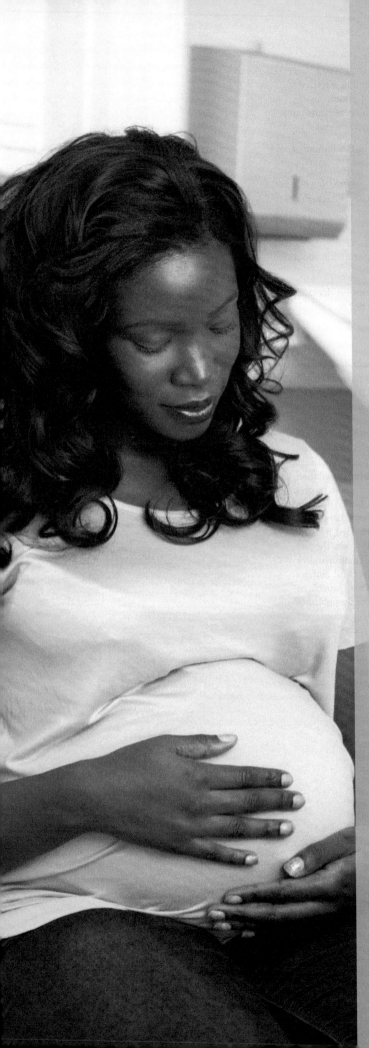

Midwifery Skills

at a Glance

Edited by

Patricia Lindsay
RN, RM, MSc, PGCEA, DHC
Registered Midwife

Carmel Bagness
MA, RN, RM, ADM, PGCEA
Professional Lead for Midwifery & Women's Health
Royal College of Nursing
London, UK

Ian Peate OBE
FRCN, EN(G), RGN, DipN (Lond), RNT, BEd
(Hons), MA (Lond) LLM
Editor in Chief British Journal of Nursing
Visiting Professor of Nursing St George's
University of London and Kingston University
London
Head of School
School of Health Studies
Gibraltar

WILEY Blackwell

Registered Offices: John Wiley & Sons, Inc., 111 River Street, Hoboken, NJ 07030, USA
John Wiley & Sons, Ltd., The Atrium, Southern Gate, Chichester, West Sussex, PO19 8SQ, UK

Editorial Office: 9600 Garsington Road, Oxford, OX4 2DQ, UK

For details of our global editorial offices, customer services, and more information about Wiley products visit us at www.wiley.com.

Wiley also publishes its books in a variety of electronic formats and by print-on-demand. Some content that appears in standard print versions of this book may not be available in other formats.

Limit of Liability/Disclaimer of Warranty

Library of Congress Cataloging-in-Publication Data

Names: Lindsay, Patricia, 1951- editor. | Bagness, Carmel, editor. |
Peate, Ian, editor.
Title: Midwifery skills at a glance / edited by Patricia Lindsay, Carmel Bagness,
Ian Peate.
Description: Hoboken, NJ : Wiley, 2018. | Series: At a glance series |
Includes bibliographical references and index. |
Identifiers: LCCN 2017025965 (print) | LCCN 2017026824 (ebook) | ISBN
9781119233985 (pdf) | ISBN 9781119235125 (epub) | ISBN 9781119233916 (pbk.)
Subjects: | MESH: Midwifery | Handbooks
Classification: LCC RG950 (ebook) | LCC RG950 (print) | NLM WQ 165 | DDC
618.2--dc23
LC record available at https://lccn.loc.gov/2017025965

Cover design: Wiley
Cover image: © Monkey Business Images/Shutterstock

Set in Minion Pro 9.5/11.5 by Aptara

10 9 8 7 6 5 4 3 2 1

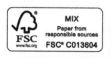

Contents

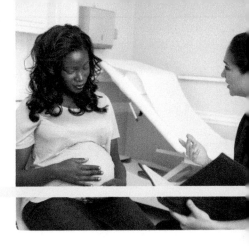

Part 3 The woman or neonate with different needs 111

Induction/stimulation of labour

Care skills for the woman with complex needs

Care skills for the baby with complex needs

Wound care

Prevention of venous thromboembolism

Part 4   Drug administration in midwifery   149

Routes of administration

Pain relief

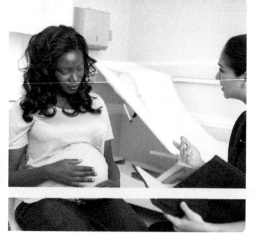

Contributors

Adelaide Aduboffour RN, RM, MSc, Fellow HEA, ITEC
Chapters 30, 67
Midwifery Lecturer
University of West London;
Perineal Specialist Midwife
Chelsea and Westminster and West Middlesex University
    Hospital;
Director
Peri Health Limited, London, UK

Andrea Aras-Payne MA, PGDip, BSc (Hons), RM, RGN, FHEA fe
Chapter 27
Senior Lecturer
University of West London
London, UK

Carmel Bagness MA RN RM ADM PGCEA
Chapters 10, 17, 20, 21
Professional Lead for Midwifery and Women's Health
Royal College of Nursing
London, UK

Karen Bartholomew RN, RM, BA (Hons) MSc, PGCEA
Chapter 33
Senior Lecturer/Course Leader
Anglia Ruskin University
Chelmsford, Essex, UK

Marcia Bartholomew RN, RM, MSc Health Promotion, PgDip
Teaching and Learning in Health Care
Chapters 28, 78, 79
Senior Lecturer
University of West London
London, UK

Judy Bothamley RN, RM, ADM PGCEA, MA
Chapter 81
Senior Lecturer (Midwifery)
University of West London
London, UK

Maureen Boyle RN, RM, MSc, PGCEA
Chapter 50
Senior Lecturer (Midwifery)
University of West London
London, UK

Jenny Brewster RN, RM, BSc (Hons), MEd, PGCEA
Chapter 26
Senior Lecturer in Midwifery
University of West London
London, UK

Alison Busby BNurs, RN, RM, ADM, MSc, PGDE
Chapter 43
Senior Lecturer Midwifery
School of Health Sciences
University of Manchester
Manchester, UK

Helen Crafter RN, RM, FP Cert, PGCEA, MSc
Chapter 18
Senior Lecturer in Midwifery
University of West London
London, UK

Doreen Crawford MA, PGCE, BSc (Hons) SRN, RSCN
Chapter 1
Consultant Nurse Editor Nursing Children and Young
    People
Crawford-McKenzie Healthcare Consultancy
Nurse Advisor, Independent Healthcare Consultancy

Helen Donovan BSc (Hons) Med, RGN, RHV, RM
Chapter 77
Professional Lead for Public Health Nursing
Royal College of Nursing;
Visiting Senior Lecturer
University of Hertfordshire;
Independent Nurse Lead
NHS Barnet CCG Governing Body
London, UK

Sarah Emberley RM, BSc, MSc, PGDPE
Chapters 6, 22, 47
Midwifery Lecturer/Clinical Skills
Bournemouth University
Bournemouth
Dorset, UK

David Foster PhD, MSc, RN, RM, FCIPD
Chapters 14, 15, 16
Registered Midwife, formerly Head of the Nursing,
    Midwifery and Allied Health Professions Policy Unit
    and Midwifery Advisor at the Department of Health
London, UK

Sophie French RN, RM, MSc, PGCEA, Senior Fellow HEA
Chapters 41, 42, 59, 60
Midwifery Lecturer
King's College London University
London, UK

Rose Gallagher
Chapters 1, 5, 9, 51, 52
Professional Lead for Infection Prevention and Control
Royal College of Nursing
London, UK

Shauna Gnanapragasam BSc (Hons), MSc
Chapters 48, 76
Midwifery Clinical Skills Tutor
Anglia Ruskin University
Cambridge, UK

Clare Gordon RM, SCPHN–SN, BSc (Hons), MSc, PG Cert Academic
Practice
Chapters 32, 73
Senior Lecturer in Midwifery
Programme Leader Berkshire Midwifery
University of West London
London, UK

Caroline Hunter RM, MSc, FHEA
Chapter 44
Senior Teaching Fellow, Midwifery
Florence Nightingale Faculty of Nursing, Midwifery and
    Palliative Care
King's College London
London, UK

Louise Jenkins RN, RM, BSc (Hons), MSc, PGDip, SFHEA
Chapters 57, 61
Deputy Head of Department Midwifery, Child and
    Community Nursing
Anglia Ruskin University
Essex, UK

Julie Jones RM, Dip HE, BSc (Hons) Mid, BSc (Hons) Psych, PG Cert
Academic Practice, MMedSci
Chapters 24, 53
Senior Lecturer in Midwifery
University of West London
London, UK

Lyn Jones RMN, RGN, RM, MSc
Chapters 54, 55, 56
Senior Lecturer Midwifery
Anglia Ruskin University
Cambridge, UK

Patricia Lindsay RN, RM, ADM, MSc, PGCEA, DHC
Chapters 11, 12, 13, 29, 37, 40, 45, 49, 62, 75
Registered Midwife

Jayne E Marshall PHFEA, PhD, MA, PGCEA, ADM, RM, RGN
Chapters 70, 71
Foundation Professor of Midwifery
NMC Lead Midwife for Education
School of Allied Health Professions
University of Leicester
Leicester, UK

Marianne Mitchell MA, BSc (Hons), DipHE, RM, RN, FHEA
Chapter 19
Senior Lecturer, Midwifery
University of Hertfordshire
Hertfordshire, UK

Martha Murtagh RM, RGN, RNT, MSc Ed
Chapter 80
Clinical Skills Facilitator
Regional Hospital Mullingar
Co. Westmeath, Eire

Kate Nash RGN, RM, BSc Hons, MSc
Chapter 72
Senior Lecturer in Midwifery
University of West London
London, UK

Ian Peate OBE
FRCN, EN(G), RGN DipN (Lond), RNT BEd (Hons), MA (Lond) LLM
Chapters 2, 4
Editor in Chief British Journal of Nursing;
Visiting Professor of Nursing St George's University of
    London and
Kingston University, London;
Head of School
School of Health Studies
Gibraltar

Elisabeth Podsiadly RN, BScN, MSc, PGCEA, Cert in Perinatal
Nursing
Chapters 63, 64, 65, 66
Senior Lecturer, Neonatal Nursing
Faculty of Health, Social Care and Education
Kingston University and St George's University of London
London, UK

David Quayle PGC, RGN, FETC
Chapter 58
Clinical Services Manager
Air Alliance Medflight UK
Birmingham Airport
Birmingham, UK

Hazel Ransome RM, BSc (Hons), PGCLTHE, HEA Fellow
Chapters 68, 69
Senior Lecturer in Midwifery
Kingston University
Kingston Upon Thames
Surrey, UK

Maureen D Raynor RMN, RGN, RM, ADM, PGCEA, MA
Chapter 36
Senior Midwifery Lecturer
Leicester School of Nursing and Midwifery
De Montfort University
Leicester, UK

Lindsey Rose MSc, RM, HEA Fellow
Chapter 39
Senior Midwifery Lecturer
Anglia Ruskin University
Cambridge, UK

Jancis Shepherd RN, RM, ADM, MTD, PGCEA, MA, Senior Fellow of the Higher Education Academy
Chapter 31
Lead Midwife for Education and Head of Midwifery
University of West London
London, UK

Antonio Sierra RN RM MSc
Chapter 74
Lead Midwife for Midwifery Education
West Hertfordshire NHS Hospitals
Hertfordshire,UK

Helen Simpson RN, RM, RSCPHN, HEA Fellow
Chapter 23
Senior Lecturer in Midwifery
University of West London
London, UK

Sheena Simpson RN, RM, 405 Course, BSc (Hons), PGDip in Education, MA, HEA Fellow
Chapter 25
University of West London
London, UK

Sara Smith RM, BSc, MSc, PGCE
Chapter 34
Senior Lecturer in Midwifery
Anglia Ruskin University
Essex, UK

Tina South RM, BA (Hons), BSc (Hons), PGCert (Research), PhD(c)
Chapter 38
Midwifery Lecturer
University of West London
London, UK

Kim Sunley CMIOSH
Chapters 7, 8
National Officer (Health and Safety)
Royal College of Nursing
London, UK

Maxine Wallis-Redworth RN, RM, BSc, MSc, PGCEA, IBCLC
Chapters 48, 76
Course Leader BSc (Hons) Midwifery
Anglia Ruskin University
Cambridge, UK

Helen Williams RN, RM, DPSM, MSc
Chapters 14, 15, 16
Associate Director and Head of Midwifery
Yeovil District Hospital NHS Foundation Trust
Somerset, UK

Nicola Winson MA, PGCEA, RN, RM
Chapter 3
Senior Lecturer in Midwifery
University of West London
London, UK

Sandy Wong MSc (Midwifery), ADM, RM, RGN, PgCert (HE), FHEA
Chapters 35, 46
Senior Lecturer Midwifery
University of Hertfordshire
Hertfordshire, UK

Foreword

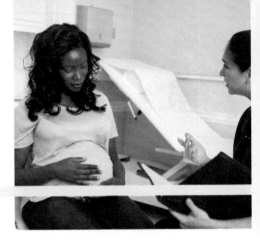

I am delighted to have been asked to write the foreword for this text. The *At a Glance* series has supported nursing practice for many years; to have a *Midwifery Skills* text is a bonus for practitioners.

Midwives and student midwives are faced with a plethora changes and challenges in practice and finding relevant and up to date information, which is accessible to support practice, is essential.

Maternity care and services are provided in a variety of settings through different models of care, resulting in midwives and student midwives working in varied surroundings and situations; consequently, keeping current with practices and procedures can sometimes seem overwhelming. This text provides an easy access resource to fundamental aspects of practice.

The *At a Glance* series provides information in easy to digest bite-size pieces, practitioners can dip in to particular aspects of practice as needed. The text gives key messages supported by illustrations to provide clear guidance for practice.

The book is divided into four parts with further subdivisions and chapters, which makes navigation of themes and topics easy and the presentation of complex skills is made simple.

This text will be of great value to all student midwives, midwives and mentors who will appreciate the importance of the book when undertaking new midwifery skills and in preparation for practice assessment, for example OSCEs (Objective, Structured Clinical Examination) and professional conversations.

Midwives can be reassured that the content is appropriate for practice; many of the authors are renowned for their expertise in their midwifery practice and education as well as expertise provided by professionals from outside of midwifery care, for example in supporting safe practice in the work environment.

The editors bring their own experience to support the gravitas of the text. Dr Patricia Lindsay is an experienced midwife, midwife teacher and academic, who has supported the development of students and midwives throughout her career. Patricia is passionate about safe and effective care for women and families and appreciates the importance of ensuring that professionals have access to contemporary, relevant information for care. Professor Ian Peate shares his nursing experience and the application to midwifery practice. In addition, Ian has a long-established academic career and has produced excellent resources for professional development. Carmel Bagness is an experienced practitioner and academic and brings to the text her wide experience of midwifery practice and issues relating to women's healthcare and health policy.

I have no doubt that this book will prove to be an invaluable resource for midwives, student midwives and other practitioners working in maternity services. Professionals will find themselves dipping in to the text to support their daily practice. The clear concise approach will provide midwives with the confidence to address practice safely as well as signposting to further information or evidence where appropriate.

Gail Johnson
Professional Advisor for Education
Royal College of Midwives

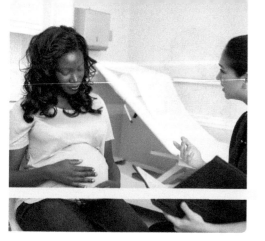

Preface

At the time of writing, midwifery as a profession, and the context of practice, are undergoing some changes. However, the needs of women, their babies and their families remain the same and midwives have a unique and privileged role in providing care to this client group. A high level of competence and confidence in skills ensures care is safe and of a high quality. In addition, the use of evidence and local knowledge, as well as understanding policy and services available, must be drawn on to provide the best care possible. Multiprofessional working and the judicious use of voluntary and other services are also required to provide a complete service to the childbearing woman and her family.

This text has been written with the student midwife in mind but is equally useful for others providing care, for example maternity support workers, registered midwives or medical students. It offers educational support for practitioners in the application of midwifery knowledge to clinical practice in relation to women, their babies and their families through the childbearing continuum. It follows the familiar *At a Glance* format, which has been shown to be beneficial to the success of student groups' knowledge of many topics. This volume is unique in that it is related to midwifery practice, but demonstrates links with other relevant healthcare professionals across many disciplines who may also care for women during the childbearing period. The text therefore draws on the wisdom of expert practitioners in midwifery, or in fields pertinent to

midwifery, and offers readable, easily digestible information, supported with illustrations to enhance application to practice. Wherever possible the voice of service users has been included to add a different, and important, perspective, one which is often absent from skills books.

The chapters reflect a variety of skills, ranging from fundamental personal care skills to more complex matters such as ECG monitoring or assessment of clinical deterioration. In addition, topics related to risk management and quality assurance are also addressed. When using the book, and carrying out clinical care, practitioners must remain aware of and abide by standards set and published by the regulatory bodies such as NMC Code (*The Code,* 2015. London: Nursing and Midwifery Council. Available at: https://www.nmc.org.uk/globalassets/sitedocuments/nmc-publications/nmc-code.pdf). They must also remain aware that psychosocial care skills are equally important.

While the information in the chapters provides guidance and insight, the reader must ensure that they are competent to carry out the care and, where necessary, have had their competence assessed and confirmed. Everyone has a duty to ensure that care provided is safe and effective at all times, is based on the best available evidence and the woman must be central to every interaction.

Patricia Lindsay
Carmel Bagness
Ian Peate

The basics of care

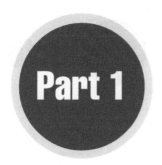

Part 1

Infection prevention and control

Box 1.1 Infections may:

- Be transmitted person to person (e.g. mother to baby, staff to patient, baby to mother)
- Be as a result of a communicable disease/infection in pregnancy e.g. chickenpox
- Originate as a direct result of a healthcare intervention
- Occur naturally as a result of displacement of bacteria present on or in the body (endogenous infection)
- Be as a result of an outbreak or infection in a healthcare setting e.g. Group A Streptococcal infection

Box 1.2 Common infections associated with childbirth.

- Urinary tract infections
- Mastitis
- Wound infections (LSCS and perineal)
- Epidural site infection
- Vascular access device related infections
- Bacteraemia/fungaemia
- Respiratory infection/pneumonia
- Influenza

Box 1.3 Key recommendations for best practice around infection prevention and control.

- Compliance with organisational policies
- Documentation of the need for practices in place to mitigate the spread of infection
- Information to the woman and visitors re precautions required
- Specimens as required and action on results
- Attention to cleanliness of the physical environment (room or incubator)
- Focus on hand hygiene before and after leaving the room/incubator/cot
- Observation of any negative psychological effects of isolation

Box 1.4 Signs and symptoms of neonatal sepsis.

- An infant who is irritable, continuously crying, has a weak cry or is lethargic and difficult to rouse
- Poor tone, flat frog-like posture/hypotonic, the so called 'Floppy baby'
- Not interested in feeds, or who has feeding difficulties, infants who are vomiting and not tolerating their feeds
- Hypoglycaemia or hyperglycaemia
- Hypothermia or hyperthermia measured at lower than 36°C or higher than 38°C
- Cold peripheries and prolonged capillary refill time (greater than 2 seconds)
- Tachypnoea: rate over 60 breaths per minutes and signs and symptoms of respiratory distress, grunting, sternal and intercostal retractions – pneumonia is much more common in early onset sepsis
- Deviation from expected heart rate
- Bradycardia, is a sign unique to neonates and infants who were developing septic shock when compared to older children
- Hypoxia: saturations less than 90% in air
- Infant a poor colour appears ashen, has cyanosis, a non-blanching rash or has skin mottling
- There may be local signs of infection such as septic spots, omphalitis, umbilical flare, sticky eyes
- Oliguria, few or no wet nappies
- Diarrhoea and distended abdomen sometimes clinically suggestive of necrotising enterocolitis

Key points

- The midwife has a key role to play in preventing and controlling infection.
- Midwives should always deem the development of infection as an adverse event, whilst monitoring and investigating and managing all infections as part of good practice.

Midwifery Skills at a Glance, First Edition. Edited by Patricia Lindsay, Carmel Bagness and Ian Peate.
© 2018 John Wiley & Sons, Ltd. Published 2018 by John Wiley & Sons, Ltd.

The prevention of infection is a core element of safe and effective midwifery practice. Midwives and other healthcare professionals should consider the development of infection as an 'adverse' event, and monitor and investigate all infections as part of their organisation's patient safety systems and learning culture. Box 1.1 indicates how infections may occur.

As knowledge of microbiology and the epidemiology of multiresistant organisms has increased, prevention now also includes the avoidance of colonisation of bacteria of clinical importance including (but not limited to):

- *Staphylococcus aureus* (including PVL strains)
- Meticillin-resistant *Staphylococcus aureus* (MRSA)
- *Pseudomonas aeruginosa*
- Multidrug-resistant Gram-negative bacteria (MDR GNB) such as *Klebsiella pneumonia* and *Escherichia coli* (*E. coli*)
- *Mycobacterium tuberculosis*
- Fungi and yeasts.

Viruses can also be problematic, in particular blood-borne viruses (hepatitis B and C, HIV) and chickenpox.

Box 1.2 provides examples of common infections associated with pregnant and postnatal women.

A number of different practice interventions are described supporting the midwife to prevent or interrupt the development of infection or colonisation, which may lead to risks specifically in-patient care setting. They are:

- The use of standard precautions (see Chapter 4)
- Knowledge and compliance of organisational infection prevention and control policies and guidance
- Active laboratory surveillance and reporting of cases of infection
- Screening of women/babies
- Vaccination of staff, women and babies
- High standards of cleanliness
- Education and information on hygiene, infection and prevention methods.

Many women and babies who develop an infection recover well; a small proportion go on to develop sepsis, a potentially life-threatening condition (Chapter 5). The importance of sepsis as a cause of maternal death has been recognised in reports such as MBRRACE UK.

Sepsis cannot be transmitted from person to person. It is a condition that occurs due to overwhelming infection, resulting in an immune cascade leading to septic shock. It can affect both mothers and neonates. Information on neonatal sepsis is detailed below. See Chapter 5 for the management of sepsis in adults.

Isolation: Physical (source) isolation has traditionally been used to separate people receiving hospital care from others due to a risk of spread of infection. In midwifery and neonatal care, isolation may be through the provision of single room accommodation (for mother or mother and baby) or an incubator/cot in the neonatal setting.

The route of transmission for the infection must always be known; this identifies which specific practice precautions are required. Box 1.3 indicates the requirements when source isolation is used.

Identifying neonatal infection, and preventing and managing neonatal sepsis

Midwives are uniquely placed to identify deviations from the normal in the newborn they care for as part of holistic family-centred care. There are some factors that can predispose to a higher risk of early-onset neonatal sepsis. The neonate may be exposed to organisms from the mother during pregnancy as well as vaginal delivery and in many cases of early-onset neonatal sepsis there have been intrapartum complications identified. Identifying these babies and providing the appropriate management will save lives.

Assessment of the neonate

NICE (2014a) recommends that all infants born to women who had prelabour rupture of the membranes at term are closely observed for the first 12 hours of life (at 1, 2, 6 and 12 hours).

The assessments recommended are:

- Temperature
- Heart rate
- Respiratory rate
- Presence of respiratory grunting
- Significant subcostal recession
- Presence of nasal flare
- Presence of central cyanosis, confirmed by pulse oximetry if available
- Skin perfusion assessed by capillary refill
- Floppiness, general wellbeing and feeding.

If any of the above are present, a neonatologist assesses the baby and advises the family of any need for transfer to appropriate neonatal services if required. In the absence of a neonatal assessment (e.g. non-hospital settings) an urgent referral or transfer to a hospital will be required.

Neonatal sepsis can present with subtle and non-specific symptoms. By the time sepsis is considered the infant may already be very ill. NICE recommendations (2014b) include the use of the red flag to support clinical decision making and British Association of Perinatal Medicine (BAPM) have developed a Newborn Early Warning Trigger and Track (NEWTT) framework to alert midwives to babies who need further help. The framework provides a visual prompt, aiding the identification of abnormal parameters by using a colour code.

Signs and symptoms of sepsis are provided in Box 1.4.

The diagnosis of shock does not require that a neonate be hypotensive. This is a late finding in septic shock and when it occurs confirms progression towards decompensated shock (Robinson *et al.* 2008). A tense or bulging anterior fontanelle is suggestive of meningitis, common in late-onset sepsis. The assessment of the infant's fontanelles should be made with the infant held and supported in an upright position.

Temperature instability can be an indication of infection. An neonate who is difficult to keep warm is a concern, as too is a baby who develops pyrexia due to pyrogens secreted by the bacteria.

2 Hand hygiene

Figure 2.1 The chain of infection.

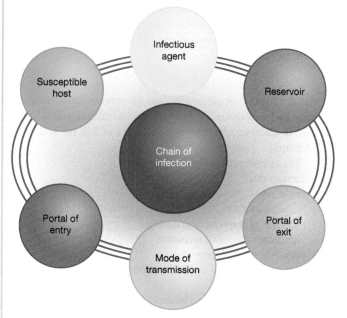

Key point
Hand hygiene is the single most important activity for minimising the likelihood of infection, in every setting.

Figure 2.2 Hand-washing technique.
Source: *Nursing Practice: Knowledge and Care*, First Edition. Edited by Ian Peate, Karen Wild and Muralitharan Nair. © 2014 John Wiley & Sons, Ltd. Reproduced with permission of John Wiley & Sons.

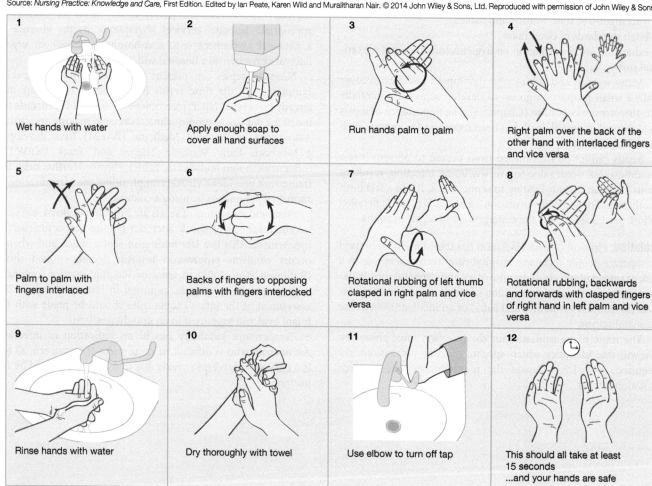

1 Wet hands with water	**2** Apply enough soap to cover all hand surfaces	**3** Run hands palm to palm	**4** Right palm over the back of the other hand with interlaced fingers and vice versa
5 Palm to palm with fingers interlaced	**6** Backs of fingers to opposing palms with fingers interlocked	**7** Rotational rubbing of left thumb clasped in right palm and vice versa	**8** Rotational rubbing, backwards and forwards with clasped fingers of right hand in left palm and vice versa
9 Rinse hands with water	**10** Dry thoroughly with towel	**11** Use elbow to turn off tap	**12** This should all take at least 15 seconds ...and your hands are safe

Midwifery Skills at a Glance, First Edition. Edited by Patricia Lindsay, Carmel Bagness and Ian Peate.
© 2018 John Wiley & Sons, Ltd. Published 2018 by John Wiley & Sons, Ltd.

Healthcare-associated infections (HCAIs) cost the health service millions of pounds per year, as well as causing women and their families unnecessary suffering and concern.

In the mid 1800s, Semmelweis established that hospital-acquired diseases were transmitted via the hands of healthcare workers. He observed that maternal mortality rates, predominantly attributed to puerperal fever, were higher in one clinic than another. As a consequence, Semmelweis recommended that hands be scrubbed using chlorinated lime solution before every contact.

Healthcare-associated infections

An HCAI is described by the 2006 Health Care Act as any infection to which a person may be exposed or is made susceptible (or more susceptible) in circumstances where healthcare is being, or has been delivered, to that or any other individual, and the risk of exposure to the infection, or susceptibility (or increased susceptibility) to it, is directly or indirectly attributable to the provision of healthcare.

HCAIs are the most common complication affecting those in hospital; the problem does not just affect people in hospital and hospital workers. HCAIs occur in any healthcare setting, including the general practice setting, clinics and long-term care facilities. HCAI is a potentially preventable adverse event, as opposed to unpredictable complications. Anybody working in or entering any healthcare facility can transmit infection or become infected. This risk can be significantly reduced when effective infection prevention and control procedures are implemented.

It is acknowledged that not all infections are preventable. Managing infection control and ensuring best practice can improve care outcomes and service user safety significantly.

Transmission of infections can occur through contaminated hands of a healthcare worker, equipment and medical devices used.

All healthcare workers will come into contact with people who have infections and/or contagious diseases; they must know how to prevent or reduce the transmission of infection.

The National Institute for Health and Care Excellence has produced evidence-based guidelines regarding management and how to prevent and control HCAIs.

Hand hygiene

Hand hygiene is seen as the single most important activity for minimising the likelihood of infection. Pathogens on the hands of midwives can be removed by hand washing if transmission is to be prevented. Infection involves a cycle of events that permits the spread (transmission) of infection occurring (Figure 2.1).

Healthcare workers, including midwives, have the greatest potential to spread micro-organisms that can result in infection; this is related to the number of times that they have contact with people in the care environment. Hands, therefore, are very efficient vehicles for the transmission of micro-organisms.

Hands should be decontaminated before direct contact with women and after any activity or contact that contaminates the hands; this includes after gloves have been removed. Alcohol hand gels and rubs are a practical alternative to soap and water; however, alcohol is not a cleaning agent. Hands that are visibly dirty or potentially grossly contaminated must be washed with soap and water and dried thoroughly. Hand preparation increases the effectiveness of decontamination. Whenever feasible, staff should have access to the means to clean their hands at the point of care; where possible soap and water should be used. However, this is not always possible with the placement of sinks or access to sinks in the home. The ability to clean the hands is possible when the midwife uses alternative methods.

Detergent wipes should be used if soap and water is not available and this should be followed by drying the hands thoroughly with paper towels or air drying; then alcohol gel can be used. Only use alcohol gel if the hands are visibly clean; using alcohol gel on contaminated hands renders the solution ineffective. Detergent wipes and hand rubs should be readily available at the point of care; if not, the chance of using them will be lost and hands will retain potentially dangerous microbes. Alcohol gel should be used between different care activities with the woman or baby.

The midwife should keep nails short, clean and polish free and should avoid wearing wristwatches and jewellery, particularly rings with ridges or stones. Artificial nails must not be worn and any cuts and abrasions must be covered with a waterproof dressing.

Wristwatches and any bracelets should be removed and long sleeves rolled up before washing the hands and wrists. The NHS has implemented a 'naked below the elbows' rule that has banned healthcare workers from wearing long sleeves, wrist watches and jewelry to promote effective hand and wrist washing; this includes the avoidance of wearing ties when carrying out clinical activity.

Hospitals are unique places that differ considerably in terms of the risk of potential infection spread when compared to a 'normal' home environment. While risks occur wherever direct contact between people or equipment happens, inpatient hospitals have a large number of people who are living in a small physical area. Moreover, those being cared for may have direct contact with a large number of people as a result of their on going care needs, allowing for many more opportunities for micro-organisms to be spread from one person to another than would normally occur at home. Some of these micro-organisms may be resistant to antibiotics.

Figure 2.2 demonstrates the correct technique for hand washing.

The five moments of hand hygiene (Figure 2.3, which can be found in the Appendices at the end of the book) define the key times, providing a standardised approach to hand washing that is simple and straightforward.

Along with an understanding of hand hygiene, the midwife must also understand how infection is transmitted. Knowing how and when to apply the fundamental principles of infection prevention is key to controlling infection.

Service user's view

'I was scared of coming in as you hear all sorts about infection but my midwife made a point of washing her hands each time she touched me and she made sure everyone else did as well!'

Comment from mother of twins

3 Infectious diseases in pregnancy

Table 3.1 Infectious organisms and diseases caused.

	Disease	Route of spread	Incubation period	Specific signs	Effect in pregnancy
Viruses	Chicken pox (Varicella)	Droplet inhalation; contact with fluid from blisters	10–21 days	Spots on face and chest, becoming blisters, fever	Fetal varicella syndrome; fetal loss; after 36 weeks the baby may be born with active chicken pox
	Glandular fever	Saliva	2–7 weeks	Sore throat, fever, lymphadenopathy	Possible association with low birthweight
	Cytomegalo-virus	Body fluids: saliva, urine, genital fluids	28–60 days	Fever, tiredness, sore throat, hepatitis, joint pain, anorexia	Congenital cytomegalovirus infection, low birthweight, neural impairment, fetal loss
	Mumps	Droplet infection; saliva	12–25 days	Fever, malaise, swollen parotid glands	Possible miscarriage if infected in first trimester
	Measles	Droplet infection	10 days. Rash appears 14 days	Cough, runny nose, fever, conjunctivitis, blotchy rash, Koplik's spots in mouth	Miscarriage, stillbirth, preterm birth
	Rubella	Droplet infection	12–23 days	Low fever, sore throat, blotchy rash, swollen glands	Congenital rubella syndrome
	Hepatitis A (HAV)	Faecal-oral via food or water; occasionally blood	14–28 days	Fever, nausea, anorexia, jaundice, abdominal pain, dark urine, pale stools	Vertical transmission rare. Possible premature rupture of membranes; possible preterm birth
	Hepatitis B (HBV)	Blood, body fluids	30–180 days	Nausea, vomiting, abdominal pain, fatigue, jaundice, dark urine, liver failure	Possibly low birthweight, preterm birth. Fetal infection during birth
	Hepatitis C (HCV)	Blood, body fluids	2 weeks-6 months	Fever, fatigue, nausea, vomiting, abdominal pain, jaundice, dark urine	Possible low birthweight and preterm birth. Infection at birth
	HIV	Blood, body fluids	Primary stage 2–4 weeks; AIDS develops over years	Fever, headache, rash, sore throat; may be asymptomatic	Transmission to fetus in utero, during birth or breastfeeding
	Dengue	Mosquitoes	4–10 days	High fever, headache, swollen glands, rash	Stillbirth, low birthweight, preterm birth
	Zika	Mosquitoes; sexual contact	3–12 days	Fever, rash, headache, joint pain, conjunctivitis	Microcephaly in offspring
Bacteria	Tuberculosis	Droplet infection	2–12 weeks	Fever, cough, weight loss, night sweats	Possible preterm labour and low birthweight; neonatal infection, perinatal death
	Pertussis (Whooping cough)	Droplet infection	7–14 days	Mild fever, runny nose, frequent coughing with a 'whoop', cyanosis	Fetal effects of infection unlikely; vaccination in pregnancy advised to protect the neonate
	E. coli	Faecal-oral via food or faeces (animal or human)	3–4 days	Vomiting, bloody diarrhoea, abdominal cramps	Main risk is dehydration due to infection; may cause miscarriage or preterm birth if severe
	Salmonella		6–72 hours	Diarrhoea, abdominal cramps, fever	Pregnancy loss if organism enters the blood stream and fetal infection occurs
	Listeria	Contaminated food; also found in soil and water	3–70 days	Maternal symptoms may be mild. They include fever, nausea, diarrhoea, muscle pains; septicaemia, meningitis (rare)	Intracellular organism; crosses the placenta causing fetal listeriosis. In pregnancy, may cause fetal loss; neonatal listeriosis includes sepsis and meningitis
	Chlamydia	Sexually transmitted; genital fluids	1–3 weeks	Dysuria, vaginal discharge, abdominal pain. May be asymptomatic in some people	Miscarriage, stillbirth, preterm birth; neonatal infection may cause pneumonia, conjunctivitis
	Gonorrhoea	Sexually transmitted; genital fluids	2–5 days on average	Yellow/green vaginal discharge, dysuria; asymptomatic in some people	Neonatal infection at birth may cause conjunctivitis (ophthalmia neonatorum) and blindness
	Syphilis	Sexually transmitted; genital fluids	3 weeks to 3 months	Chancre (ulcer(s) at the site of entry); secondary syphilis: rash, fever	Miscarriage, stillbirth, preterm birth, low birthweight; congenital syphilis in newborn
Parasites, protozoa	Malaria	Transmitted via mosquitoes	9–40 days (dependent on type of organism)	Fever, headache, vomiting, chills, sweating	Miscarriage, stillbirth, preterm birth, low birthweight
	Toxoplasmosis	Ingestion via raw meat, unwashed vegetables, cat faeces	5–23 days	Fever, muscle pain, headache, nausea, swollen glands	Miscarriage, stillbirth, congenital toxoplasmosis, fetal malformation
	Helminths (intestinal parasitic worms)	Ingestion of / exposure to ova	Variable – approximately 2 weeks	May be asymptomatic; may produce nausea, diarrhoea, abdominal pain; worms in stool	Limited impact unless heavy or chronic infestation, then anaemia and malnutrition may be apparent

Midwifery Skills at a Glance, First Edition. Edited by Patricia Lindsay, Carmel Bagness and Ian Peate.
© 2018 John Wiley & Sons, Ltd. Published 2018 by John Wiley & Sons, Ltd.

The midwife's responsibilities start with familiarity with which pathogens to consider and awareness of where to refer women. In the unwell woman, knowledge of symptoms as well as investigations that should be instigated at appointments are critical.

Organisms

Non-pathogenic organisms are essential to health. They can be found in the large intestine, referred to as 'gut flora', synthesising vitamins and controlling pathogenic organisms. They can be found in the vagina, where lactobacilli cause the mucoid secretions to be slightly acidic thereby preventing the growth of pathogenic organisms. Pathogenic organisms are ones that affect the woman's health and wellbeing. They could be viruses, bacteria, fungi, protozoa or worms. Pathogenic organisms enter the body by different routes: some will enter via the lungs (respiratory transmission, inhalation); by the gastrointestinal tract (ingestion); into the blood circulation via the skin (inoculation); or through mucosa in the throat or vagina (direct contact). The incubation period is the length of time between the organism entering the body and symptoms appearing.

Physiology

The body has defences against the invasion of pathogens. Skin, sebum, (which contains antibacterial and antifungal properties), normal flora (non-pathogenic organisms) and mucous membranes prevent entry into the body. Ciliated epithelial cells waft unwanted material away. Saliva contains IgA and the stomach produces hydrochloric acid, which kills many swallowed pathogens. The lowered pH of the vaginal mucosa renders the environment hostile to pathogenic organisms.

The main defence against infection is the immune system. It produces phagocytic cells, enzymes and proteins that destroy pathogens.

There are various leucocytes (white blood cells) in the blood. B and T lymphocytes identify pathogens and mark them with a specific protein, indicating that cells with this protein need to be destroyed. Other leucocytes are neutrophils, monocytes, eosinophils and basophils. These are measured in haematological tests and identified by the levels and the ratio of each to the others. Bacterial or viral infections can be identified.

The immune system will, when identifying a specific pathogen, produce antibodies to that pathogen such that if it invades the body a second or subsequent time the antibodies are present to prevent illness occurring.

Pregnant women are vulnerable

Physiological changes in the anatomy in pregnancy make women vulnerable. Gut motility is slower. The pH of the stomach is less acid, so ingested pathogens will not be destroyed so effectively. Non-pasteurised cheese would not cause a problem in the non-pregnant state but in pregnancy the gut may not be able to neutralise the bacteria. The pH of the vagina is changed and pathogens are more able to grow in this less hostile environment. There is a higher risk of infectious disease transmission.

Immune response

In pregnancy, the maternal immune response is altered to permit tolerance of the semiallogeneic fetal–placental unit. This is achieved through the activity of uterine macrophages and regulatory T cells, and effectively protects the fetus from rejection by the maternal immune system. While the changes between T1 and T2 helper cells protect the fetus, this has implications for maternal protection from infection. The maternal immune response is not suppressed but is

---

> **Box 3.1** Some signs of infection.
>
> - Lethargy, tiredness
> - Loss of appetite, nausea, vomiting
> - Rapid respirations, cough
> - Raised body temperature, raised heart rate
> - Generalised 'body pain' or malaise, headaches
> - Rashes, ulceration of mucosa
> - Signs of possible fluid imbalance: diarrhoea, thirst, sweating, reduced urinary output

> **Key point**
>
> Working with the multidisciplinary team to discuss care and management will ensure better care for the woman and baby.

moderated to accommodate the fetus. This means that pregnant women have increased susceptibility to infections and may suffer more severe consequences if infected. For example, pregnant women with influenza have a higher risk of developing pneumonia. Maternal infection during pregnancy has been linked to an increased risk of brain disorders in the offspring, such as schizophrenia.

Signs and symptoms of infection in women

Table 3.1 lists some common infections and Box 3.1 indicates some signs of infectious disease in women. It is important to note where the rash is, where it started and were it spread to. The same applies if ulceration is present. These observations help with diagnosis.

The midwife should be aware of local or national outbreaks of infectious diseases and needs to be aware of how to prevent the spread of an infectious condition.

At every visit check whether the woman has travelled or lived in a high-risk area. If the woman has a rash, it is advisable that she separated from other pregnant women.

Give advice regarding the prevention or spread of infection. Demonstrate and maintain good practice such as hand washing, wearing of gloves where appropriate and use of Standard Precautions. The midwife should liaise with the infection control specialist nurse in the hospital.

The midwife must screen the woman appropriately. This may mean taking blood or urine samples. The results must be obtained and followed up.

Refer appropriately

If a positive diagnosis is made, the woman may now be considered to have a high-risk pregnancy so more frequent antenatal checks are required. Obstetric input together with skills from the virologist, fetal medicine specialist, neonatologist and GP are required. The woman (and partner) need to be informed of the risks of suspected or diagnosed infections.

A multidisciplinary meeting should be convened to discuss management of the woman and baby.

The midwife should remain up to date on diagnosis and vaccines that are becoming available. Postnatally the woman can be vaccinated against some infectious diseases but the midwife must check the suitability of vaccines if the woman is breastfeeding.

Modes of transmission

4

Box 4.1 Modes of transmission.

Contact infection
Pathogens that are transmitted directly or indirectly, mainly via hands, occur when there is direct physical contact between an infected person and a non-infected person. There is no intermediate host. Herpes simplex virus uses this route to infect the host.
Indirect contact infection occurs between a non-infected person and the environment, for example objects. Pathogens can reach the host via open wounds or mucous membranes. Pathogens (norovirus for example) transmitted via the faecal-oral route (is one example) may lead to severe diarrhoea.

Infection via blood and tissue
Pathogens transmitted from the environment to humans is known as indirect contact infection, e.g. via needle stick injuries. Hepatitis C or B or HIV can be passed on this way. Disease-causing microorganisms can also be transmitted via body secretions, such as saliva, sweat, pus, or semen.

Infection via droplet or particles in the air
Droplet and airborne infections are part of direct transmission. Droplets produced during speaking, sneezing or coughing reach the mucous membranes of the upper respiratory tract, where they spread. Larger droplets can only travel short distances. Influenza is transmitted this way. *Mycobacterium tuberculosis* is an example of a disease spread by much smaller droplets and is passed on in the air; this is referred to as airborne transmission.

Infection via contaminated water and food
Indirect contact transmission happens when there is no direct contact between carriers of infection and newly infected people, for example, via contaminated water or contaminated food. This mode of transmission occurs predominantly in areas with poor hygiene; bacteria, for instance, reach the drinking water via excretions or colonise animal products. The cause of typhus is *Salmonella typhi* and is transmitted this way.

Box 4.2 The principles underpinning asepsis.

- The place in which the procedure is to take place should be as clean as possible
- During the procedure there should be as little disturbance as possible as this may cause air turbulence and the distribution of dust i.e. bed making, floor sweeping or buffing
- Hand hygiene must be performed prior to and during the procedure
- Sterile equipment must be used
- Lessen contamination of the vulnerable site by using forceps or sterile gloves, do not touch any sterile parts of the equipment

---

Figure 4.1 Transmission of pathogens.

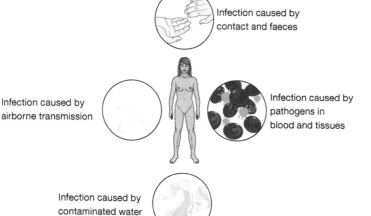

Infection caused by contact and faeces

Infection caused by airborne transmission

Infection caused by pathogens in blood and tissues

Infection caused by contaminated water

Key point
Infection prevention and control is required to prevent the transmission of communicable diseases in all healthcare settings and is a key role of the midwife.

Midwifery Skills at a Glance, First Edition. Edited by Patricia Lindsay, Carmel Bagness and Ian Peate.
© 2018 John Wiley & Sons, Ltd. Published 2018 by John Wiley & Sons, Ltd.

When micro-organisms have been transferred from one person to another, from equipment or the environment to people or between staff, infection can occur. If there are any disorders of the person's 'normal bacterial flora' this may predispose that person to infection. A woman is put at risk when bacteria are transferred from one part of her body to another where they are not usually resident, such as the movement of faecal bacteria from the perineum to the face during washing, or the administration of medication without performing hand hygiene or failing to change gloves in between caring for women.

Modes of transmission

Infectious agents are biological agents that have the potential to cause disease or illness in their hosts. Women and healthcare workers are often the most likely sources of infectious agents and are usually the most common susceptible hosts. Visitors and those working in healthcare may also be at risk of both infection and transmission.

Box 4.1 outlines the modes of transmission. Figure 4.1 illustrates the transmission of pathogens.

Disease prevention

Standard precautions

Standard precautions refer to those work practices applied to everyone, despite their perceived or confirmed infectious status; they aim to ensure a basic level of infection prevention and control. Standard precautions should be applied as a first-line approach to infection prevention and control, minimising the risk of transmission of infectious agents from person to person, even in high-risk situations.

Transmission-based precautions

The use of standard precautions is the first line of prevention of infection.

Transmission-based precautions are additional work practices for specific situations where standard precautions are inadequate to interrupt transmission. These precautions are adapted to the particular infectious agent and its mode of transmission.

Personal protective equipment

Personal protective equipment (PPE) is a requirement of health and safety legislation and is used to protect healthcare workers and women from risks of infection. The risk of infection is reduced by preventing the transmission of micro-organisms to the woman via the hands of staff or visa versa. The common types of PPE include items such as gloves, aprons, masks, goggles or visors. The decision to use PPE is based on a risk assessment.

Sharps

The safe handling and disposal of sharps are essential features of infection prevention and control. Sharps will include needles, scalpels, stitch cutters, glass ampoules and any sharp instrument. The chief hazards of a sharps injury are blood-borne viruses, such as hepatitis B, hepatitis C and HIV.

Unsafe or poor practice can cause injury to the individual or others, for example laundry workers who experience injuries as a result of sharps being misplaced in used linen. Sharps injuries

can be prevented and learning after an incident can help to avoid recurrence. It is essential that sharps are used safely and disposed of carefully and staff must work to agreed policies regarding the use of sharps to reduce the risk of injury and exposure to blood-borne viruses.

Disposal of waste

Waste created by staff in the line of their work can include sharps, hazardous, offensive, municipal (household) and pharmaceutical (medicinal) waste. Reducing waste, segregation and disposal is key to maintaining a healthy environment and reducing the risk of ensuing public health implications.

Healthcare organisations and local authorities have policies on waste segregation and disposal, offering guidance on all aspects, including special waste, pharmaceutical waste and segregation of waste. This includes the colour coding of bags used for waste.

Spillage

When blood and bodily fluids have been spilt these must be dealt with quickly and with adherence to local policy and procedure for dealing with spillages. Policy and procedure dictate the chemicals to be used, ensuring that any spillage is disinfected correctly, taking into account the surface where the incident occurred.

Asepsis and asepsis technique

The aim of asepsis is to prevent or reduce micro-organisms from entering a vulnerable body site such as a surgical wound, an intravenous catheter or during the insertion of an invasive device, for example a urinary catheter. Asepsis reduces the risk of an infection developing as a result of the procedure that is being undertaken.

Aseptic technique includes a series of specific actions or procedures carried out under controlled conditions. The ability to control conditions varies according to the care setting; the principals are summarised in Box 4.2. These should be applied in all cases.

Indwelling devices

Intravascular or invasive devices, for example urinary catheters, IV cannulae or central venous catheters, are often responsible for healthcare acquired infections (HCAIs) such as urinary tract, insertion site infections or bloodstream infections. When these devices are used correctly they offer valuable assistance in providing care to the woman along with positive care outcomes. However, these devices are not without risk and the development of infection can occur as they bypass the body's natural defence mechanisms such as skin and mucous membranes.

In order to ensure that the device is functioning effectively and to detect any signs or symptoms of infection, day to day management is essential and local policies and procedures must be adhered to. This includes, at a minimum, a documented daily review assessing the continuing need for the device, and regular documented checks for patency of the device, signs of infection and condition of the dressing. Implementation of hand hygiene prior to any contact with the device or associated administration sets must occur, and also cleaning/disinfection of any add-on devices/attachments and the replacement of peripheral intravascular devices after 72 hours (or as per local policy) or sooner depending on the woman's individual needs.

5 Asepsis and sepsis

Figure 5.1 An example of a hand-washing technique to support aseptic technique.

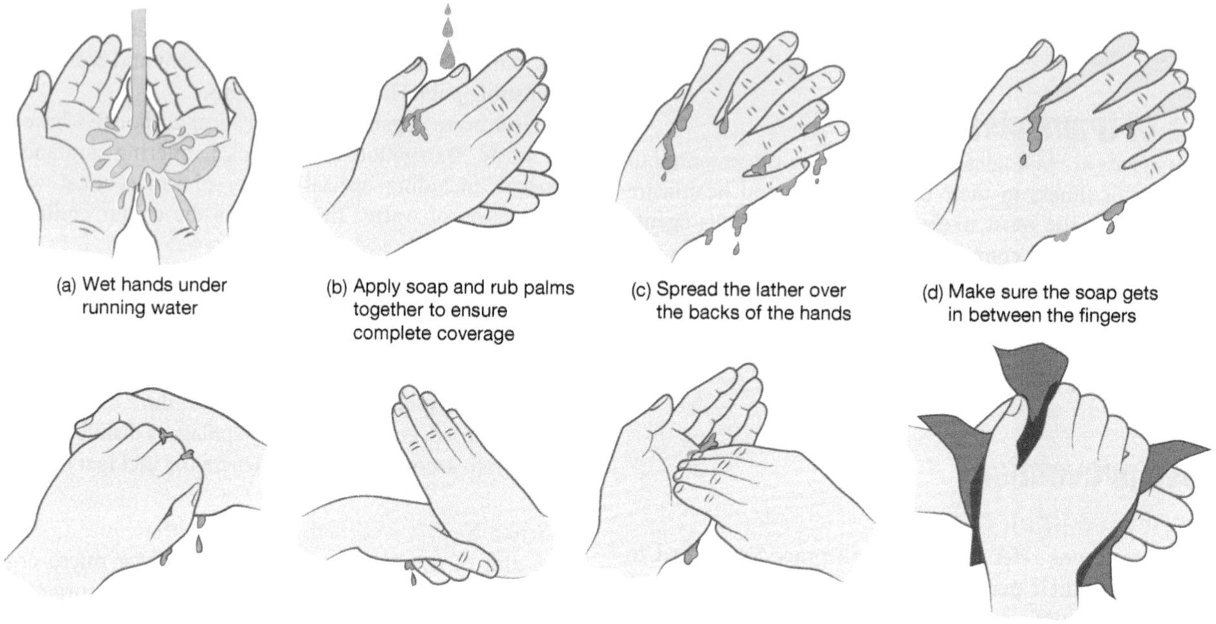

(a) Wet hands under running water

(b) Apply soap and rub palms together to ensure complete coverage

(c) Spread the lather over the backs of the hands

(d) Make sure the soap gets in between the fingers

(e) Grip the fingers on each hand

(f) Pay particular attention to the thumbs

(g) Press fingertips into the palm of each hand

(h) Dry thoroughly with a clean towel

Figure 5.2 A traditional dressing trolley.

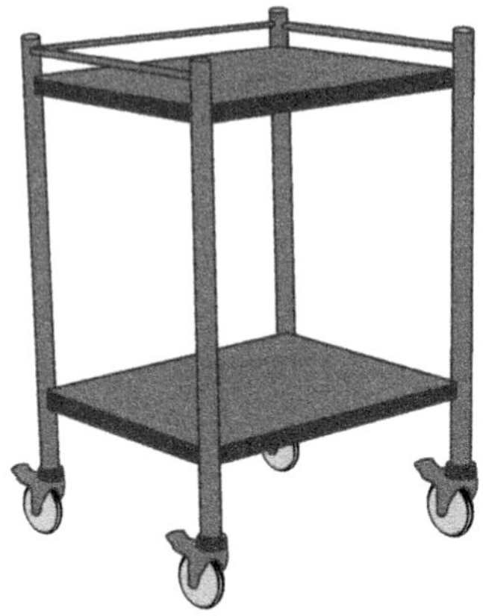

Figure 5.3 A dressing tray.

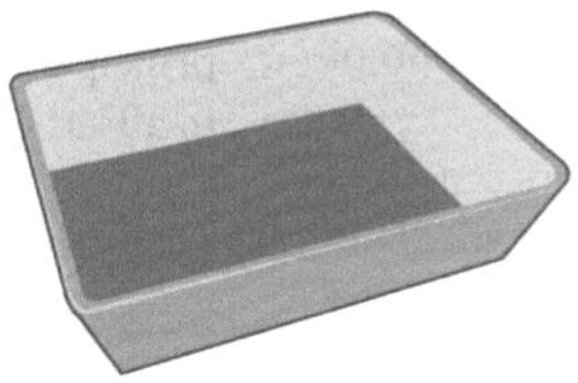

Figure 5.4 Example of a pre-prepared sterile dressing pack.

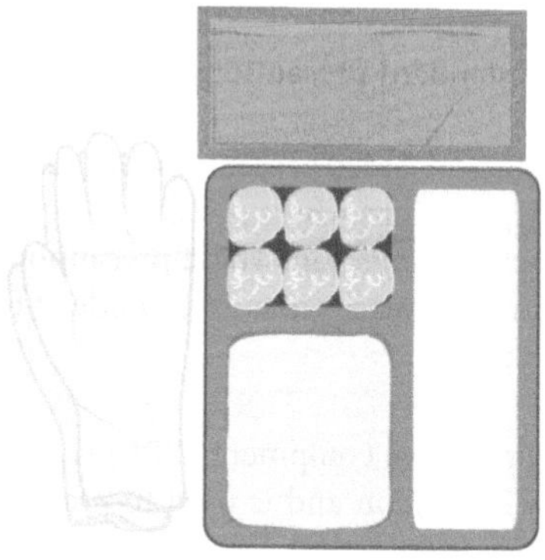

Key points
- Healthcare professionals must be assessed as competent to undertake aseptic technique.
- Local organisational polices and guidelines should always be understood and adhered to.

Originating in the operating theatre, aseptic technique is now commonly used to reduce the risk of infection. Aseptic technique avoids contamination of susceptible body sites or sterile equipment/specimens by micro-organisms (Figure 5.1).

Contamination may occur via contact with hands of healthcare professionals or the women or equipment. Contamination via the environment may also occur (for example dust on a sterile dressing pack).

Midwifery Skills at a Glance, First Edition. Edited by Patricia Lindsay, Carmel Bagness and Ian Peate.
© 2018 John Wiley & Sons, Ltd. Published 2018 by John Wiley & Sons, Ltd.

Aseptic versus clean technique

These techniques are different; however, confusion occurs as the language is used interchangeably.
• Aseptic technique – avoids contamination with micro-organisms during a procedure.
• Clean technique – reduces the number of micro-organisms present (commonly used on chronic wound dressings as these are often heavily colonised with bacteria).

How to undertake aseptic technique

There is no evidence that any specific technique results in better outcomes for the woman or neonate. Aseptic technique reduces risks by interrupting the chain of infection. Traditionally, use of a dressing trolley (Figure 5.2) has enabled midwives to meet the requirements of an aseptic technique in hospital settings by providing a structure to enable both carriage of equipment and a surface to support a sterile field. Midwives working in community settings will need to adapt to meet requirements and may find the use of dressing trays (Figure 5.3) of help. All techniques should meet the following principles:
• Healthcare professionals must be assessed as competent to undertake the procedure.
• Explain the procedure to the woman, and gain her informed consent.
• Hand hygiene is undertaken before any contact with the woman/neonate, sterile equipment and following the procedure.
• Gloves are only used when needed. Sterile gloves are only required in specific circumstances where the woman is severely immunocompromised or for specific procedures where maximum sterile precautions are required, e.g. insertion of central line.
• Personal protective equipment (PPE) such as gloves and aprons should be worn if contact with blood or body fluids is anticipated.
• Assess the procedural requirements before undertaking it, ensuring all equipment is available; avoid interruptions.
• Where large wounds are exposed, avoid undertaking aseptic technique if cleaning or bed making is occurring due to risk of airborne contamination to the vulnerable site.
• Consider the use of analgesia prior to the procedure.
• Remove/loosen soiled dressings before creating a sterile field.
• Ensure only sterile items come into contact with a susceptible site.
• Ensure sterile and non-sterile items do not touch.
• Dispose of waste in line with the risk assessment.
• Preprepared dressing packs are available (Figure 5.4).
   Following the procedure:
• Perform hand hygiene.
• Make the woman/neonate comfortable.
• Document procedure and any findings.

Asepsis and specimen collection

The collection of specimens without contamination is essential for accurate laboratory interpretation and antibiotic recommendations (where required).

Not all specimens are free from contamination (e.g. faeces). Particular care should be taken with urine samples, wound swabs and blood cultures to avoid contamination.

Top tips for quality specimens are:
1 Is there a need for the specimen? 'Just in case' specimens are not of value and are costly.
2 Identify the woman/neonate correctly.
3 Obtain the specimen without contamination.
4 Document specimen collection.

5 Ensure all clinical information is recorded on the specimen and laboratory form including any antibiotic therapy.
6 Store appropriately – do not leave at room temperatures for long periods to preserve any micro-organisms present and/or avoid overgrowth of 'contaminants'.
7 Check and act on results.

Sepsis

Sepsis is a life-threatening condition, and is also known as blood poisoning or septicaemia. It occurs when the body's immune system is triggered by the presence of an infection. Instead of the immune system successfully combatting the infection, an uncontrolled immune (complement) cascade occurs, leading to shock and organ failure and in some cases death. Sepsis cannot be predicted – any infection can trigger it. Rapid identification of possible cases of sepsis is key to avoiding poor outcomes for the mother or baby.

Sepsis is a leading cause of maternal death globally. In 2012–14, sepsis was the second leading cause of maternal mortality in the UK after cardiovascular disease.

Postpartum sepsis occurs within the postpartum period – historically, the identification of puerperal sepsis associated with a lack of hand hygiene led to the implementation of hand washing by Semmelweis (Chapter 2). Within the maternity setting, causes of sepsis may be pregnancy related or entirely unrelated.
• Pregnancy or delivery related:
  • Sepsis in pregnancy from miscarriage or abortion
  • Post-delivery infection – for example genital tract, uterine or perineal infection
  • Following caesarean section
  • Mastitis
  • Urinary tract infection
  • Obesity
  • Instrumental vaginal delivery.
• Non-pregnancy related
  • Respiratory infection – pneumonia, influenza
  • Wound or skin infection.

Signs and symptoms of sepsis

Early indications of sepsis can be vague, appearing as flu like symptoms. As sepsis develops the following symptoms can occur – action is must be taken immediately to assess if the mother or baby may have sepsis.
• For the mother:
  • Slurred speech
  • Shivering and/or muscle pain
  • Reduced urine output
  • Severe breathlessness
  • Mottled skin/blotching
  • Complaining of feeling 'like I might die'.
• For the baby:
  • Tachypnoea
  • Seizures or convulsions
  • Skin appears mottled, pale or blue
  • Lethargic, difficult to rouse
  • Feels cold to the touch.
More details of neonatal sepsis are given in Chapter 1.

Service user's view

'She deserved to have her baby and live to see him grow up.' *Hayley's story by her mother describing how Hayley dies of sepsis after delivering her baby.*

UK Sepsis Trust. Available at: http://sepsistrust.org/story/hayley/

6 Moving and handling

Figure 6.1 Biomechanics of moving and handling.

Source: Adapted from Health and Safety Executive (2012). *Moving and Handling: A Brief Guide*, p. 5–6.

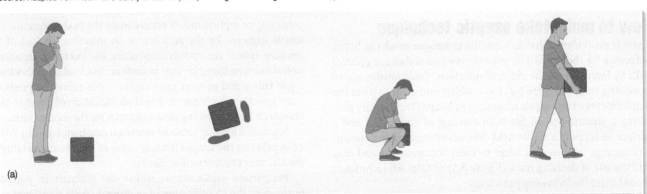

(a)

(b)

- Think before moving and handling
- Adopt a firm and stable base (can be changed depending on task performed)
- Get a good hold
- Start in a good posture
- Keep back in straight alignment and upright
- Bend knees
- Keep load close to waist
- Be aware of own centre of gravity
- Lift using the stronger leg muscles

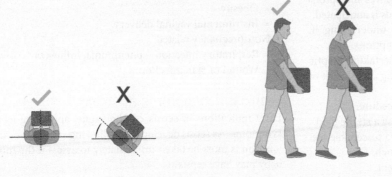

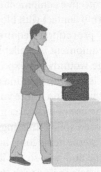

(c)

(d)

- Avoid twisting the back or leaning sideways, especially while the back is bent
- Keep head up
- Move smoothly
- Don't lift or handle more than can be easily managed
- Ask for help
- Put down load and then adjust

Key point

Take no 'short cuts'. Think and plan to reduce the risk of individual injury and provide safe moving and handling at all times.

Midwifery Skills at a Glance, First Edition. Edited by Patricia Lindsay, Carmel Bagness and Ian Peate.
© 2018 John Wiley & Sons, Ltd. Published 2018 by John Wiley & Sons, Ltd.

In the *Manual Handling Operations Regulations* 1992, manual handling is defined as:

…any transporting or supporting of a load (including the lifting, putting down, pushing, pulling, carrying or moving thereof) by hand or bodily force.

This definition is inclusive as it effectively covers any activity where an individual is required to lift, move or support a load (whatever that load may be). In the workplace an individual can be at risk of injury from these activities and the employer and employees have a responsibility to reduce that risk. Musculoskeletal injury occurs in over a third of all workplace injuries and this is caused by bad manual handling techniques, especially in relation to back injuries.

See Figure 6.1a–d for an overview of the biomechanics of moving and handling.

Although the women and families that midwives predominantly care for are mobile and independent, there are times when there is a need to support a woman with reduced mobility, for example women with epidurals, caesarean section or a disability, women who are overweight or obese (including bariatric women), and maternal collapse. Any activity has to be carried out with informed consent, comfort, privacy, dignity and respect.

As midwives work in a variety of environments (community and hospital) an understanding relating to safer 'moving and handling' in all these environments is paramount. The moving of equipment (homebirth kit, various equipment, trolleys, dry and fluid stores and beds – this list is not exhaustive) is a daily occurrence. Working at computers can also increase the risk of personal injury with the use of repetitive movements and static positions. Therefore regular workstation assessment is a legal requirement. Consideration of car driving is required (e.g. correct seat positioning and times of rest).

Principles

When considering and planning a manual handling activity it is a recommended requirement that a risk assessment is performed. This may have been carried out previously with local guidance already set or this may occur at the time, depending on the task. Several acronyms can be used to assist with the recall of this process. These include AARR and TILE.

AARR:
- **Avoid** – does the task need to be performed?
- **Assess** – if it does, assess how it can be performed?
- **Reduce** – reduce the risk to the individuals involved
- **Review** – review the whole process assessing the potential to develop the procedure with ongoing risk assessment.

TILE: These are important factors to consider as issues relating to these could cause potential for harm for the individuals involved (Figure 6.1a–d).
- **Task**
- **Individual capability**
- **Load**
- **Environment.**

Task

What is the task? Does it require repetitive movements, stooping or twisting, stretching upwards, holding a load away from the trunk (this increases stress on the lower back), insufficient rest or recovery, demanding pushing and/or pulling, changeable movement of an object or individual. This may also require the midwife assuming an awkward position to support a woman in labour or facilitate a birth (water birth, standing position, birthing on the floor). The task may involve the potential for twisting (e.g. monitoring of vital signs, monitoring of the fetal heart or venepuncture). Adopting a 45 degree angle or less of positioning will reduce that risk ensuring that shoulders are in alignment with feet with correct positioning of equipment. To change position move your feet and body, do not just twist your trunk.

Individual capability

This involves consideration of physical and mental capabilities, health status, current knowledge base, confidence and competence and age range (younger and older) of the person performing the task. The Health and Safety Executive (2004) state 'employees in their teens and fifties and sixties' have an increased risk of injury from manual handling activities. An individual also has a responsibility for their own competence (attending training and updates) and to inform their employer of any change in health.

Load

Several questions need to be considered – is the load heavy, bulky, difficult to hold or harmful? An affirmative to any of these should trigger the need for assistance, whether that is the use of appropriate equipment or an individual. Within the provision of midwifery care, the load can be a woman, baby, equipment, bags, beds and so on. In relation to the woman, several factors can also impact, for example mobility, pain, understanding (language or deafness), and pre- or postsurgery (urinary catheters/dressings/intravenous infusions). These can be seen to affect the unpredictability and sometimes complexity of the load and therefore need to be considered.

Environment

This may be within a home or hospital situation but the principles are similar. These are: constraints of posture, floor surface (wet/ carpeted, other hazards, e.g. bags, wires), poor lighting and variation of levels – be that floor or bed and other furniture.

Equipment to assist lifting and handling

Equipment to assist lifting and handling includes PAT slide, slide sheets, hoists and pneumatic hoists. Ensure the equipment is checked, intact and fit for purpose, and that individual users are updated with knowledge and understanding of its use.

Other considerations are:
- Ensure adequate numbers of staff are involved.
- Work as a team with appointment of a 'leader'.

> **Service user's view**
>
> '…she placed herself in such a position that all her equipment for putting my drip in was in easy reach and she did not need to twist at all…'
>
> Verbal communication, service user, London

7 The control of substances hazardous to health

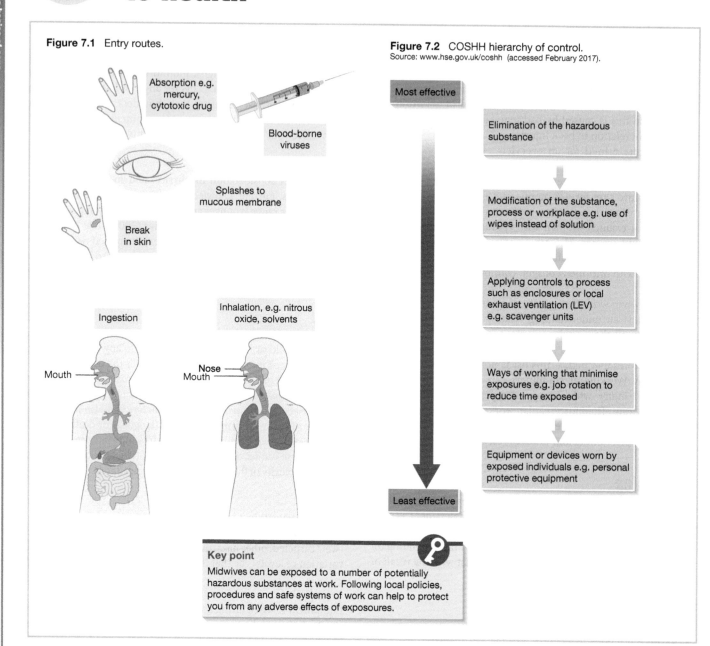

Figure 7.1 Entry routes.

Absorption e.g. mercury, cytotoxic drug

Blood-borne viruses

Splashes to mucous membrane

Break in skin

Ingestion

Mouth

Inhalation, e.g. nitrous oxide, solvents

Nose
Mouth

Figure 7.2 COSHH hierarchy of control.
Source: www.hse.gov.uk/coshh (accessed February 2017).

Most effective

Elimination of the hazardous substance

Modification of the substance, process or workplace e.g. use of wipes instead of solution

Applying controls to process such as enclosures or local exhaust ventilation (LEV) e.g. scavenger units

Ways of working that minimise exposures e.g. job rotation to reduce time exposed

Equipment or devices worn by exposed individuals e.g. personal protective equipment

Least effective

Key point

Midwives can be exposed to a number of potentially hazardous substances at work. Following local policies, procedures and safe systems of work can help to protect you from any adverse effects of exposoures.

Midwifery Skills at a Glance, First Edition. Edited by Patricia Lindsay, Carmel Bagness and Ian Peate.
© 2018 John Wiley & Sons, Ltd. Published 2018 by John Wiley & Sons, Ltd.

The Control of Substances Hazardous to Health Regulations (COSHH) is a key health and safety law introduced in the 1990s to protect employees from exposure to a range of hazardous substances. A hazardous substance is one that has the potential to cause harm and can be a solid, liquid, gas, fume, vapour, dust or micro-organism and can endanger health by being absorbed or injected through the skin or mucous membranes, inhaled or ingested (Figure 7.1)

In addition to frequent exposures to biological agents through blood and body fluid, there are a number of other hazardous substances that healthcare workers may be exposed to, including cleaning agents, anaesthetic gases, cytotoxic agents, natural rubber latex proteins, diathermy/surgical smoke fumes and formaldehyde.

Under the COSHH regulations, employers have a duty to reduce the risk of ill health from exposure to hazardous substances at work and follow a hierarchy of controls (Figure 7.2). Employees have a duty to follow safe working practices and should report any concerns relating to exposure to hazardous substances to their manager and/or their union safety representative.

Furthermore, certain hazardous substances can be harmful to new or expectant mothers and child through exposures in utero or through breast feeding.

Common hazardous substances in midwifery

Latex and gloves

Proteins found in natural rubber latex (NRL) can cause serious allergies, whether through direct contact with the skin or through inhalation of powders in the gloves. Type I or immediate hypersensitivity reactions to NRL can lead to anaphylaxis.

Other materials in latex and non-latex gloves known as accelerators can also cause skin irritation and type IV allergic reactions, a less severe and more localised skin reaction. This can lead to the skin condition, dermatitis.

For these reasons, it is important that glove selection is subject to a thorough risk assessment. Important issues to consider include the suitability of the glove (does it protect against exposures); the fit and comfort (does it allow dexterity); and whether there are any individuals, including service users, with existing latex allergy who may be exposed. Where staff are allergic to latex, suitable alternative gloves must be provided.

While the use of latex gloves hasn't been banned by the regulator, the Health and Safety Executive (HSE) recommend that if latex gloves are selected they must be powder free and low protein. A number of NHS organisations have gone 'latex free' to protect both the public and staff who may have an existing latex allergy.

Overuse of examination gloves in healthcare settings has also been observed and this can lead to additional problems such as breakdown of the skin's natural barrier. Deciding whether gloves are required for the task alongside appropriate selection is key.

As frequent hand washing and glove use are known to increase the risk of irritant contact dermatitis, employers should carry out regular skin surveillance on the hands of healthcare workers. Midwives should also regularly check their hands and report signs of dermatitis to their employer.

Nitrous oxide

Often referred to as 'gas and air', nitrous oxide has the potential to be harmful to the health of midwives, especially through frequent and prolonged exposures in poorly ventilated environments. The HSE has set a daily exposure limit for nitrous oxide and employers need to monitor staff exposures to ensure that limits are not exceeded and ventilation and scavenger systems are effective. Cylinders to be used in home or other less controlled environments may also be fitted with portable scavenger units. Where cylinders are transported in vehicles, midwifery staff must be trained in the safe transport of medical gasses.

Chemical disinfecting agents

Disinfecting agents, such as hypochlorite solutions, used to clean equipment such as birthing pools, surfaces and spillages of blood and body fluids, can cause respiratory, skin and eye irritation.

Incidents can occur when different cleaning agents are mixed, resulting in toxic fumes, or tablet-based hypochlorite agents are mixed with hot rather than cold water.

It is important that all staff are trained in safe use and that solutions are prepared and used as per manufacturer's instructions. While being mindful of infection control needs, employers also need to take steps to reduce exposures following the hierarchy of controls. For example, by using a disinfecting wipe to reduce the risk of splashes.

Biological agents

The most common type of exposure to biological agents in healthcare is through potentially infected blood and body fluids. HIV and hepatitis B and C are examples of biological agents that can be transmitted to healthcare workers from sharps or needle-stick injuries and splashes to the mucous membranes or non-intact skin. Standard precautions, including the use of personal protective equipment (PPE) such as gloves, aprons, googles and visors, can reduce the risk of exposures. The type of PPE used will depend on an assessment of the risks presented by the procedure. Immunisation against hepatitis B should be offered to all workers at risk of exposure to blood and body fluids.

New regulations to protect midwives and other healthcare workers from the risk of needle-stick injuries were recently introduced in the UK and are covered in more detail in Chapter 9.

Healthcare worker's view

'Knowing that my employer and my colleagues look out for my health and safety at work makes a big difference to my morale.'

Verbal communication, RCN member with latex allergy, London

8 Safety in the working environment

Table 8.1 Colour-coded segregation proposed for the safe management of healthcare waste in the UK.
Source: Royal College of Nursing (2014). *The Management of Waste from Health, Social and Personal Care.* https://www.rcn.org.uk/-/media/royal-college-of-nursing/documents/publications/2014/april/pub-004187.pdf (accessed April 2017). Reproduced with permission of the Royal College of Nursing.

Colour coding	Waste description and disposal/treament type	Container type	Examples
Yellow	Infectious waste which must be sent for incineration at a suitable authorised facility. It must not be sent for alternative treatment.	Yellow bag or rigid yellow-lidded container or sharps receptacles.	Waste which is classified as infectious (contaminated with bodily fluids where the assessment process leads you to believe the waste poses a potential infection risk, and there are also medicines or chemicals present). Examples are: • infectious waste contaminated with chemicals • chemically contaminated samples and diagnostic kits • infectious waste contaminated with medicines • laboratory specimens.
Orange	Infectious waste which can be sent for alternative treatment to render it safe prior to disposal.	Orange bag or orange-lidded, rigid yellow sharps receptacles.	Waste which is classified as infectious (contaminated with bodily fluids where the assessment process leads you to believe the waste poses a potential infection risk), such as: • dressings • bed pads • bandages • protective clothing (for example, gloves or aprons). Note: If you do not believe the waste presents an infection risk and there are no medicines or chemicals present, use the offensive waste stream.
Purple	Cytotoxic or cytostatic medicine waste or any items contaminated with these must be sent for incineration at a suitably authorised facility. For unused/redundant medicines, refer to The *Safe Management of Healthcare Waste* manual (Department of Health 2013).	Yellow/purple bag, purple bag or rigid yellow purple-lidded medicine container or right yellow purple-lidded sharps receptacles.	Waste consisting of, or contaminated with, cytotoxic and/or cytostatic medicines, such as: • medicine containers with residues of cytotoxic or cytostatic medicines (bottle, infusion bags or syringe barrels) • items contaminated with cytotoxic or cytostatic medicines (swabs) • used sharps from treatment using cytotoxic or cytostatic medicines.
Tiger	Offensive/hygiene waste which may be sent for energy recovery at energy from waste facilities. These wastes can also be sent to landfill if no other recovery or recycling option is available.	Yellow and black striped bag.	Healthcare waste classified as non-hazardous, ie where the assessment process leads you to believe the waste does not pose an infection risk. These can be items contaminated with bodily fluids such are: • stoma or catheter bags • incontinence pads • hygiene waste • gloves, aprons, maternity waste where no infection risk exists • blood contaminated items from screened community.
Red	Anatomical waste sent for incineration at a suitably authorised facility.	Red-lidded, rigid yellow receptacles.	Anatomical waste, which includes: • recognisable body parts • placenta.
Blue	Non-hazardous medicinal waste for incineration at a suitably authorised facility. Refer to The *Safe Management of Healthcare Waste* manual (Department of Health 2013).	Blue-lidded, rigid yellow receptacles.	Waste medicines such as: • unused non-cytotoxic/cytostatic medicines in original packaging • part empty containers containing residues of non-cytotoxic/cytostatic medicines • empty medicine bottles.
Black	Domestic/municipal waste to be sent to energy from waste facilities or landfill.	Usually a black bag.	Items which you would find in the normal household waste stream, such as: • food waste • tissues.

The biobin may also be used in accordance with colour coding system, where provided.

Key point

Reporting near misses, incidents and faults promptly is key to preventing more serious incidents to healthcare workers and service users.

Midwifery Skills at a Glance, First Edition. Edited by Patricia Lindsay, Carmel Bagness and Ian Peate.
© 2018 John Wiley & Sons, Ltd. Published 2018 by John Wiley & Sons, Ltd.

The health sector is covered by a robust legislative framework aimed at ensuring a safe working environment for healthcare staff and, in turn, contributing to the safety of women.

Employers have a duty to ensure, so far as is reasonably practicable, the health, safety and welfare at work of all employees. They must also ensure that non-employees, including women, babies, visitors and contractors, are protected from harm whilst on their premises. Employees have a duty to take reasonable care of themselves and others and to cooperate with their employer on health and safety matters.

Moreover, the Nursing and Midwifery Council code expects midwives to preserve safety, including the requirement to take all reasonable personal precautions necessary to avoid any potential health risks to colleagues, people receiving care and the public and to raise and escalate concerns.

Risk assessment is the foundation of health and safety management and is also underpinned by a legal requirement. Employers must: identify health and safety hazards; decide who may be harmed and how; evaluate the risks; and decide on precautions to reduce the risk. They must also record the findings and review and update the assessments as necessary.

Accidents

In 2009, a review into the health and wellbeing of NHS staff found a greater propensity for NHS staff to incur a work-related accident than other comparative groups of workers. Work in healthcare is both physically and psychologically demanding, with staff carrying out diverse activities in pressurised environments. According to the Health and Safety Executive (HSE) over half a million days are lost per annum in the health and social care sector due to workplace injuries.

Procedures, safe systems of work and risk assessments, regular inspections and safety audits of the working environment, in addition to policies, can help prevent and detect problems. It is also essential that midwives are encouraged and supported to report near misses and incidents promptly so that preventative action can be taken before harm occurs.

Slips and trips

Slips and trips are the single most common cause of injuries at work and make up over a half of reported injuries in the health and social care sector. Wet floors, trailing leads, poor lighting, uneven surfaces and icy car parks all contribute to slips and trips in the sector. Workplace conditions can also be a contributory factor in falls, resulting in death or serious injury to already vulnerable women. In midwifery units, slips and trips can be caused by spillages of liquids (e.g. amniotic fluid, water from birthing pools) and trailing wires from equipment such as fetal heart monitors. Working in the community can also present a risk, particularly when working at night and entering poorly lit premises.

In addition to the selection of floor surfaces that are slip-resistant, easily cleanable and have an impervious finish, simple steps can be taken to reduce the risk of slips and trips. These include clear policies for promptly dealing with spillages, including outlining responsibilities and having readily accessible cleaning equipment or spill stations (a 'see it sort it!' mentality can reduce the risk, e.g. dealing with a spillage instead of waiting for someone else to do it). Floors should be free from trip hazards and obstructions, for example avoiding trailing wires and ensuring equipment is stored away when not in use rather than left in walkways. Providing torches for community staff to use when carrying out home visits at night can help reduce their risk of falls. Much of this is common sense but in a pressurised environment these steps can be overlooked.

Equipment safety

According to the HSE there are a number of serious and sometimes fatal accidents each year to employees and service users from faulty equipment. Examples of equipment in use in healthcare environments include hoists, electric profiling beds and diathermy machines. Incidents occur when the equipment hasn't been maintained, the wrong type of equipment has been used or the user hasn't been trained in safe use. The selection, use and maintenance of equipment is governed by regulations that suppliers and employers must follow. Staff must be trained in the safe use of equipment and equipment should be inspected and maintained by a competent person.

Certain types of work equipment are regulated by the Medicines and Healthcare Regulatory Authority (MHRA). The MHRA ensures that medical equipment is safe to use and advises on maintenance and disposal, and provides alerts on reported faults.

Midwives should ensure that they have been trained and are familiar with the safe use of equipment and report any faults immediately.

Waste disposal

The management of healthcare waste is governed by a complex regulatory framework encompassing environmental, transport and health and safety legislation. Healthcare organisations produce many different types of waste from domestic to cytotoxic. In order to protect human health, the environment and to reduce the cost of waste disposal, it is important that the correct waste stream is used (Table 8.1). Midwives should familiarise themselves with the different types of waste streams.

In 2011, an RCN report identified that organisations and individuals are not fully utilising the 'offensive' waste stream preferring a 'just in case' approach and using the more costly 'infectious' waste stream. The RCN recommends improved training for healthcare workers to assess waste and ensure that the appropriate waste streams are used.

As well as employer duties, individual practitioners have a duty of care to ensure the safe disposal and transport of healthcare waste, including waste produced by a midwife working in the community.

Service user's view

'As anyone can imagine, these easily avoidable accidents have had a horrendous effect on my life.'

Alison Hockaday, NHS Occupational Therapist who lost a limb following two serious slip incidents. Health and Safety Executive 2012 autumn newsletter. Available at: www.hse.gov.uk

9 Sharps injuries

Figure 9.1 The hierarchy of controls applied to prevention of sharps injuries.

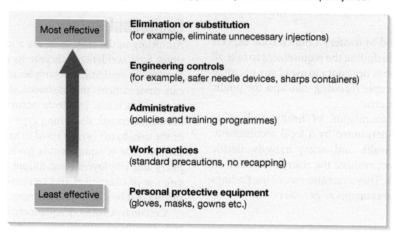

Most effective

Elimination or substitution
(for example, eliminate unnecessary injections)

Engineering controls
(for example, safer needle devices, sharps containers)

Administrative
(policies and training programmes)

Work practices
(standard precautions, no recapping)

Least effective

Personal protective equipment
(gloves, masks, gowns etc.)

Figure 9.2 (a, b and c) A number of engineering controls are available, some examples are shown here.

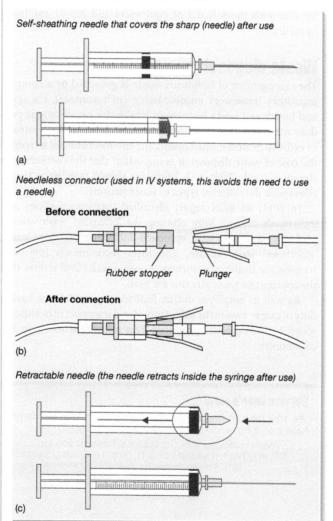

Self-sheathing needle that covers the sharp (needle) after use

(a)

Needleless connector (used in IV systems, this avoids the need to use a needle)

Before connection

Rubber stopper   Plunger

After connection

(b)

Retractable needle (the needle retracts inside the syringe after use)

(c)

Figure 9.3 Nurse disposing of sharps directly into a sharps container.

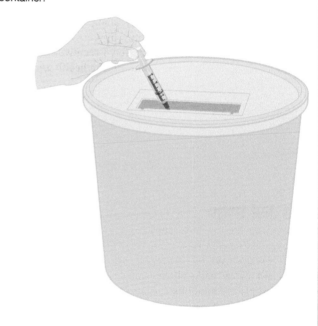

Key points

- For some staff the experience of sharps injury may have emotional and occupational consequences.
- Organisational polices and guidelines should always be adhered to.

Midwifery Skills at a Glance, First Edition. Edited by Patricia Lindsay, Carmel Bagness and Ian Peate.
© 2018 John Wiley & Sons, Ltd. Published 2018 by John Wiley & Sons, Ltd.

The use of sharps is common in healthcare and therefore healthcare workers (HCW) and others are particularly at risk. Injuries frequently occur through accidental cutting or penetration of the skin or when disposing of sharps.

Sharps injuries are also referred to as percutaneous injuries. The greatest risk to healthcare workers is the transmission of blood-borne viruses (BBV).

Vaccination can be offered to protect staff from hepatitis B virus (HBV); however, not all staff respond to the vaccination and therefore cannot be guaranteed full protection. There is currently no vaccination to protect healthcare workers against hepatitis C (HCV) and human immunodeficiency virus (HIV).

Since 1997, 21 healthcare workers in the UK have experienced seroconversion as a result of exposure to HCV in blood/body fluids from infected patients. A further 1478 healthcare workers were exposed to an HIV-infected source patient. The risks to healthcare workers after injury with a needle contaminated by a BBV is estimated to be:
1 in 3 for hepatitis B
1 in 30 for hepatitis C
1 in 300 for HIV.

Percutaneous injuries are the most commonly reported injury, with hollow bore needles the most commonly reported device involved. Sharps used in midwifery care include:
- Hollow bore needles
- Intravenous cannulas
- Suture needles
- Scalpels/surgical blades
- Glass ampoules
- Vaccination needles
- Butterfly needles
- Lancets.

Injuries may occur:
- During use
- After use, before disposal
- Between steps in procedures
- During disposal
- Whilst resheathing or recapping a needle.

Healthcare workers can also be injured as a result of poor practice of others – for example sharps disposed of in waste bags can injure domestic staff and others.

Some procedures carry a higher risk of causing a sharps injury, such as insertion of intravascular (IV) cannulas, venepuncture, making an episiotomy, perineal suturing, surgery (e.g. caesarean section).

Reducing the risk of sharps injuries

Reducing the risk of sharps works best when staff consider the problem from the perspective of the 'hierarchy of controls'. This framework, which can be applied across all employment sectors, guides staff to consider risks and how they can be manages by planning actions in an ordered way rather than jumping to what might seem to be the simplest option. The hierarchy of controls as applied to sharps injuries can be found in Figure 9.1.

A number of simple good practices, when used consistently, can help the midwife avoid the risk of sharps injury and the potential consequences. These include:
- Ensuring all healthcare workers are offered vaccination to prevent hepatitis B
- Having organisational policies in place to support staff to use and dispose of sharps safely
- Use of safer needle devices for procedures involving sharps (Figure 9.2)
- Providing education to all staff on safe sharp practices
- Encouraging staff to report all cases of sharps injuries, including those where a patient is not thought to pose a risk so that learning can be identified and future injuries potentially prevented.

Good practice to reduce the risk of sharps injuries:
- Handling of sharps is kept to a minimum.
- Syringes or needles are not dismantled by hand and are disposed of as a single unit straight into a sharps container for disposal.
- Sharps containers are readily available as close as possible to the point of use (sharps trays with integral sharps boxes are a useful resource to support this practice point) (Figure 9.3).
- Needles are never resheathed/recapped.
- Needles are not broken or bent before use or disposal.
- Arrangements should be put in place to ensure the safe disposal and transport of sharps used in a community setting such as patients' homes.
- All single use sharps containers should conform to BS EN ISO 23907.
- Sharps containers are not filled to more than two-thirds full.
- Never dispose of sharps in waste bags.
- Sharps boxes are signed on assembly and disposal.
- Sharps bins are stored safely away from the public and out of reach of children (in other words, not stored on the floor or at low levels.
- Staff attend training on the safe use of sharps and safety engineered devices.
- Staff are aware and comply with their local sharps or inoculation injury policy.

Actions to take following a sharps injury

The most important action after sustaining a sharps injury is to perform first aid. Only after this has taken place should the injury be reported.
- Encourage the wound to bleed, ideally holding it under running water.
- Wash the wound using running water – do not scrub the wound whilst you are washing it.
- Do not suck the wound.
- Dry the wound and cover it with a waterproof plaster or dressing.
- Seek urgent medical advice as per organisational policies.
- Report the injury as per local policies.

Healthcare worker's view

'I couldn't even sleep. I couldn't perform my tasks properly, fearing that it would happen again ... I just hesitated about things that I had usually performed without any problem.'

Jeong et al. 2016

10 Working safely in the community

Table 10.1 Self-assessment for working safely in the community.
Source: Adapted from NHS Employers (2013). Improving Safety for Lone Workers. http://www.nhsemployers.org/case-studies-and-resources/2013/10/improving-safety-for-lone-workers-a-guide-for-lone-workers. Reproduced with permission of NHS Employers.

Self-assessment for Working Safely in the community	Comments
Do you feel safe working in the community?	
Do you know and understand your own responsibilities?	
Do you risk assess visits to community centres, GP surgeries and home visits?	
Do you know your manager's responsibilities?	
Are you aware of lone working policies and local procedures?	
Do you discuss safety and working in the community with colleagues, students or others you may be working with?	
Do you have sound techniques for prevention and management of violence (e.g. conflict resolution and personal safety)?	
Do you plan before a visit and be aware of the risks and do everything you can in advance to ensure your own safety?	
Do you have access to appropriate safety equipment (for example lone worker alarm devices, method of informing your manager/buddy of where you are)?	
Do you know how to use and maintain lone worker safety equipment?	
Do you know how to report an incident?	
Do you leave an itinerary with your manager or your colleagues?	
Have you been given all the information about the risks of aggressive and violent behaviour by women, their partners and families and the appropriate measures for controlling these risks?	
Do you keep in regular contact with your base?	
Do you carry out risk assessments during your visits?	
Are you aware that you should never put yourself or colleagues in danger and that, if you feel threatened, you should withdraw immediately?	
Do you understand the circumstances under which a visit can be terminated?	

Key point

The midwife has a duty to care for childbearing women wherever they are situated; however, the midwife also has a responsibility to ensure their own and colleague's personal safety.

Midwifery Skills at a Glance, First Edition. Edited by Patricia Lindsay, Carmel Bagness and Ian Peate.
© 2018 John Wiley & Sons, Ltd. Published 2018 by John Wiley & Sons, Ltd.

The majority of the time, working in the community is a safe and rewarding part of midwifery practice. However, as a healthcare professional who may be working alone and throughout the day and night, it is important that midwives take reasonable steps to ensure their safety, both for themselves, students and colleagues.

Employers also have a responsibility to ensure all employees work in a safe and secure environment, and all organisations should have clearly understood processes in place to maximise the safety of their employees. Such polices should be communicated to lone workers, and the team around them.

In a member survey (of nurses, midwives and healthcare assistants) carried out in 2012, the Royal College of Nursing reported that over 62% had either very rarely or rarely felt unsafe or at risk in the last 12 months; however, that does leave nearly 30% who did not always feel safe.

Providing care in the community environment does require a local knowledge of the area and a need to be realistic about the possibility of dangerous situations, which may escalate. The safety issues will vary, whether it is an urban or rural location, and the responsibility rests with the individual midwife to identify risks, discuss them with their manager and use their skills to remain safe and secure. The midwife also needs to take account of students or colleagues joining them for short periods of time, and should not be nonchalant about concerns expressed as they may not have local knowledge, worked in isolation before or may be unclear about polices around working outside of major acute units.

Most midwives are well aware that when entering a woman's home, there is a need for respect and not being critical of the home, being aware of others there and their attitude to health and social care staff, which may be influenced by previous experiences or concerns about an authority figure entering their home.

Midwives also use GP surgeries and other community centres, which may not have many staff around, and care must be taken when considering entering or leaving premises, as well as being on their own between appointments at clinics, waiting for women and their partners for parent education or other supporting activities.

The midwife needs to:
• Assess the risks to personal safety realistically, initially, and then as often as the circumstances change, or at least as the seasons change. (Table 10.1 provides a self-assessment form that could be used and then shared with a manager for further discussion.)
• Discuss the risks with their manager.
• Know about lone working policy – employers should have policies in place, and the midwife needs to be familiar with these, including recommendations or equipment available to increase their safety and peace of mind.
• Access training and education – be prepared, be alert to possible risks, be responsible, be safe; this may include training on conflict resolution, which would cover risk assessment, de-escalation techniques and post-incident support.
• Review the risk assessment, especially for different times of the year and different locations.
• Know how to escalate a concern.

• Lone worker alarm systems are an important part of best practice for safe working in the community. These may include
  • a buddy system, which should be structured and provide details of information required and when workers are scheduled to be alone;
  • use of electronic monitoring systems, such as Identicom (SoloProtect), or similar devises, which enable transmission of the user's location and a professional security response when an alarm is raised. They are discreet; the midwife's identification card fits into the front, making it more covert and easy to use, should the midwife become concerned. Generally, they are easier to activate than a personal alarm or mobile phone; however, some of them rely on the midwife using them effectively, as some need whereabouts inputted before they enter premises, whilst others have GPS locating systems.
  • The NHS provides further details on safe use of devices, including panic alarms and mobile phone usage (NHS 2017).
• Equipment, including mode of transport should be serviced and working.
• Be aware of changing timetables for buses and trains.
• Use technology (such as satellite navigation systems and mobile phones) to the midwife's advantage, but do not rely on them.
• Consider how you might keep in contact with colleagues, agree beforehand how often this should be, and that there is a mechanism in place if the colleagues cannot be contacted, especially if there is a concern about safety.
• Always plan a route to and from a visit; think about lighting and ease of access.
• A torch, map of the area and telephone numbers for emergencies should be easily available.
• Be aware of animals in homes; it is reasonable to ask that they be removed and contained during the visit.
• Understand that any area can pose a risk; do not let familiarity create less vigilance.
• Midwives must take reasonable care when carrying medication, mobile phones and devices, and women's records to and from a woman's home.
• Report incidents and 'near misses'; provide details about violent individuals, unsafe environments and other important information on the risks faced.

Midwives have a responsibility to take care of themselves; self-awareness is a critical skill, especially not becoming complacent to the practice location. They should assess the risk of working in the community environment, consider any changes to their circumstances and take action to minimise the possibility of an incident occurring. It is not unreasonable to ask the manager for an escort/companion, or for help if the midwife feels alarmed – better to be safe than need to recover from an unsafe situation. Remember, the vast majority of midwifery community care is safe and enjoyable.

Healthcare worker's view

'I don't have a problem with lone working in general. If I feel at risk I always take someone with me. If there are any complaints or abuse it gets reported to management and we leave the visit immediately.'

RCN 2012

Personal hygiene care for women

Table 11.1 Bed bathing procedure.

Action	Rationale
Explain what you are about to do, noting any personal preferences.	To gain consent
Collect the equipment.	To avoid interruption to the procedure
Ensure that the room or ward area is warm.	To maintain the woman's comfort
Screen the bed or close the door.	To maintain privacy and dignity
Wash hands and apply an apron and gloves. Raise bed to a comfortable working height. Apply the brakes.	To reduce the risk of cross infection For patient and employee health and safety
Remove the top bedding and cover the woman with a towel or blanket. Remove spectacles and wristwatch if worn. Dirty linen is placed in the laundry skip.	To avoid injury and maintain warmth, privacy and dignit
Fill the bowl and check the temperature of the water. It should be 'hand hot'. Ask the woman to confirm that the temperature is satisfactory for her.	To maximise comfort and avoid injury
Ask if the woman wishes to wash her own face and if she wishes to use soap. If she declines, wash her face, rinsing using a cloth wrung out in clean water. Dry her face.	To maintain hygiene and comfort, promote autonomy and maintain independence
Remove the woman's upper garments then wash the upper limbs, starting with the arm furthest away. Place a towel underneath the arm in order to avoid wetting the sheets. Cover the area that is not being washed. Dry the arm and wash the other in the same way.	The woman's dignity and warmth is maintained if only the area to be washed is exposed at any time If there are any spills, they will not dampen the part of the body that have already been washed and dried
Wash the chest, washing and drying under the breasts carefully.	To promote comfort
Repeat the above procedure for the lower limbs (legs and feet).	To promote wellbeing and cleanliness
Roll the woman on to her side. Ensure correct manual handling techniques and/or equipment are used.	To assist in the cleaning of the woman To remove the risk of the woman or you receiving an injury
While the woman is on to her side wash her back and buttocks (wear gloves). Check her pressure areas.	To promote cleanliness To maintain skin integrity; to prevent / treat pressure sores
Change the water and use new gloves. Ask the woman if she wishes to wash her own genitalia. If not, the area is washed using the second flannel. If she has a urinary catheter, catheter hygiene should be carried out.	To reduce the risk of infection
Reposition the woman comfortably and assist to dress in clean clothing. Apply sanitary pad if needed.	To maintain privacy and dignity and ensure the woman remains warm
Make the bed, using clean bed linen. Dispose of used bed linen.	Soiled or contaminated linen must be disposed of according to local policy to avoid infection risk
Carry out or assist the woman with oral hygiene.	To promote comfort and wellbeing
Comb or brush her hair.	To promote wellbeing
Wash hands; dispose of equipment appropriately. Ensure the woman's possessions are replaced in her locker.	To minimise the risk of infection
Document in the woman's care plan. Condition of pressure areas must be recorded.	For good communication and to promote continuity of care

Key point

Personal hygiene has an impact on health. Attention to a woman's personal hygiene is an essential component of competent midwifery care.

Midwifery Skills at a Glance, First Edition. Edited by Patricia Lindsay, Carmel Bagness and Ian Peate.
© 2018 John Wiley & Sons, Ltd. Published 2018 by John Wiley & Sons, Ltd.

Good personal hygiene is of paramount importance in maintaining good health. Maternity clients are not usually ill but are vulnerable to infection. In addition, the maternity population is becoming increasingly high risk, with rising numbers of women entering pregnancy with a pre-existing medical condition and/or requiring delivery by caesarean section. Sepsis in pregnant or newly delivered women can have fatal results.

General advice

Personal hygiene care addresses care of the whole woman, including oral hygiene, nail care and hair care. It may also include cleanliness of clothing. Women who are self-caring should be advised to shower or bathe regularly and also change their clothes regularly. Hand washing before and after using the toilet or changing sanitary pads is essential. The woman should be made aware of the signs of infection so that she can seek help early. Midwives who suspect infection in a pregnant or newly delivered woman should refer her for medical attention as soon as possible.

Women who are unable to attend to their own personal hygiene should be offered assistance with this aspect of care.

Bed bathing

Purpose: To maintain comfort, reduce infection risk and maintain morale.

Procedure: Two people are required if the woman is unable to move herself. The woman should be offered a bedpan and analgesia before the procedure and any specific personal or cultural requirements are noted (Table 11.1). In the interests of comfort and dignity, if the woman can wash herself she should be encouraged to do so, the assistant passing clean flannels and towels as needed. Equipment such as washing bowls should be disposable if possible. If not disposable, they should be thoroughly cleaned before and after use. The water should be changed at least once during the procedure to maintain warmth and cleanliness. During the procedure any vaginal loss such as amniotic fluid, or blood/lochia should be noted and recorded.

Equipment:
- Clean nightwear/clothing
- Sanitary pads if needed
- Clean bed linen, including disposable bed pads
- Laundry skip
- Apron, gloves and clinical waste bag
- Washing bowl
- Soap and two disposable cloths or flannels
- Toiletries as requested by the woman
- Two towels
- Hairbrush or comb.

Additional equipment may include oral care items, nail care items, slide sheet or other manual handling equipment, and antiembolism stockings, as necessary.

The procedure is outlined in Table 11.1.

Once the bed bath is completed the woman should be asked about her comfort level and if she has any other care needs. All personal care is documented in the notes.

Oral hygiene

Purpose: To promote comfort and wellbeing, remove food particles and protect the health of oral tissues.

Procedure: The assistance may be limited to be offering the required equipment; if the woman is not able to carry out her own oral care this should be done for her to avoid oral infections such as candidiasis (thrush). Poor oral hygiene has an impact on general health and wellbeing. Women who are nil by mouth, who are vomiting, who have a nasogastric tube in situ or who are having oxygen therapy are in particular need of attention to oral hygiene.

Key points:
- Maintain privacy and dignity – screen the bed.
- Use the woman's own toothbrush and toothpaste if possible.

Equipment: toothbrush, toothpaste, towel, water to rinse, receiver to spit into.

Emollients such as lip balm may help if the lips are dry or cracked. Petroleum-based products must *not* be used if the woman is having oxygen therapy as there is a theoretical risk of burns. Water-based products are safer and the pharmacist will advise on which is suitable.

If the woman is unable to self-care

Equipment: towel, small, soft-bristled toothbrush, toothpaste, water to rinse, lip balm, receiver to spit into, clinical waste bag, disposable gloves and apron. A small torch and a spatula are useful to inspect the oral cavity. Foam sticks are not recommended as they do not clean the mouth effectively. If they detach from the holder they are a choking hazard.

Procedure:
- Collect equipment, ensure privacy, wash hands and put on gloves and apron.
- Inform the woman and gain consent.
- Position her on her side, with the towel beneath her head.
- Observe the state of the oral tissues.
- Apply a small (pea-sized) amount of paste to the (dry) toothbrush and gently clean the teeth, gums and tongue.
- Ask the woman to rinse her mouth with water and spit into the receiver. If she is unable to, rinse the toothbrush and use the wet brush to rinse the mouth.
- Dry the lips and face.
- Apply lip balm if required (and if not receiving oxygen therapy).
- Reposition the woman.
- Clean and dry the toothbrush; dispose of equipment.
- Document.

> **Service user's view**
> 'Other patients can hear even with the curtains round. Curtains are a visual but not a hearing barrier.'
> Bailey 2009

12 Perineal and vulval hygiene; use of bedpans and commodes

Box 12.1 Procedure for giving a bedpan.

- Screen the bed and ask visitors to leave
- Raise the bed to a safe working height and apply brakes
- Wash hands
- Don gloves and apron
- Offer hand-washing equipment
- With the woman semirecumbent, remove the top bedding to knee level
- Ask the woman to raise her buttocks off the bed and slide the bedpan under her, with the widest area under her buttocks and the narrow end between her thighs
- Remove sanitary pad
- Assist her to sit more upright with legs slightly apart if she can as this makes urination easier
- When she has finished offer toilet paper
- Assist into a semirecumbent position; ask her to raise her buttocks and remove the bedpan carefully
- Offer hand-washing equipment
- Apply clean sanitary pad and disposable bed pad
- Replace top bed clothes and check her comfort level
- Dispose of bedpan and contents according to Trust policy
- Remove gloves and apron, wash hands and document

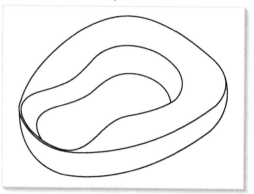

Figure 12.1 Metal bedpan.

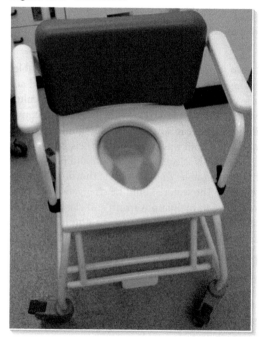

Figure 12.3 Commode.

Figure 12.2 Slipper bedpan.

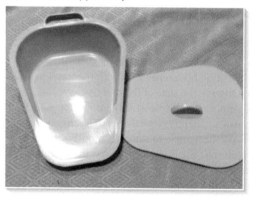

Key point

Attending to the genital hygiene and toileting needs of women requires a tactful and compassionate approach to avoid causing distress to women who are already vulnerable.

Midwifery Skills at a Glance, First Edition. Edited by Patricia Lindsay, Carmel Bagness and Ian Peate.
© 2018 John Wiley & Sons, Ltd. Published 2018 by John Wiley & Sons, Ltd.

Most women in maternity care do not require assistance with genital hygiene care or toileting but those who are bedbound may need some help. It is essential that this is skilful, carried out in private and preserves dignity as much as possible. All personal hygiene cares must be carried out with informed consent and documented fully. The midwife must wash hands before and after assisting with perineal hygiene and toileting.

Perineal care

Care of the perineum after birth is important to assist healing. Most women are able to attend to this themselves and only need advice about using maternity sanitary pads, changing them regularly and attention to hand hygiene before and after toileting or changing pads. The perineal area should be washed at least daily, in the shower or bath. Alternatively a bidet can be used (avoiding the 'jet' setting), or the vulval area rinsed with warm water poured over while she is sitting on the toilet. The area should be patted dry, from front to back. Hair dryers should not be used to dry the perineum. The midwife should inspect the perineum regularly to assess healing. The woman should be advised of the signs of infection and the need to report any concerns to the midwife.

Vulval hygiene

Women who are bed-bound will need assistance with vulval hygiene to maintain comfort and dignity, to assist perineal healing and prevent infection.

Equipment: gloves and apron, bedpan, jug, warm water, absorbent bed pad, clean sanitary pad, and dry wipes or disposable towels.

Procedure: Explain the procedure and gain consent. Ensure privacy. Wash and dry hands and don gloves and apron. Help her onto the bedpan. With the woman semirecumbent and knees flexed and apart, pour warm tap water over the vulva until it is clean. The area is gently dried with wipes or disposable towels and a clean sanitary pad applied. The woman is made comfortable and all equipment disposed of in accordance with local policy. Wash and dry hands.

Giving a bedpan

Purpose: To assist in emptying the bladder for women who do not have an in-dwelling catheter; to assist in managing defecation. Requests for a bedpan must be met promptly. The woman should be asked if she requires analgesia first. Correct moving and handling techniques must be used if the woman is unable to move herself.

Equipment: Gloves and apron, wash bowl with soap and towel or wet-wipes for hand cleaning before and after using the bedpan, clean, warm bedpan and cover, toilet tissue, clean sanitary pad, and clean disposable bed pad.

Procedure: See Box 12.1

Some bedpans are metal (Figure 12.1) but most are disposable pulp liners placed in a plastic support. If the woman is unable to lift her buttocks, a slipper bedpan can be used (Figure 12.2). The woman rolls onto her side, the slipper pan is slid in under her buttocks and she is rolled back onto it. A slipper bedpan is used with the wider or thicker end between the legs and the thinner portion under the buttocks.

Using a bedpan in front of another person is difficult for many women. If she asks for privacy and is stable while sitting on the bedpan, the call bell can be given while the midwife waits within earshot until she has finished.

Use of commodes

Commodes (Figure 12.3) are useful when the woman has enough mobility to get out of bed.

Equipment: Commode, with bedpan/commode liner in position below the seat, toilet paper, hand-washing equipment, gloves and apron. Moving and handling equipment may be required and a second person may be needed.

Procedure:
- Assess whether the woman needs assistance to move; check the load limit of the commode to ensure the woman's weight does not exceed this.
- Offer analgesia if required.
- Collect equipment, ensure privacy, wash hands and put on gloves and apron.
- Discuss the procedure with the woman and gain consent. Offer hand-washing equipment.
- Lower the bed to a safe height for the woman and apply the brakes.
- Position the commode by the bed, lock the brakes and assist the woman onto it. Give her the toilet paper.
- Cover her legs for warmth.
- If the woman asks for privacy she may be left with the call bell to hand. The midwife should stay within earshot.
- When the woman has finished, offer a clean maternity pad and hand-washing equipment.
- Assist her back into bed and check comfort.
- Remove equipment and dispose of bedpan contents.
- Remove apron and gloves and wash hands.
- Document.

Urine passed into a bedpan or commode can be measured and the amount recorded. Commodes and reusable bedpans must be thoroughly cleaned and disinfected between uses.

Service user's view

'They did not have any toilet tissue...I suppose at times they are busy...but they could have shown more care.'

Cohen 2009

13 Pressure area care

Figure 13.1 Common sites of pressure ulcers.

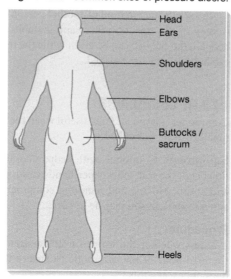

- Head
- Ears
- Shoulders
- Elbows
- Buttocks / sacrum
- Heels

Figure 13.2 Grade 1 pressure ulcer.
Source: Wicks G (2007) The treatment of pressure ulcers from grade 1 to grade 4. *Wound Essentials*, 2, 108. Reproduced with permission of Wounds UK.

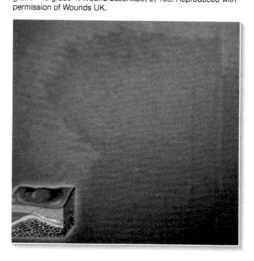

Table 13.1 Pressure ulcer risk factors.
Source: Morison B, Baker C (2001) How to raise awareness of pressure sore prevention. *British Journal of Midwifery* 9, 147-150. Reproduced with permission of MA Healthcare Ltd.

Factor	Specifics	Score	Factor	Specifics	Score
Skin condition	Dry	1	Body size	Overweight	1
	Oedematous	1		Obese	2
	Damp	1		Underweight	3
	Discolouration	2			
	Damaged	3	Continence / moisture	Incontinent of urine / faeces	1
				Ruptured membranes	1
Mobility	Restless	1	Food intake	Normal appetite	1
	Apathetic	2		Fluids only	2
	Restricted mobility	3		No oral intake / no appetite	3
	Inert / passive	4	Neurological / sensory risks	Neurological condition such as multiple sclerosis	2–6
	Chairbound / bedbound	5		Neurological deficit such as paraplegia, epidural	4–6
Tissue nutrition	Smoker	1	Scoring		
			Women: add 2 to score		
	Anaemia	2	Age 14–49 add 1 to score		
			Scores		
	Unstable diabetes	2	10+		At risk
			15+		High risk
	Surgery	2–4	20+		Very high risk

Key point

Pressure area assessment and management is an essential component of competent midwifery care.

Midwifery Skills at a Glance, First Edition. Edited by Patricia Lindsay, Carmel Bagness and Ian Peate.
© 2018 John Wiley & Sons, Ltd. Published 2018 by John Wiley & Sons, Ltd.

Pressure ulcers (also known as bed sores, pressure sores, decubitus ulcers)

A pressure ulcer is localised damage to skin and underlying tissue caused by shearing, friction or pressure forces. They may result in long-term morbidity such as pain and infection and are largely avoidable. It takes as little as 1 hour for tissue damage to begin. The National Patient Safety Agency receives around 100 reports of pressure ulcers in maternity cases each year.

Sites

The commonest sites are over bony prominences, often those with little underlying fat (Figure 13.1). These are:

- Elbows
- Heels
- Buttocks/sacrum
- Shoulders
- Head
- Hips
- Ears.

Causes

Pressure: localised pressure on a small area, pushing the tissues down onto a hard surface will reduce or stop capillary blood flow. The resultant tissue ischaemia leads to damage.

Shearing forces: damage occurs when tissue layers are forced to slide over each other. This may occur when a woman slides down the bed, or is pulled into another position. The skeleton moves in one direction but the soft tissues may stay in place, exerting a mechanical shearing force.

Friction: superficial damage occurs when the skin resists movement and is more likely if the skin is damp. Friction injury may occur if a woman is moved up the bed incorrectly.

Any person can develop a pressure ulcer but they are more likely to occur under the following conditions:

- Immobility/reduced mobility
- Neurological deficit resulting in impaired sensation
- Damp clothing/bedding (sweat, amniotic fluid, urine, faeces, blood)
- Poor posture
- Poor moving and handling techniques
- Poor nutritional status
- Obesity.

The European Pressure Ulcer Advisory Panel (EPUAP) recognises four grades of pressure ulcer:

Grade 1: skin discoloration, which does not blanch on light finger pressure (Figure 13.2).

Grade 2: the skin may appear chafed or blistered. The wound is shallow and there is damage to the dermis and epidermis.

Grade 3: the wound is deep and crater-like and there is full-thickness skin loss. The wound may undermine adjacent tissues.

Grade 4: the wound is deep, with necrotic tissue and underlying structures such as muscle and bone may be exposed.

Signs and symptoms

- Skin damage or abrasions: this may look like slightly grazed or roughened skin.
- Non-blanching erythema: light finger pressure on the reddened/darkened area should cause it to blanch (go white). The area should return to the normal colour once the pressure ceases. Failure to blanch is a sign of underlying tissue damage
- Soggy-looking skin: the skin looks damp and may feel slightly boggy
- Localised warmth
- Localised soreness.

The underlying damage is always more extensive than the skin signs would suggest. Women with darker skin tones are at higher risk as identification of superficial tissue damage such as non-blanching erythema is harder to determine.

Prevention

The skin should be checked at least every 2 hours to assess:

- Integrity, looking for signs of breaches, chafing
- Colour, looking for changes/discoloration
- Changes in local skin temperature
- Texture: pliability, elasticity and firmness.

Use of the Plymouth Score for Maternity may help to assess risk of pressure ulcer development (Table 13.1).

Bedding must be kept dry and wrinkle free. Barrier creams may be useful if the membranes are ruptured and bedding is persistently damp. The pressure areas must be assessed and the woman's position must be changed regularly, at least every 2 hours, using appropriate moving and handling techniques and equipment. The skin should not be rubbed or massaged. Use pressure relieving devices where appropriate. A pillow between the knees may relieve pressure between these joints and the overlying skin. The pillow must not be placed lengthwise between the lower legs as this may produce pressure on the calf muscles and reduce venous return from the legs.

Neonates are at risk of pressure ulcers if they are immobile as may be the case with a sick baby in the neonatal intensive care unit. The occiput is a common site of pressure sores in neonates.

Service user's view

'They give me pain killers and sleeping tablets but I wake up with it.'

Hopkins *et al.* 2006

14 Risk management, liability and avoidable harm

Figure 14.1 Evidence-based practice and good record keeping is essential.

Key point

Proactive risk management frameworks reduce the incidence of avoidable harm and promotes the provision of safe high-quality maternity care through effective multidisciplinary team working.

Midwifery Skills at a Glance, First Edition. Edited by Patricia Lindsay, Carmel Bagness and Ian Peate.

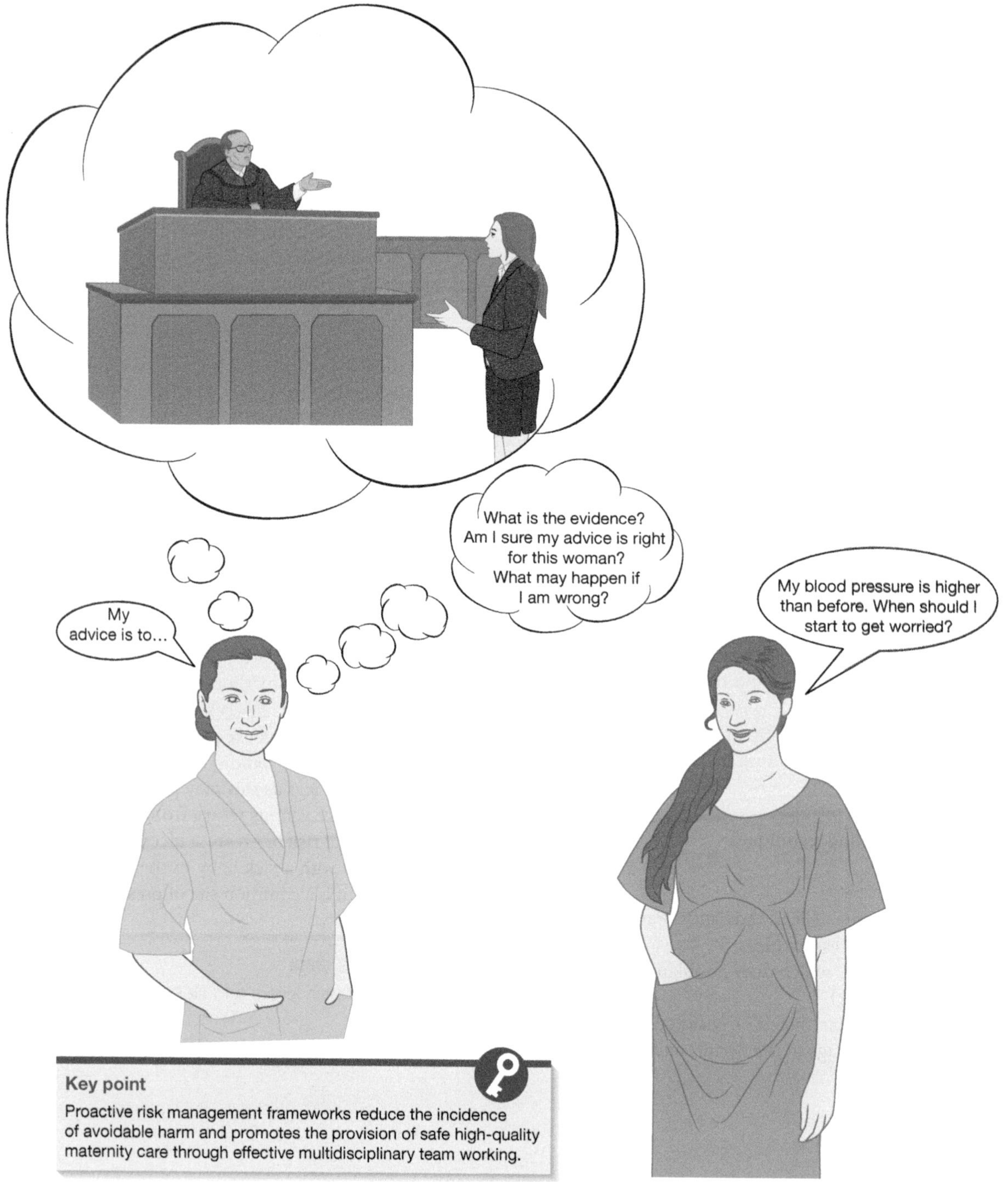

Reducing harm, promoting safety, quality and being accountable for the standard of care given are important aspects of risk management. These interconnected topics can generate fear and result in cautious practice but by creating a culture of proactive risk management, lower levels of harm will result.

Managing risks is intended to reduce harm and promote safety, which impacts across every aspect of life not just in professional practice, ranging from crossing the road to preventing postpartum haemorrhage. As a systematic way of reducing harm, risk management processes rely on the identification, assessment, and prioritisation of real or potential problems.

In general, practitioners do not set out to cause harm. In managing risk, the distinction needs to be made between committing intentional harm and unintentional mistakes. Humans make errors so it is not possible to eradicate all risks but steps can be taken to minimise them. Consequently, organisations will focus on those risks that are likely to have the most impact on them or women in their care. Commonly, organisations will give priority to risks that carry the highest potential for harm, including those that expose them financially and have implications for their reputation.

NHS Resolution handles clinical negligence claims against NHS organisations. From their data, 70% of total obstetric claims are caused by three (overlapping) categories. These are mistakes in fetal heart rate interpretation, mistakes in the management of labour and the development of cerebral palsy.

Clinical negligence, litigation and compensation are issues that organisations might look at corporately. Of course women accessing services would want catastrophic and rarely occurring risks to be minimised but they also want more common risks such as medication incidents and the occurrence of infection to be minimised too.

In considering human factors in relation to risk management, the aim is to optimise human performance and reduce human failures. Where possible, systems and processes should be created that design out the potential for human failure and design in the potential for recovery should human failure occur. This includes the design of equipment, environments and tasks, and takes into account the needs and capabilities of practitioners. Although important, reliance on procedures and training alone are unlikely to be sufficient.

Elements of risk management are related to relationships between professionals and the women accessing services. Multiprofessional teams often practice skills and drills together to ensure that when a problem happens in reality they are well rehearsed in what to do; teams who train together tend to work well together. A fundamental skill in this is listening to each other – and the women – when concerns are raised.

Harm can be avoided. Catastrophic harm has a high profile partly because it is rare and partly because it has become a political ambition to minimise the risks associated with stillbirths, infant deaths and maternal deaths. There are now targets to reduce the number of stillbirths, neonatal and maternal deaths and intrapartum brain injuries to babies by 20% by 2020 and by 50% by 2030 to ensure England is one of the safest places to have a baby. It is intended to achieve this in part by funding better equipment and training and also through the use of agreed pathways of care such as the Saving Babies Lives care bundle. There is also a need to ensure women can access appropriate and timely antenatal, intrapartum and postnatal care, which promotes wellbeing and reduces the risk of their babies coming to harm through smoking, drinking alcohol, obesity and diabetes for example.

The action plan for the NHS in England to make maternity services safer is *Safer Maternity Care: next steps towards the national maternity ambition*, which is being implemented.

Effective communication and strong clinical and managerial leadership within teams is crucial – thus teams who train together tend to work well together. Avoidable harm is usually not the result of staff failing their duty of care, it can be caused by competing priorities, pressures of work and not being able to keep up-to-date with training and new clinical developments. There is therefore a relationship between the wellbeing of teams (and their individual members) and the quality of care to women and babies.

Empowered women are now much more vocal about the quality of the services they are provided with. They are supported by apps and electronic access to information, which is ever growing and gives them confidence to have conversations with practitioners as equal partners in their care. The dynamics of these relationships are extremely important when it comes to avoiding harm.

Liability

All midwives are accountable to the Nursing and Midwifery Council (NMC) and are bound by the NMC Code. It is a legal requirement to have in place an indemnity arrangement that provides appropriate cover relevant to personal scope of practice. For midwives working in the NHS, their employer will be vicariously liable provided their practice follows the guidelines, protocols and processes expected by the employer. Some midwives practice independently, and have to demonstrate personal indemnity or insurance cover.

It is important to consider any conflict of interest when caring for a friend or relative, where a separate indemnity or insurance arrangement will be required.

Liability, when something goes wrong, could be judged long after the event, so contemporaneous records are crucial to tell the story years hence (Figure 14.1).

In organisations providing maternity services, the chief executive is the accountable officer with responsibility for risk including health and safety. However, this does not diminish practitioners' personal and professional accountability.

Healthcare worker's view

'[We should be] putting the mother and baby at the heart of all protocols and procedures.'

Smith *et al*. 2009

15 Types of incident, incident reporting, record keeping and duty of candour

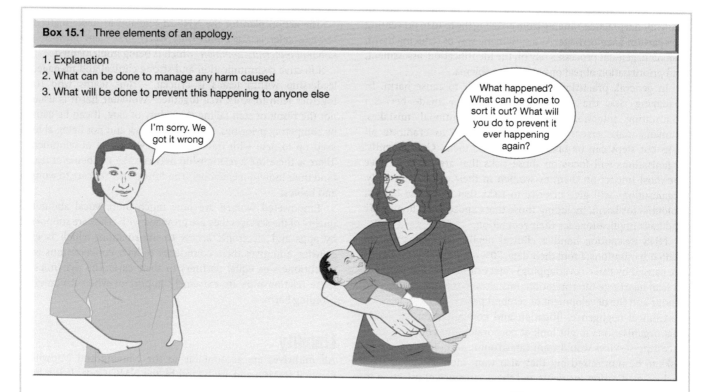

Box 15.1 Three elements of an apology.

1. Explanation
2. What can be done to manage any harm caused
3. What will be done to prevent this happening to anyone else

Key point

A culture of high incident reporting, low harm and openness and transparency in maternity services supports the identification of trends and remedial action to learn from errors.

Midwifery Skills at a Glance, First Edition. Edited by Patricia Lindsay, Carmel Bagness and Ian Peate.
© 2018 John Wiley & Sons, Ltd. Published 2018 by John Wiley & Sons, Ltd.

This chapter draws together:
- Incidents
- Record keeping
- The duty of candour.

Incidents can take a number of forms and might be clinical, operational or near misses. They are situations from which learning takes place and some of that learning comes from examining the contemporaneous records, which can be looked at in retrospect with a critical but objective view without seeking to find blame for mistakes. However, errors and incidents do happen and practitioners should be clear about what is said, being candid with women and families when explaining the incidents and their consequences.

Types of incident

Incidents in maternity services can fall into two groups: maternity triggers and wider incidents. Maternity triggers include postpartum haemorrhage (PPH), massive obstetric haemorrhage (MOH), third- and fourth-degree tears, cord prolapse, and an Apgar score of less than 7 at 5 minutes. Wider incidents include operational incidents relating to the running of the organisation, staffing levels and complaints, for example.

Reporting incidents

All incidents or near misses must be reported. Most organisations have an electronic system of recording and reporting incidents or near misses. The purpose of reporting incidents is to improve care so those reporting incidents should have feedback about what is going to be done to address the consequences of the incident. Readily reporting incidents drives a culture of openness and transparency, change and reducing risk. Organisations with high levels of reporting tend to have low levels of harm – but only if they do something about the incidents that are reported.

Midwives should know their organisation's top five incidents. Analysing incidents, spotting trends and implementing targeted actions to reduce incidents all serve to raise the awareness of the risks and what can be done to mitigate them. Acting on incidents could include a one-off investigation, including findings from a review in a clinical audit programme, a documentation audit or surveying staff and service users for their views and input.

In serious incidents, such as maternal or neonatal death or traumatic shoulder dystocia, it is good practice to hold a debriefing session for those involved as soon as practically possible after the event. This gives those involved a chance to reflect and discuss what happened, expose the possible reasons why and examine the team dynamics at play during the incident.

If a midwife is involved in an incident, they should seek support. This might come from a senior and experienced colleague, a clinical leader or a professional organisation.

For more information on reductions in incidents see the National Patient Safety Agency and NHS Resolution websites.

Record keeping

The Nursing and Midwifery Council (NMC) have said that good record keeping is an integral part of practice, and is essential to the provision of safe and effective care. It is not an optional extra and is the mark of a skilled and safe practitioner.

Contemporaneous records are best with dates and times, but make clear if they are written some time after an event with the date and time that the records were actually written.

Records must be kept secure and respect confidentiality. Information can be shared appropriately for investigations into incidents or other situations, which are in the best interests of high-quality care.

Records should be written as though they are being read long after the event, especially if there is a complaint, investigation or hearing. If it is not written down, there is no evidence that something took place.

Avoid using abbreviations and use black ink if they are handwritten. They must be legible when photocopied or scanned. Any corrections should be made by striking through the discarded text with a single line only, signed and dated.

The objective of record keeping is to provide a factual account of care and offer protection to the woman and the midwife. Good documentation can help reduce risks, harm and litigation, and improve the quality of care.

Regular audits of documentation are essential to ensure that a good standard of record keeping is maintained with action taken to improve practice.

Duty of candour

The duty of candour imposed on all practitioners is part of the Health and Social Care Act 2008 (Regulated Activities) Regulations 2014: Regulation 20. The NMC and the General Medical Council have produced joint guidance on the professional duty of candour, which reinforces the need for practitioners to be open and honest when things go wrong. It is covered in section 14 of the NMC Code.

The principles are that practitioners must:
- Tell the woman (or, where appropriate, her advocate, partner, carer or family) when something has gone wrong
- Apologise to the woman (or, where appropriate, her advocate, partner, carer or family)
- Offer an appropriate remedy or support to put matters right (if possible)
- Explain fully to the woman (or, where appropriate, her advocate, partner, carer or family) the short- and long-term effects of what has happened.

Women expect to be told three things as part of an apology (Box 15.1):
- What happened
- What can be done to deal with any harm caused
- What will be done to prevent someone else being harmed.

Apologising to a woman does not mean admitting legal liability for what has happened. This is set out in legislation and NHS Resolution also advises that saying sorry is the right thing to do. And when there is an investigation the woman (or, where appropriate, her advocate, partner, carer or family) should be kept informed of its progress, findings and remedial actions.

Healthcare worker's view

'Healthcare workers are often impacted by medical errors as "second victims", and experience many of the same emotions and/or feelings that the "first victims" – the patient and family members'.

Wu and Steckelberg 2012

16 Audit and quality assurance in maternity care

Figure 16.1 The focus of audit is the people we serve.

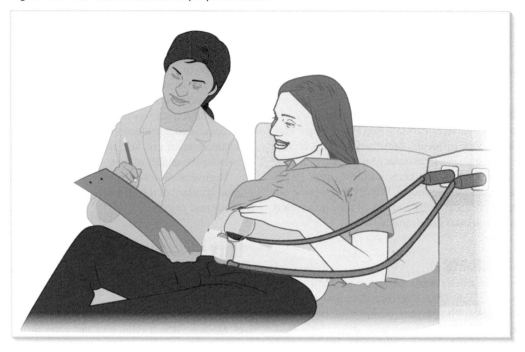

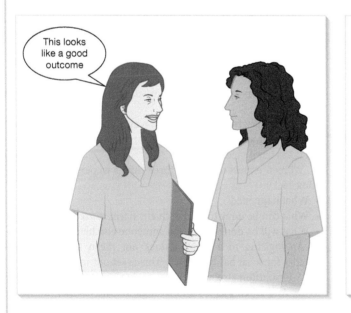

This looks like a good outcome

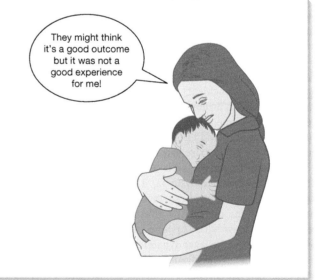

They might think it's a good outcome but it was not a good experience for me!

Key point

Effective audit and quality assurance processes are integral parts of the clinical governance framework within maternity services.

Midwifery Skills at a Glance, First Edition. Edited by Patricia Lindsay, Carmel Bagness and Ian Peate.
© 2018 John Wiley & Sons, Ltd. Published 2018 by John Wiley & Sons, Ltd.

Audit is a process of quality improvement. This chapter considers clinical audit, that is audit directly related to clinical care, but audits of other integral parts of service delivery, such as staffing, education and training, sickness absence, bed occupancy and activity levels, are also important as part of the infrastructure that enables high-quality care to be given.

Clinical audit contributes to quality assurance, which in turn contributes to clinical governance. Clinical governance is a set of processes that examine clinical outcomes alongside risk management and user feedback, particularly to provide evidence of service outcomes and quality. In considering quality assurance, there is also a distinction to draw here between assurance and reassurance. Assurance is best thought of as a positive declaration that something is guaranteed, whereas reassurance will confirm an impression. Assurance is based on objective evidence in a way that reassurance is not necessarily, because it can be based on a subjective opinion and give false confidence that standards and quality are being met.

For this reason, audits or clinical audits are used to improve care and outcomes by systematically examining systems and processes against explicit criteria. These criteria might be standards that are set nationally by, for example, the National Institute of Health and Care Excellence (NICE), royal colleges, service regulators, professional regulators, commissioners of services or organisations (or teams within them) themselves. The standards set the baseline against which to audit and measure how well services are being run, and to discover what needs to be changed to improve them. This process should be ExACT: based on examining, analysing, changing and testing.

Examining

The topic to be examined should be clearly defined so that robust data can be collected. In maternity services it is common that certain issues are regularly audited so that trends and areas of concern can be addressed, and areas where improvement has been made can be celebrated. Such regular audits include, for example, breast feeding rates, normal births, caesarean section rates, vaginal births after caesarean section, instrumental deliveries, postpartum haemorrhage and third- and fourth-degree tears. Mandatory training, such as cardiotocograph (CTG) interpretation for all organisations that use CTG monitoring, should be in place. Whatever form that training takes, whether it is face-to-face, e-learning or multiprofessional review of CTG interpretation, its purpose is to reduce the risk of human error in interpreting a trace. Audit should therefore not be confined, in this example, as to whether the training has taken place and who accessed it, but should also examine its effectiveness: have risks, errors and harm been reduced as a consequence?

A comprehensive series of maternity audit indicators was produced collaboratively in 2008 by the Royal College of Obstetricians and Gynaecologists, the Royal College of Midwives, the Royal College of Anaesthetists and the Royal College of Paediatrics and Child Health. These standards and audit indicators cover the whole maternity pathway from looking forward to pregnancy to the postnatal period.

NHS Resolution has also produced an audit template for maternity services.

With so many resources available it is important, in conducting personal audit, not to reinvent the wheel. There may be situations in organisations and in teams where a specific issue needs close examination because of the systems and processes employed and where outcomes, because of feedback from women or other sources, can be improved. It is important, in deciding what to examine, to engage with women and their families who have direct experience of the service to gauge what they think is important to audit; their perspective might be different from the perspective of the professionals (Figure 16.1) and audit should focus on the people we aim to serve.

Analysing

Analysis of the data collected is important so that it is not accepted at face value. There should be objective scrutiny so that the constituent parts of a service or the issue under examination can be understood. This analysis can be focussed on individual elements of a service or take a wider view. There are now examples of a number of services pooling their data for analysis to gain a broad picture of quality, including safety, effectiveness and experience, which can be used regionally to benchmark services against each other as a strategic clinical network dashboard. This is an area highlighted as good practice in *Better Births* (NHS 2016).

Changing

Analysis will generate findings from which recommendations for change can be derived. Recommendations made from the audit findings should be SMART (specific, measurable, achievable, realistic and timely). This enables re-audit and subsequent examination to be clear what improvements have been made and where more work needs to be done. A timetable for change and a process for ensuring teams are stimulated and motivated to drive the change is essential. Audit results will not bring about change by telepathy so a systematic implementation plan needs to be constructed and monitored.

Testing

To test the effectiveness of improvements each maternity service should have an audit programme reviewed on an annual basis linked to national and regional benchmarking data. Local indicators for the audit programme arise from trends and analysis of clinical outcome data, incident reporting and findings from investigations. Local audit can be indicated when there is a need to test a deeper understanding of contributory factors related to practice issues, organisational processes and the subsequent impact on clinical outcomes and the quality of care. It is imperative to test the impact against the criteria and standards set at the beginning of the process. Involving users of the services is important when testing out each component of the audit: the findings are not just about the professionals and their practice; it is also about the outcomes for and the experiences of the women, babies and families in our care.

17 Safeguarding vulnerable women

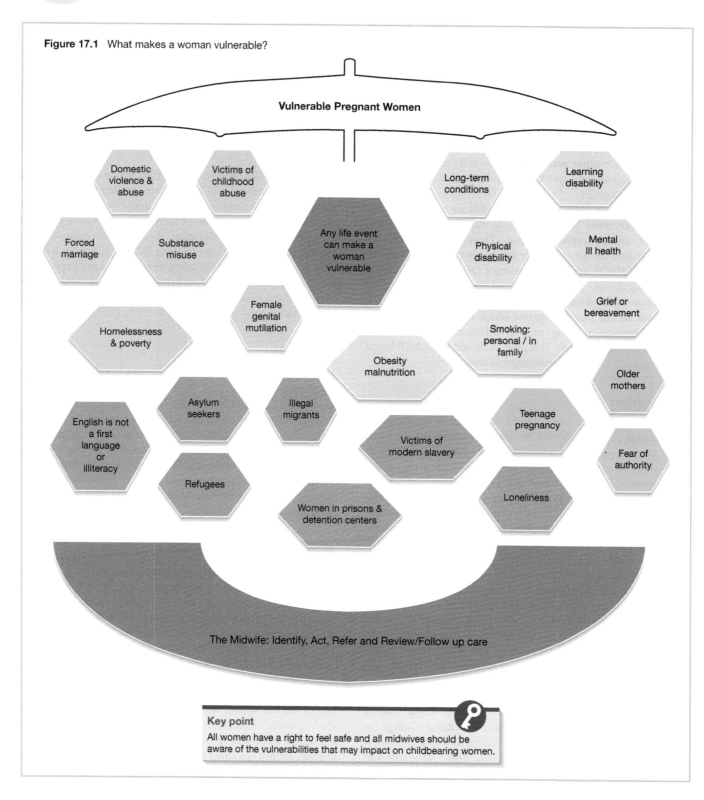

Figure 17.1 What makes a woman vulnerable?

Key point

All women have a right to feel safe and all midwives should be aware of the vulnerabilities that may impact on childbearing women.

Midwifery Skills at a Glance, First Edition. Edited by Patricia Lindsay, Carmel Bagness and Ian Peate.
© 2018 John Wiley & Sons, Ltd. Published 2018 by John Wiley & Sons, Ltd.

Anyone can feel vulnerable, and any pregnant woman may feel some vulnerability even when attending for care. Feeling at risk of harm, physical or psychological, social or economic, makes one less able to manage, whilst being safe is a basic human right, based on dignity, respect, fairness and equality. These principles should be applied to maternity care, where all women should be treated with respect and kindness. Some women fear authority, which may be extreme in some cases, and the midwife needs to understand this in order to focus her compassion and care appropriately.

Women should feel safe, be able to express concerns without prejudice and feel they are working in partnership with the maternity team towards informed decisions about their childbirth. Midwives are obliged to see all pregnant women and have a responsibility to identify vulnerability, and facilitate the best care possible. Figure 17.1 outlines some of the reasons that may make women vulnerable. Midwives also have a role in ensuring the right services are commissioned to meet the needs of all women in their area, working with health and social care to have clear referral paths to enhance continuity of care.

The midwife needs to understand who may be at greater risk of being vulnerable (Figure 17.1), and how they might identify these women. This may mean asking difficult questions, not making judgments based on appearance or language skills or attitude. It demands treating everyone equally, whilst being prepared to probe carefully, with sensitivity (in private) and with a sound knowledge of the signs to consider. Their duty of care involves taking reasonable steps to identify and reduce risk whilst respecting the woman's right to make choices; however, if the midwife believes the woman is at risk, she may require referral through the local safeguarding processes, which the midwife should be familiar with.

Vulnerable women come with different needs:
• Women who have physical or learning difficulties, or long-term conditions may require different services or ongoing contact with services they are already familiar with to make the best choices that suit them.
• Women experiencing mental health issues need support and good links with local mental health services, as well as voluntary groups, who may be able to provide help such as cognitive behavioral therapy.
• Women who are in poverty or homeless, or those in prison or detention centres, may have real concerns about whether they will be able to keep their baby.
• Pregnant women with complex social needs are more likely to require additional support. Social isolation has been identified as a significant factor with regards to vulnerability.
• Women who are suffering domestic abuse need access to safety information; all midwives should know referral pathways and sources of support.
• Midwives need to understand the strategies to employ should they be concerned. Safelives (2016) showed that 85% of victims sought help on average five times the year before they received effective help. The midwife is a key person in recognising and supporting those suffering domestic abuse.
• Many women who come from abroad, especially asylum seekers, refugees, migrants or victims of modern slavery, may not know how to access services, or indeed if they are entitled to care within the NHS.

• For women who do not speak English or English is not their first language extra care must be taken to ensure they understand the services and that the midwife understands their expectations. Their previous experiences may be very different, so assumptions cannot be made about their understanding of systems and processes.
• If it is felt that a woman does not have the capacity to make decisions, this may be a safeguarding issue, and further help should be sought through the safeguarding lead. Any actions taken by the midwife without informed consent must be justifiable and recorded.

Women may face more than one challenge in their lives; they may be in a cycle of deprivation, where they have complex issues to manage during pregnancy. Some women come with chaotic lives meaning they may not be able to attend or afford to access services. Being pregnant may be a vulnerability that can be avoided going forward so effective family spacing is also a critical part of the midwife's role.

Partners and families are also an important part of care provision, particularly so when a woman is vulnerable, with the possible exception of when the midwife is concerned that the women is being abused or at risk from family members or community members.

There are voluntary groups and charities that campaign on behalf of vulnerable people (for example homelessness, FGM survivors, domestic abuse), which the midwife should have knowledge of, especially any working locally that can be used as ongoing support mechanisms.

The quality of the midwife's communication skills are key when supporting vulnerable women; the need to be able to converse and listen are essential. This combined with evidence-based care, collaboration across multiple agencies and the need to provide culturally appropriate services, whilst acknowledging they may have to be balanced with the reality of available services and support mechanisms, can be challenging.

Top tips for midwives

• Knowing how to recognise the range of vulnerabilities
• Compassion towards all women (and their partners)
• Open questioning
• Active listening
• Private safe environment
• Believe the woman
• Non-judgmental attitude
• See the woman on her own at least once
• Coordinating care across a range of services
• Knowing what to do when you identify the vulnerability.

Service user's view

'Women who are homeless are among the most marginalised people in society. Sadly, women's homelessness often occurs after prolonged experiences of trauma, including physical, sexual and emotional abuse, frequently within the home. It often follows from and results in a cycle of mental ill health and substance use, and a myriad of other problems.'

Hutchinson *et al.* 2015

18 Safeguarding of children: key issues

Figure 18.1 Potential situations and action.

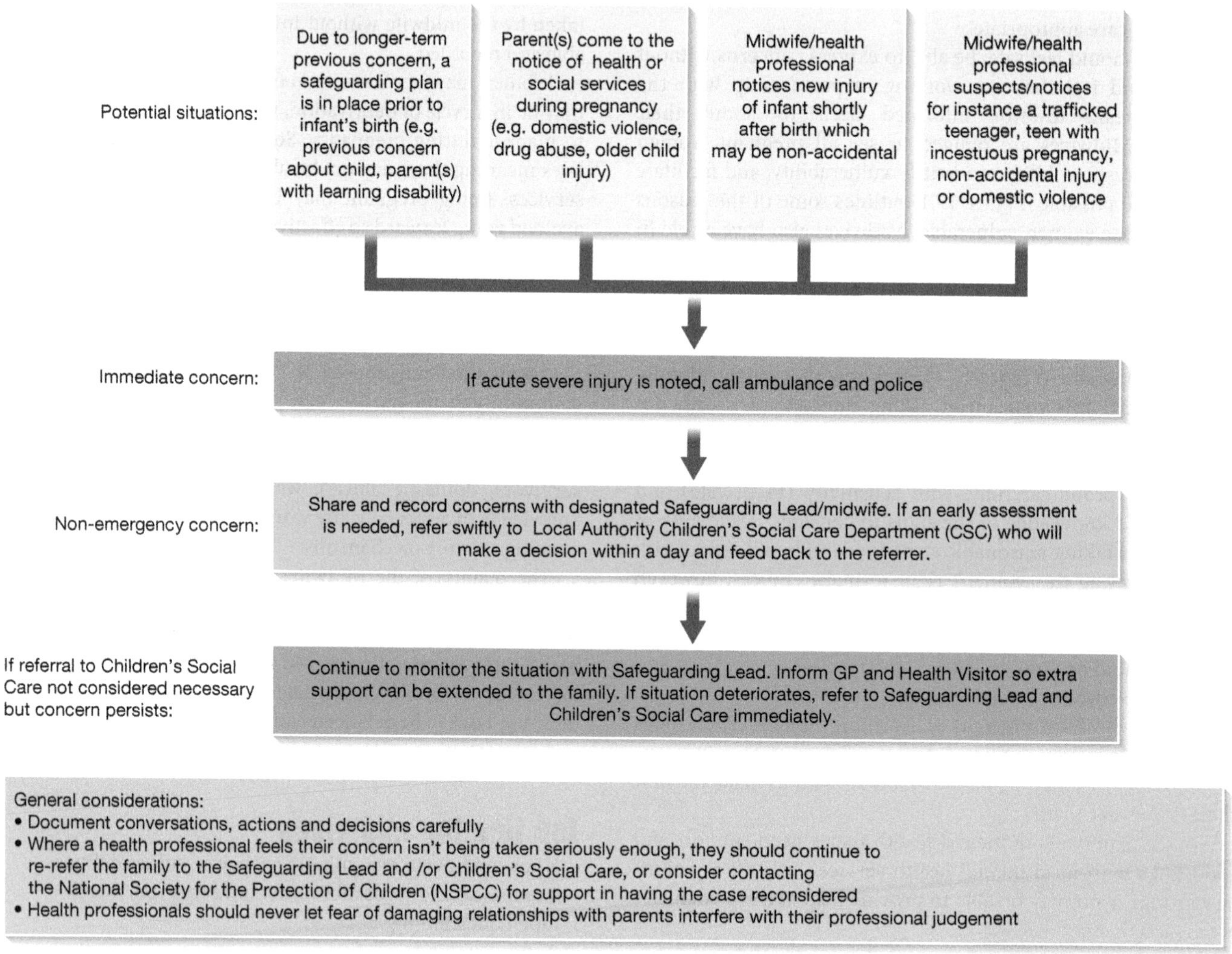

Potential situations:

| Due to longer-term previous concern, a safeguarding plan is in place prior to infant's birth (e.g. previous concern about child, parent(s) with learning disability) | Parent(s) come to the notice of health or social services during pregnancy (e.g. domestic violence, drug abuse, older child injury) | Midwife/health professional notices new injury of infant shortly after birth which may be non-accidental | Midwife/health professional suspects/notices for instance a trafficked teenager, teen with incestuous pregnancy, non-accidental injury or domestic violence |

Immediate concern:

If acute severe injury is noted, call ambulance and police

Non-emergency concern:

Share and record concerns with designated Safeguarding Lead/midwife. If an early assessment is needed, refer swiftly to Local Authority Children's Social Care Department (CSC) who will make a decision within a day and feed back to the referrer.

If referral to Children's Social Care not considered necessary but concern persists:

Continue to monitor the situation with Safeguarding Lead. Inform GP and Health Visitor so extra support can be extended to the family. If situation deteriorates, refer to Safeguarding Lead and Children's Social Care immediately.

General considerations:
- Document conversations, actions and decisions carefully
- Where a health professional feels their concern isn't being taken seriously enough, they should continue to re-refer the family to the Safeguarding Lead and /or Children's Social Care, or consider contacting the National Society for the Protection of Children (NSPCC) for support in having the case reconsidered
- Health professionals should never let fear of damaging relationships with parents interfere with their professional judgement

Key points

Safeguarding involves both supporting the wellbeing of children and child protection, and covers:
- Protecting children from maltreatment
- Preventing impairment of children's health or development
- Ensuring that children are growing up in circumstances consistent with the provision of safe and effective care, and
- Taking action to enable all children to have the best life chances.

Midwifery Skills at a Glance, First Edition. Edited by Patricia Lindsay, Carmel Bagness and Ian Peate.
© 2018 John Wiley & Sons, Ltd. Published 2018 by John Wiley & Sons, Ltd.

Health and social care professionals have a role in both promoting positive practices in health and social care of children and young people, and protecting and reporting individuals where they are at risk of abuse. Each of these lie within a continuum of professional practice referred to as safeguarding. Unborn infants are not legally defined as children in the UK but they may need protection from harm.

The UN Convention on the Rights of the Child lists four core principles at the heart of children's safety and wellbeing:

* Non-discrimination
* Devotion to the best interests of the child
* The right to life, survival and development
* Respect for the views of the child.

The role of health and social care professionals in safeguarding unborn babies, children and young pregnant adolescents

* The role starts before birth, by offering expectant parents evidence-informed information and an opportunity to discuss their beliefs, values and wishes for their child. The provision of two-way information should include the principles of emotional attachment and parenting skills, and coping with a persistently crying baby.
* Where a health professional has concerns about a child's safety and wellbeing, they should discuss this with their manager and designated Safeguarding Lead. The family should be referred to services they may benefit from, for instance a supportive play group or registered organisation providing respite care.
* If a child is in acute danger the police should be informed immediately as well as the Local Authority Children's Social Care Department.
* Where meetings, or a Child Protection Conference is convened, involved health professionals should attend and be prepared to give evidence and, when asked, their opinion.
* With pregnant teenagers, health professionals should consider the possibility of coercive and other forms of abuse, especially if no partner is acknowledged or the partner is much older.

Potential situations and actions are outlined in Figure 18.1.

Where child abuse occurs, it can take a number of different forms.

Physical abuse or 'non-accidental injury' includes pinching, slapping, punching, burning, throwing, scalding, burning, poisoning or stabbing. Shaking babies and young children can cause brain damage, and 'Chinese burns' can cause friction burns and long bone fractures to very young children.

An unusual form of physical abuse is fabricated or induced illness (FII, formerly known as Munchausen's syndrome by proxy), where a parent presents the child to health professionals as ill, for instance having starved the child while claiming s/he eats well, or giving a noxious substance. Female genital mutilation (FGM) is also a form of child abuse.

Generally, the midwife should look for both damage to a baby's skin, abnormal movement (head injury or fractured bones), and note the parents' history and current behaviours in considering their diagnosis. Sometimes a partner or family member will attempt to physically abuse an unborn baby by attacking the expectant mother's abdomen or causing her to come to physical harm herself, thereby damaging the fetus.

Emotional abuse of children can take the form of lack of kindness or emotional warmth, excessive teasing and verbal cruelty, criticism or control, verbal aggression, conditional love and affection, persistent unrealistic expectations and/or rejection. This type of abuse is often difficult to recognise but the midwife should take into account any family history of abuse with previous children, or an apparent lack of caring and emotional warmth in either parent. Physically abused children are almost always emotionally abused, but emotionally abused children may not be physically abused.

Child sexual abuse involves any sexual contact with a child under 16 years old, usually by an adult. It may also take the form of a child being looked at, groomed or photographed for indecent purposes, and images being circulated to others. Child sexual abuse does not necessarily involve contact or violence, and a child may not realise it is happening or wrong. The midwife should be alert to any damage to the external genitalia or femur fractures in a baby, which should be immediately reported and investigated. Although less common, women and other children can be perpetrators. Affected children can develop mental ill health and/or behaviour issues.

When caring for a pregnant girl under 18 years old incest should always be considered, especially if the girl is reticent about giving details about the baby's father.

Child exploitation is usually for sexual and/or housekeeping purposes (modern slavery), often involving young teenagers, sometimes with a controlling man (or woman) 'minder' when they access health services. This is thought to be an under-reported crime in the developed world with children being brought from other countries, sometimes sold by their parents. Western children who have been in care are also at risk, particularly of sexual exploitation.

Neglect

Neglect of babies and young children can cause serious harm, as they may be poorly fed, supervised or protected.

Expectant mothers can also neglect their unborn baby by substance misuse or excessive alcohol consumption.

Other forms of abuse include online abuse (for instance bullying, 'sexting', revenge pornography) and young children observing domestic abuse and violence in the home.

Midwives should always be alert to this possibility as they interact with new mothers and observe their behaviour around the baby and any other children.

Service user's view

'I didn't know what to do! How do I know when to change her, how do I know when to feed her? And the worker said to me, "You'll just know don't worry." She told me, "You can do it." …Knowing somebody, especially a professional, believed in me helped me believe in myself.'

Sixteen-year-old participant, Dumbrill 2006

19 Female genital mutilation

Box 19.1 World Health Organization: Definition and classification of FGM.
Source: Adapted from WHO (2016) *FGM Fact Sheet* http://www.who.int/mediacentre/factsheets/fs241/en/ (accessed February 2017). Reproduced with permission of World Health Organisation.

'FGM comprises all procedures that involve partial or total removal of the external female genitalia, or other injury to the female genital organs for non-medical reasons.'

Type 1: Clitoridectomy: Part or all of the clitoris is removed, or more uncommonly the removal of the clitoral hood only.

Type 2: Excision: Part or all of the clitoris and labia minora are removed; can involve the labia majora as well.

Type 3: Infibulation: The opening of the vagina is narrowed by the labia minora or the labia majora being cut and repositioned to form a seal over the vaginal entrance. The clitoris may or may not be removed.

Type 4: Any other methods carried out for non-medical reasons which damage the female genitalia. Can include the following: pricking, piercing, incising, scraping and cauterisation.

Key point

On assessment of the woman's genitalia, if you are able to visualise the urethral meatus easily, this means the woman has an adequate introitus for a vaginal birth and will not require a deinfibulation procedure.

Figure 19.2 Type 2 FGM with key genitalia identified.

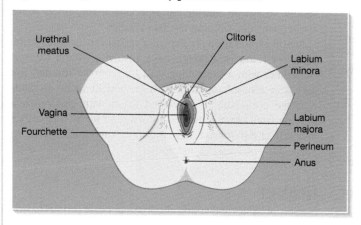

Figure 19.3 Type 3 FGM – infibulation.

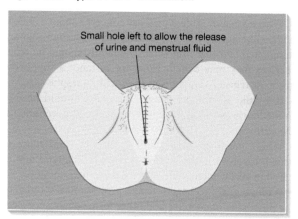

Figure 19.4 Type 4 FGM example – stretched labia.

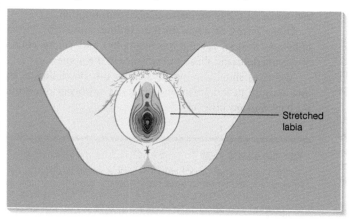

Figure 19.5 Anterior episiotomy (deinfibulation) procedure.

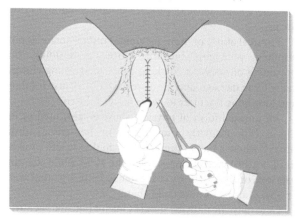

Midwifery Skills at a Glance, First Edition. Edited by Patricia Lindsay, Carmel Bagness and Ian Peate.
© 2018 John Wiley & Sons, Ltd. Published 2018 by John Wiley & Sons, Ltd.

Female genital mutilation (FGM), also known as female genital cutting, is an unjustifiable practice that damages the health of girls and women. It is mainly performed by certain ethnic communities in Africa, some areas of the Middle East and Asia, but due to immigration it is an issue in the UK, where it has been categorised as a form of child abuse. Safeguarding procedures must be initiated if a girl or vulnerable adult is thought to be at risk. As a midwife, knowledge and skills need to be developed in order to provide effective care for a pregnant woman with FGM. A focus on both the woman's health needs, alongside the safeguarding aspects, must be considered carefully and sensitively within the care provided.

Identification and assessment of FGM

A woman with FGM should be identified early in the antenatal period (preferably at booking) and referred to a consultant obstetrician or midwife specialising in FGM, so that a full assessment and plan of care is put in place. Effective communication is key, as women should be asked about FGM in a culturally sensitive way and be given time to discuss this issue. In turn, the midwife needs to understand FGM to be able to help facilitate the conversation, identifying individual needs and remaining nonjudgmental. Information on how to communicate with women and girls with FGM is available in the Government's multiagency guidance on FGM and the FGM e-learning programme by Health Education England.

Many health problems result from FGM and a good understanding of these will assist a midwife in identifying a woman's needs. For example, urinary tract infections, HIV or hepatitis B, complications in labour and birth and the psychological trauma a woman may face will all have a direct impact on a woman and her pregnancy. Assessing a woman thoroughly will enable her to be cared for in a holistic manner, which takes account of physical, psychological, psychosexual and social needs.

It is important to assess (if possible) the type of FGM a woman has (Box 19.1; Figures 19.1–19.4); however, in maternity care, what needs to be ascertained is whether the woman has an adequate introitus for the birth of her baby. If, on inspection, the urethral meatus can be easily visualised, the woman has the potential for a normal vaginal birth and to receive midwifery-led care, although the Royal College of Obstetricians and Gynaecologists advise that this may be dependent on the history of previous births. In all cases, the midwife should always be vigilant for any vaginal or perineal scarring that could affect progress in the second stage of labour. If the urethral meatus cannot be visualised, as in type 3 FGM, then a deinfibulation procedure is required (also known as anterior episiotomy).

Deinfibulation is where the scar tissue concealing the entrance of the vagina is cut open. This should be offered in the antenatal period at around 20 weeks or, if preferred, during the labour itself, either in the first stage to enable procedures to be performed or in the second stage, just prior to the fetal head crowning. If performing an anterior episiotomy for deinfibulation in labour, infiltrate with lidocaine 1% (as per local policy) along the midline of the scar. Use of forceps behind the scar can help prevent damage by the needle to the area beneath. An orange (25 gauge) needle may be used if the area is thin and weak. The anaesthetic should be allowed to infiltrate, then with the forefinger inserted as a guide, straight scissors should be used to perform an incision along the middle of the scar, going no further than the urethral meatus (Figure 19.5). This is to avoid excessive bleeding, which could occur if the more vascular clitoral region was cut. Pressure may be applied to the cut, although bleeding is often minimal. Aseptic technique must be used throughout. If the clitoris is felt, a skilled practitioner may carefully extend the cut to that region.

Promoting normality

Girls may be held down by force for FGM to take place and the psychosocial trauma and post-traumatic stress that can result from the procedure is significant. This highlights how a woman with FGM must be empowered to have the birth that she desires, so that she feels in control of her body and any decisions made. By offering and performing deinfibulation in the antenatal period, if appropriate, the woman could be transferred to midwifery-led care and be more in control of her labour and birth by having less intervention than if she were placed on a high-risk regimen due to the FGM.

Legislation and safeguarding

The UK does not tolerate FGM, as it remains illegal through the FGM Act 2003 and the revised Serious Crime Act 2015. A midwife must be fully aware of the responsibility with regard to the safeguarding aspects surrounding FGM and the recording of cases through the FGM Enhanced Dataset. Guidance is provided by the Government, which includes information about the FGM **mandatory reporting duty** for girls under 18 years and assessing risk for a female child or woman, with guidance on the most appropriate safeguarding route for different scenarios. Legislation and health issues relating to FGM must be discussed, so that parents are made aware of the severity of FGM and the legal consequences (breaching the law) if they are considering FGM for their child or reinfibulation following the birth. Pressure from family members may also influence decisions made, therefore continuing support and education for the whole family may be necessary.

Service user's view

'I know that female circumcision is practised in my community, but I do not know whether I have experienced this myself.'

Verbal communication, service user, Berkshire

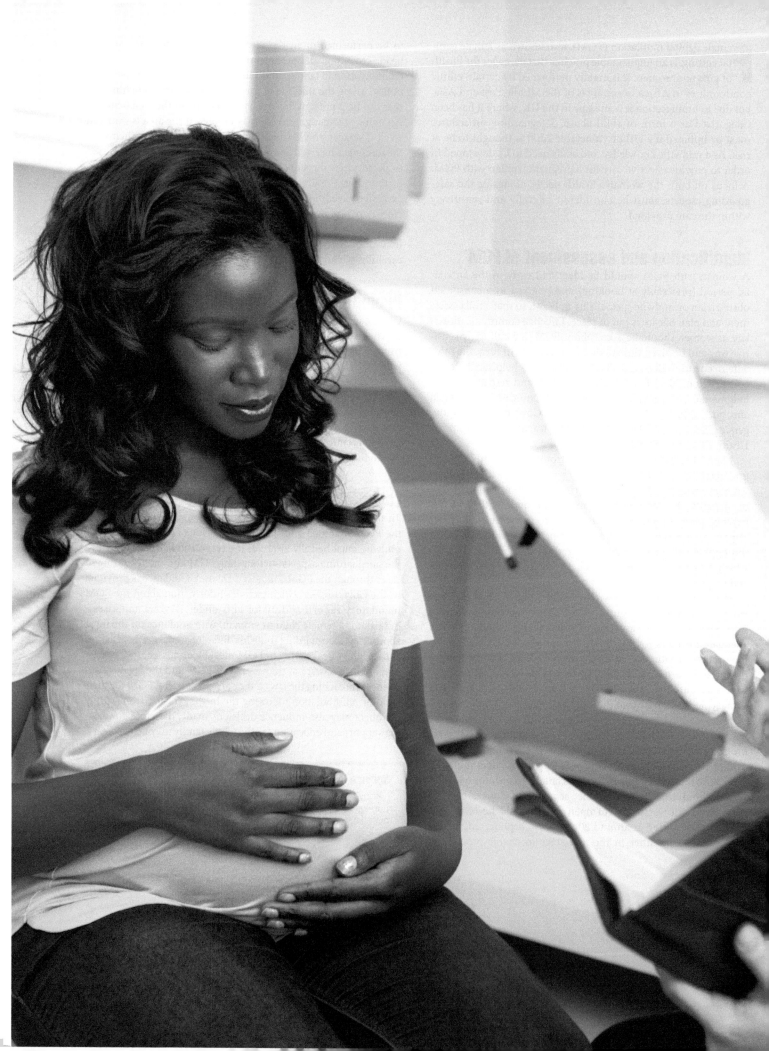

Assessment, examination, screening and care of the woman and baby

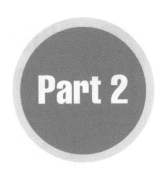

Part 2

20 'Booking': the initial consultation with the midwife

Box 20.1 The initial consultation with the midwife - Building a picture of the woman to personalise her care.
Source: Adapted from NHS Quality Improvement Scotland (2008). *Best Practice Statement August 2008: Maternal History Taking.*
http://www.healthcareimprovementscotland.org/previous_resources/best_practice_statement/maternal_history_taking.aspx (accessed February 2017).

History taking = Screening
                             Personal, Obstetric and Medical
                             Maternal and Paternal Family History
                             Family Origin Questionnaire

Information exchange = Informed decision making,
                                     Health Promotion and Advice
                                     Personal Budget options
                                     Place of Birth

Clinical examination of the woman:
- Physical & psychological assessment
- Measurement of weight & body mass index
- Female genital mutilation
- Domestic violence and abuse
- Prediction, detection and initial management of mental disorders (NICE 2016b)

- Routine screening rubella, HIV, syphilis
- Symptomatic screening for *Chlamydia trachomatis* or Group B streptococcus (GBS)
- USS for fetal growth & development or placental position
- Referral to other professionals as required
- Social circumstances assessment

Screening for clinical conditions:
- Asymptomatic bacteriuria
- Blood pressure measurement and urinalysis (pre-eclampsia)
- Gestational diabetes or underlying diabetic conditions

Haematology:
- Anaemia
- Blood grouping and red-cell antibodies
- Screening for Down syndrome
- Haemoglobinopathies

An audit for initial consultation history taking:-	✔
Details of the woman's previous obstetric history are ascertained and information recorded sensitively.	
The woman's personal physical and mental health history is comprehensive to enable informed decision making.	
The woman's social support has been discussed, including consideration of vulnerabilities and strengths she has.	
A referral for an early ultrasound scan to confirm gestational age is offered at this first appointment.	
Family health risk factors significant for the pregnancy are identified and acted upon.	
The woman is given the opportunity to define her own ethnic group, and is asked about the ethnic origin/ancestry of her and the father of her child.	
The woman is given the opportunity to discuss beliefs or customs which may affect her care.	
The appointment has been used as an opportunity to provide general health advice and promotion of health advice including immunisation opportunities and healthy living advice such as diet and exercise.	
The woman is provided with information about local antenatal education, exercise and relaxation activities.	
Information about the harmful effects of smoking. Referral for smoking cessation support is offered if applicable.	
The woman is asked about current and previous use of alcohol and other substances and appropriate information given. Referral for support to stop use of alcohol and other substances is offered if applicable.	
The woman (and her partner) have been given opportunity to ask questions throughout the exchange.	

Key points
- The midwife develops a positive relationship with the woman (and her partner), whilst applying clinical expertise to use information effectively to provide a positive childbirth experience.
- Choice and risk are elements that need to be balanced and the midwife should understand what the woman's expectations are and how they can be best supported.

Midwifery Skills at a Glance, First Edition. Edited by Patricia Lindsay, Carmel Bagness and Ian Peate.
© 2018 John Wiley & Sons, Ltd. Published 2018 by John Wiley & Sons, Ltd.

The first time a pregnant woman meets her midwife is the most important opportunity for both, and ideally takes place at 10 weeks into the pregnancy. Women (and their partners) come with a range of emotions from excitement about their forthcoming baby to anxiety about this life changing event, and/or fear about the journey ahead. The first contact is critically important to put the woman (and partner) at ease, whilst reassuring her of the clinical expertise available to have the best possible experience, balancing expectations and needs.

Effective communication skills will enable the midwife to facilitate informed choice and give the woman the sense of being in control, whilst competence and confident clinical expertise will enhance the care provided. The importance of the atmosphere (warm, friendly midwife) and environment (safe, private, quiet), within which this meeting takes place cannot be over emphasised.

Effective communication skills include:
- Being non-judgemental
- Being ready to build a relationship
- Open questioning
- Active listening
- Understanding what the woman wants
- Recognising body language and the signs that can create a compassionate caring environment
- Answering questions honestly
- Use language that is familiar
- Clarify all information given.

This 'booking' visit is an initial consultation to establish physical and mental wellbeing, recognising that pregnancy is a normal physiological life event and that any intervention offered should have evidence-based benefits, whilst being acceptable to women. It is a time for the midwife to develop a relationship with the woman (and her partner), which should enhance the whole maternity care experience. This is the opportunity to understand the woman's history and discuss screening tests (Box 20.1), with risk assessments based on shared information.

The midwife needs to work methodically to ensure all elements of this important consultation are achieved (Box 20.1), whilst ensuring the mother (and partner) have ample opportunity to express needs and questions. Whether a first or subsequent pregnancy, the woman's attitude will be influenced by previous experiences.

The midwife is equally responsible for supporting the woman's mental health, recognising mental illness, including the possible devastating effects this can have if not identified early. Using an understanding of mental wellbeing (and specific pregnancy-related mental illnesses) will help to judge the woman's mood and emotional wellbeing.

It can be easy to make assumptions and the midwife has to probe, sometimes with difficult questions, in order to provide the right care. The midwife also needs to be familiar with local and national standards/pathways of referral across the health and social care spectrum.

Screening is an essential component of antenatal care. Box 20.1 outlines usual screening; however, these and others will be employed to enable the woman to have a safe maternity care journey. The foundation for decisions made rest with the history about physical, psychological and the socioeconomic situation that the woman and her family live in. This has to be combined with calculation of the estimated date of delivery, which will then form the basis for the care offered. Together with a clinical examination, the midwife will be able to suggest the pathway that best suits her. This will be combined with the opportunity to offer lifestyle and health promotion advice such as diet, exercise, immunisation opportunities and parenthood education.

Beyond the maternity team, including obstetricians and specialist midwives, the midwife may liaise with medical teams, GPs, nurses, health visitors, mental healthcare, and those working with other organisations, such as interpreting services, parent education, smoking cessation or social care services.

If the woman has a disability or long-term condition, she may already attend other services, and the need for collaboration will be critical to how she is supported.

The voluntary sector also have a role to play and midwives should know local provision to complement NHS services, enabling women to successfully navigate them.

The midwife's responsibilities further include identifying vulnerability; for example from domestic abuse, homelessness or asylum seekers or migrants, malnutrition or self-harming lifestyles such as addictions or dependency. Once identified the midwife should be familiar with referral pathways, including local support, and how the woman can realistically be guided within her particular needs.

For some women, where English is not their first language, independent interpreting services may be required. Screening for haemoglobinopathies should be available to all women identified using the *Family Origin Questionnaire* from the NHS Antenatal and Newborn Screening Programme (2016). This tool can also be used to identify women who have been affected by female genital mutilation.

NICE (2016a) recommends all pregnant women should be offered screening for Down's syndrome, and this is a further choice for women to consider. The 'combined test' (nuchal translucency, beta-human chorionic gonadotrophin, pregnancy-associated plasma protein-A) should be offered between 11 and 14 weeks, whilst women who book later can be offered serum screening tests up to 20 weeks' gestation.

The booking visit is also an opportunity to enquire about and advise on common symptoms of pregnancy that may cause distress, such as nausea and vomiting, heartburn, backache, vaginal discharge, constipation, varicose veins or haemorrhoids.

This consultation is the time to share resources and information but many women can find this overwhelming. Being aware of this, the midwife does need to begin the process of birth planning, and the subsequent care should build on early information. This offers women time to consider the choices that best suit them, and consider how they may use their personal budget allowance. Information should be available in a range of media, including leaflets in relevant languages, access to sound internet sites and the pregnancy apps now available.

Most women anticipate a normal physiological and psychological outcome, recognising the changes that a new baby may bring; the skilled midwife should guide her though the numerous choices to be considered. The woman should feel that she has opportunities to express concerns, as well as articulate expectations. Seamless continuity of care is key to optimising this journey, with the midwife acting as professional skilled navigator.

Service user's view

'The National Childbirth Trust remind women that antenatal tests are optional, and it is your decision whether to accept or refuse any pregnancy screening.'

Verbal communication, service user, London

21 The antenatal appointment: physical and psychological assessment of the woman in pregnancy

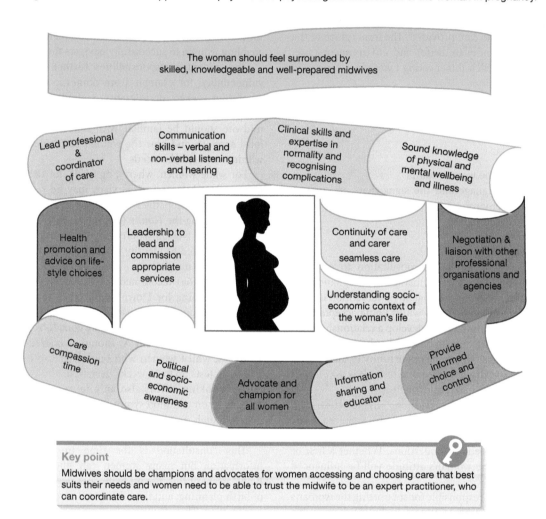

Figure 21.1 The antenatal appointment: physical and psychological assessment of the woman in pregnancy.

The woman should feel surrounded by skilled, knowledgeable and well-prepared midwives

Lead professional & coordinator of care

Communication skills – verbal and non-verbal listening and hearing

Clinical skills and expertise in normality and recognising complications

Sound knowledge of physical and mental wellbeing and illness

Health promotion and advice on life-style choices

Leadership to lead and commission appropriate services

Continuity of care and carer seamless care

Understanding socio-economic context of the woman's life

Negotiation & liaison with other professional organisations and agencies

Care compassion time

Political and socio-economic awareness

Advocate and champion for all women

Information sharing and educator

Provide informed choice and control

Key point

Midwives should be champions and advocates for women accessing and choosing care that best suits their needs and women need to be able to trust the midwife to be an expert practitioner, who can coordinate care.

Midwifery Skills at a Glance, First Edition. Edited by Patricia Lindsay, Carmel Bagness and Ian Peate.
© 2018 John Wiley & Sons, Ltd. Published 2018 by John Wiley & Sons, Ltd.

The skills of the midwife (Figure 21.1) in antenatal care focus on facilitating women to have a safe, positive experience, and enabling the new family to progress better prepared and healthier. The midwife is recognised as the lead professional in providing high-quality personalised care and co-ordinating the woman's care, using expert judgement and decision making, which should be in tune with her and her family. Women and their partners need to be able to trust the midwife in order to believe that their maternity care will meet their needs and expectations.

The main contact for the midwife with pregnant women is through the antenatal appointment, at regular intervals throughout the pregnancy. The initial booking visit (see Chapter 20) and subsequent visits should focus on ensuring women are physically and mentally prepared for their birth and postnatal period, as well as being in optimum health.

The midwife's public health role is well recognised, and women are usually receptive to healthy choices messages, including being a resource for healthy eating and exercise, smoking cessation, drug addiction or other lifestyle choices that may adversely affect health and wellbeing. As well as promoting good health, the midwife also recognises women who may be vulnerable because of physical health, mental well being or socioeconomic circumstances. This vulnerability may be life threatening or have a negative impact on them.

Sharing information with the woman will continue throughout the pregnancy, tailored to the woman's needs, based on previous assessment, including promoting normal birth and breastfeeding, as well as facilitating choice about place of birth and available care options. Choice and risk need to be balanced and the midwife should be able to facilitate the woman's expectations and how they can be best supported or considered.

Physical assessments, including abdominal examination, provide an opportunity to assess maternal and fetal wellbeing, whilst diagnosing and managing complications, should they arise. As maternity care becomes more complex, collaboration, referral and effective communication with the wider multidisciplinary care team are essential skills for all midwives.

Physical assessments, used to assess how the woman is adjusting to being pregnancy, include:

- General well being and asking about minor disorders
- Abdominal examination
- Temperature, pulse and blood pressure
- Urinalysis
- Blood tests to include blood group and Rhesus status, screening for HIV status.

Midwifery 2020 (Department of Health 2010) stated that all women need a midwife and some will also need an obstetrician. Most women will encounter a range of professionals such as health visitors, social workers, and GPs, with the midwife acting as liaison to increase continuity of care. The midwife needs to know who is working locally, both other healthcare professionals and voluntary groups who may be able to enhance care, and ensure that expectations and service provision are aligned to support all women.

Midwives are well versed in the advantages of **continuity of care and carer** and have a responsibly to champion the care provision that best suits local women. When asked about antenatal care, women want to know that they will be cared for with compassion and understanding, and the team looking after them are highly skilled professionals who will enable and facilitate choice and a safe passage through this life-changing event. *Better Births* (National Maternity Review 2016) also outline the need for the NHS Personal Maternity Care Budget for women to best support their choices, and midwives need to understand how that is managed locally.

Mental wellbeing – the majority of women will have a positive outlook, tempered with anxiety and fear, but within a normal spectrum of mental wellbeing; pregnancy is a time of emotional upheaval and adjustment to changes in lifestyle and relationships; however, for about 20% of women, this life event is affected by mental illness, recognising that severe perinatal mental health is one of the leading causes of maternal death.

The midwife will need to assess the woman's mood and emotional wellbeing at every opportunity, always being alert to changes in mood, or general wellbeing that may signify the onset of depression or a more serious mental illness.

Women may have pre-existing mental ill health, or a condition may develop or be diagnosed during pregnancy. Depression is the most prevalent illness; around 10 to 14% of mothers may be affected, which is usually mild but it can progress to a severe depressive illness that can impact on the woman and family for years after the birth, including affecting her self-esteem and family relationships.

The role the midwife plays antenatally in preparing women for the possible changes in mental wellbeing are finely balanced between informing women and partners, whilst not causing unnecessary anxiety. The midwife needs to understand the symptoms of mental ill health and to be able to articulate these to the woman and her partner, including:

- Baby blues
- Antenatal and postnatal depression
- Postnatal/ puerperal psychosis.

It is also important to acknowledge the emerging evidence that possibly 10% of new fathers may suffer anxiety and depression.

Midwifery evidence-based practice should be focused on providing seamless continuity of care, leading to better outcomes for women and their families through the whole of the childbearing experience. Antenatal care is a significant time for pregnant women, as much of the care provided will impact on the health and wellbeing of the woman and her baby; it will also impact on a partner and the wider family, making it a critical life event. Public health opportunities abound during antenatal care, which creates an ideal environment to enhance the health and well being of the entire family, providing messages and support are delivered in a positive and supportive manner to enable the mother to consider her lifestyle choices, and how they may be improved.

Service user's view

'…Women want to be able to choose the care that is right for them, their family and their circumstances, and that they want the care to wrap around them. They understand that there are finite resources, however they expect that their needs are able to be supported.'

National Maternity Review 2016, page 32

22 Abdominal examination in pregnancy

Box 22.1 Principles to consider.

Principles to consider:
- Informed consent
- Privacy
- Dignity
- Comfort
- Respect
- Universal precautions

Box 22.2 Elements of abdominal examination in pregnancy.

Elements of abdominal examination in pregnancy
- Inspection
- Palpation: Fundal, lateral and pelvic
- Auscultation

Figure 22.1 Symphysis fundal height measurement.

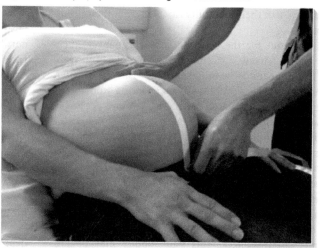

Figure 22.2 Palpation: (a) fundal, (b) lateral, (c) pelvic.

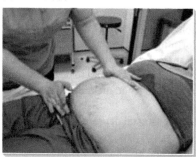

(a)

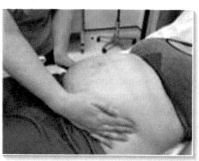

(b)

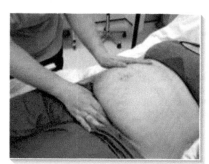

(c)

Figure 22.3 The 'position and lie' of the fetus.
Source: Johnson R and Taylor W (2016). *Skills for Midwifery Practice*, p.13. Reproduced with permission of Elsevier.

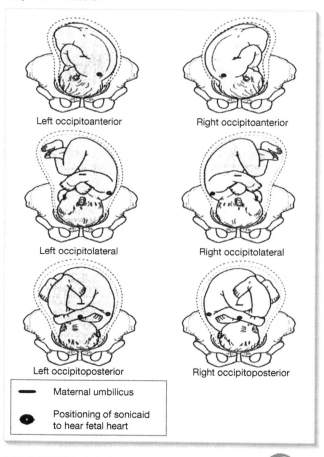

Left occipitoanterior

Right occipitoanterior

Left occipitolateral

Right occipitolateral

Left occipitoposterior

Right occipitoposterior

— Maternal umbilicus

● Positioning of sonicaid to hear fetal heart

Key point

Abdominal examination is an important element of antenatal care that requires knowledge, skill and professionalism to ensure a healthy mother and child throughout pregnancy.

Midwifery Skills at a Glance, First Edition. Edited by Patricia Lindsay, Carmel Bagness and Ian Peate.
© 2018 John Wiley & Sons, Ltd. Published 2018 by John Wiley & Sons, Ltd.

Abdominal examination is a key aspect of antenatal care and forms part of the complete antenatal assessment. From 12 weeks' gestation the uterine fundus can be palpated just above the symphysis pubis. However, an abdominal examination is carried out from 24 weeks' gestation. The aim is to assess fetal growth and wellbeing and identify any deviations from normal for both woman and fetus (Boxes 22.1 and 22.2). Ongoing conversation with the woman will inform this examination and she should be fully informed throughout, ensuring she is aware of all findings and these are accurately documented in her records.

This examination should be carried out in a warm and quiet room. Initially, assess the woman by observing her general health and wellbeing. A midwife is seeking to identify a fit and healthy woman whose pregnancy is progressing well. Ask pertinent open questions to identify any issues that may arise in conversation. This can include:

- How are you feeling?
- How is your baby moving?
- How are you sleeping?

Always seek consent prior to the examination. To reduce the risk of postural hypotension caused by aortocaval compression the woman should lie in a semi-recumbent position, with arms by her side and knees slightly bent.

For the comfort of the woman and to promote accuracy of fundal height measurement ensure she has an empty bladder beforehand. Only expose the area that needs to be viewed, ensuring privacy and dignity. The midwife should apply universal precautions throughout ensuring that her hands have been washed, are warm and her nails are short. The pads and not the finger tips are used as they are more sensitive. The skill for the midwife should be to gently apply enough pressure to gather information without making the woman feel uncomfortable or stimulate contractions.

Inspection

The midwife can use skills of observation to identify any normal or unexpected abdominal skin changes. These include striae gravidarum, linea nigra, colour changes, rashes, uterine shape, approximation of uterine size, contour, polyhydramnios, bruising, trauma and surgical scars. Identified abnormal factors such as jaundice, bruising (possible domestic abuse, clotting factors) and rashes may alert the midwife to increase surveillance or referral to the multidisciplinary team. As the pregnancy progresses the contour and shape can confirm findings found on palpation, for example transverse lie or posterior position. Fetal movements may be seen or felt. Consideration is required in relation to the care of navel piercings as the pregnancy progresses. This includes changing to a longer bar length or use of softer plastic bars or removal of jewellery until after pregnancy.

Palpation

It is recommended that from 24 weeks' gestation that the symphysis fundal height (SFH) should be measured and recorded. This has been found beneficial in identifying the 'small for gestation age' fetus and has reduced the risk of stillbirth/perinatal death.

Measuring fundal height

First identify the fundus by placing a hand just below the xiphisternum and working the hand down until the fundus is felt and secure the tape measure here (Figure 22.1). With the measurements facing downwards towards the woman's skin to reduce the potential for inaccuracies, measure the longitudinal axis of the uterus to the top of the symphysis pubis. This measure should be done only once and the result, in centimetres (1 cm for each gestational week) is plotted on a customised growth chart (if used), such as the Perinatal Institute GROW Chart, and documented in the records. If findings are potentially detrimental to the wellbeing of the fetus refer to the multidisciplinary team accordingly.

Fundal palpation (Figure 22.2a) can also be used to identify fetal parts, such as fetal buttocks or head.

Lateral palpation is used to establish the location of the fetal back. Place both hands, one on either side of the abdomen (Figure 22.2b). One hand can be used to steady the uterus while the other can apply a gentle but firm pressure as it moves up and down the side of the abdomen seeking a resistance. This is then repeated on the other side. These movements can be used to map the contours of the fetus and determine the position of the back and other body parts. If more clarity of findings is required, then the hands can be 'walked' across the abdomen to palpate the underlying fetal parts.

Pelvic palpation is recommended from 36 weeks' gestation in an uncomplicated pregnancy to identify the presenting part and its engagement in the pelvis (5ths palpable). This should not be offered prior to this as the examination can be inaccurate and uncomfortable. A two-handed manoeuvre can be used or Pawlik's grip (Figure 22.2c). Suspected malpresentations should be discussed with the woman and can be confirmed by ultrasound scan.

The findings of this whole examination will help determine the 'position and lie' of the fetus. The position is the relation of the fetal denominator to the maternal pelvic brim (Figure 22.3). The lie is the relation of the long axis of the fetus to the long axis of the uterus. Normally, this is longitudinal. Other variants include transverse and oblique, both of which will have an impact on the onset and progress of labour.

Auscultation

Routine auscultation of the fetal heart (FH) by Pinard stethoscope or fetal Doppler is not advised unless requested by the woman (NICE 2016). However, this is still carried out at most examinations. Figure 22.3 identifies the best position to locate the FH in relation to a cephalic presentation. With a breech presentation the FH should be heard clearly in the upper quadrants of the uterus informed by the abdominal examination. A normal FH is 110–160 bpm. To differentiate the FH from the maternal heart rate, the maternal pulse should be taken at the same time.

Following the examination it is important to wash hands thoroughly. Document and chart all findings accurately, and refer if appropriate. Discuss findings with the woman and answer any questions. Make arrangements for follow on appointments.

Service user's view

'...Although I knew my baby was growing, it was good to have that confirmed and so special to hear that heartbeat.'

Verbal communication, service user, Berkshire

23 Physical and emotional assessment after birth

Figure 23.1 Initial assessment by midwife.

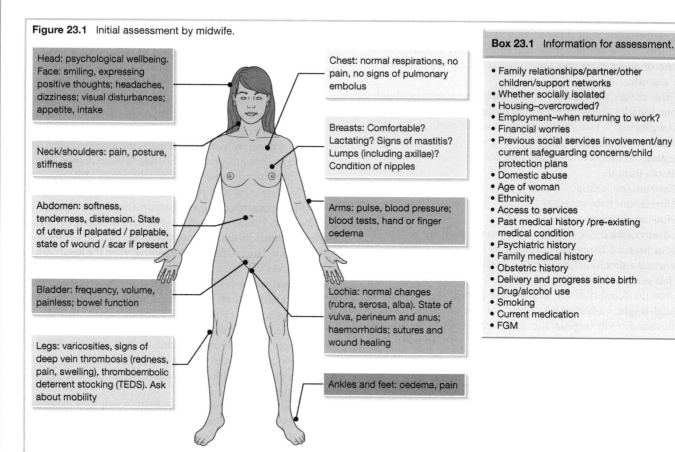

Head: psychological wellbeing. Face: smiling, expressing positive thoughts; headaches, dizziness; visual disturbances; appetite, intake

Neck/shoulders: pain, posture, stiffness

Abdomen: softness, tenderness, distension. State of uterus if palpated / palpable, state of wound / scar if present

Bladder: frequency, volume, painless; bowel function

Legs: varicosities, signs of deep vein thrombosis (redness, pain, swelling), thromboembolic deterrent stocking (TEDS). Ask about mobility

Chest: normal respirations, no pain, no signs of pulmonary embolus

Breasts: Comfortable? Lactating? Signs of mastitis? Lumps (including axillae)? Condition of nipples

Arms: pulse, blood pressure; blood tests, hand or finger oedema

Lochia: normal changes (rubra, serosa, alba). State of vulva, perineum and anus; haemorrhoids; sutures and wound healing

Ankles and feet: oedema, pain

Box 23.1 Information for assessment.

- Family relationships/partner/other children/support networks
- Whether socially isolated
- Housing–overcrowded?
- Employment–when returning to work?
- Financial worries
- Previous social services involvement/any current safeguarding concerns/child protection plans
- Domestic abuse
- Age of woman
- Ethnicity
- Access to services
- Past medical history /pre-existing medical condition
- Psychiatric history
- Family medical history
- Obstetric history
- Delivery and progress since birth
- Drug/alcohol use
- Smoking
- Current medication
- FGM

Box 23.2 Psychological assessment.

NICE (2006) recommends asking the mother these questions:
- During the past month have you often been bothered by feeling down, depressed or hopeless?
- During the past month have you often been bothered by having little interest or pleasure in doing things?
- If yes, is this something you would like help with?

If yes to depression questions, the woman is at risk or of clinical concern, then consider Edinburgh Postnatal Depression Score (EPDS)

Box 23.3 Assessing anxiety levels.

- Over the last two weeks how often have you been bothered by feeling nervous, anxious or on edge?
- Over the last two weeks how often have you been bothered by not being able to stop or control worrying?

Box 23.4 Possible indications of postnatal depression.

- Unkempt/poor personal hygiene
- Poor diet/change in appetite
- Disinterest in baby
- Negative thoughts
- Feelings of hopelessness
- Change of sleep pattern
- Worrying more than usual
- Low energy levels
- Suicidal thoughts

Table 23.1 Assessing vital signs.

Observation	Cause for concern
Pulse	over 100 beats per minute
BP – systolic – diastolic	over 160 mm/Hg under 90 mm/Hg over 80 mm/Hg
Respirations	above 21 breaths per minute
Temperature	38°C and above

Key point

A skilled and knowledgeable midwife has a crucial role in observing and monitoring mothers to identify any abnormality and potential concerns.

Midwifery Skills at a Glance, First Edition. Edited by Patricia Lindsay, Carmel Bagness and Ian Peate.
© 2018 John Wiley & Sons, Ltd. Published 2018 by John Wiley & Sons, Ltd.

Physical and emotional changes occur following the birth of a baby. Physically returning to the prepregnancy state and emotionally adjusting to parenthood can be a vulnerable time for women. A skilled and knowledgeable midwife has a crucial role in observing and monitoring mothers to identify any abnormality and potential concerns. Providing care, supporting mothers and building their confidence are equally important. Assessment will identify the potential need for treatment, referral to the multidisciplinary team, and targeted follow-up. Care will be tailored to meet the individual needs of the woman.

Assessment of the woman may vary depending on when she delivered. The number of contacts will be determined by the woman's need; some hospital guidance recommends a minimum of three home visits. NICE (2006) developed the care pathway that recommends assessment should occur within 24 hours of delivery, between 2 and 7 days postnatally and then between 8 days and 8 weeks. The rise in birth rates and reduction in midwives has led to the decrease in postnatal contacts by midwives and the offer of assessment within clinics instead of women's homes. Midwives are responsible for determining when contact will take place based on their assessment.

Each midwife will have their own way of carrying out a postnatal assessment. This may be led by their level of experience or through checklists, policies and guidance. Effective communication skills will steer this. Record keeping is an essential aspect of this too, as is ensuring knowledge and skills are up to date.

Safety of the mother and baby is paramount, as is that of the midwife. Consideration must be paid to lone working and infection prevention and control. It is essential for the midwife to carry out a risk assessment when working in the community, vigilance with effective hand hygiene is crucial. Midwives must also be prepared, ensuring they have the necessary equipment in full working order prior to visiting women at home.

As part of their initial contact, the midwife will need to undertake a full assessment. This should involve reading the records, asking open-ended and direct questions, instigating discussion and observation. Asking how the woman is feeling is a good start. Never make assumptions. Information in Box 23.1 should be solicited from the woman.

Best practice would indicate that observations should be taken to rule out ill health. Temperature, pulse, blood pressure and respirations (T, P, BP, R) will identify the need to act swiftly (Table 23.1). Vital signs should be carried out immediately postbirth. During subsequent days, these may only be taken if clinical indication identifies the need, for example palpation to determine involution of the uterus is not required unless there is abnormal lochia. Key aspects of the postnatal examination are indicated in Figure 23.1.

During the postpartum period there is an increased risk of genital tract infection. Sepsis has made a reappearance as a significant cause of maternal death. The report by MBRRACE (Knight *et al.* 2015) identified that thrombosis and thromboembolism remain the leading cause of direct maternal deaths. The report *Saving Mothers' Lives* (CMACE 2011) states that pre-eclampsia and eclampsia are the second cause of direct maternal deaths in the UK. MBRRACE (Knight *et al.* 2014) stated that postpartum haemorrhage is responsible for about 10% of all direct maternal deaths in the UK. All these conditions have the potential for early identification by a midwife following a thorough assessment.

As well as physical assessment, the midwife will be observing for emotional wellbeing. Extremes of emotions are highly probable in the postnatal period, ranging from sheer delight at the birth of a baby, to absolute exhaustion. Contributory factors influencing this could include sleep deprivation, mode of delivery, pain, whether a primigravida or multigravida, and what support networks there are available. Box 23.2 and 23.3 identify the questions the midwife should be asking women.

Postnatal depression (PND; Box 23.4) has been known to affect 10–15% of mothers and puerperal psychosis affects between 1 and 2 in 1000 women. The midwife should pay particular attention to those women with a history of mental health problems. Psychosis should be treated as an emergency and swift referral must be made.

The midwife plays an important role in reducing mortality and morbidity rates amongst new mothers. Discharge from midwifery care is usually around 10 days postnatal but could carry on to 6 weeks. A thorough handover to the health visitor is essential to enable effective transition to another provider and to allow continuity of care.

Service user's view

'I stayed in hospital for a week after giving birth to my son due to pre-eclampsia. During this time my blood pressure, temperature, respiratory and heart rate were measured regularly. I had a physical assessment to see if I had any tears. …I felt quite low for a few weeks after the birth but my mental health was not assessed until my 8 week check.'

Verbal communication, service user, Berkshire

Assessing the woman in labour

Figure 24.1 Assessment in labour.

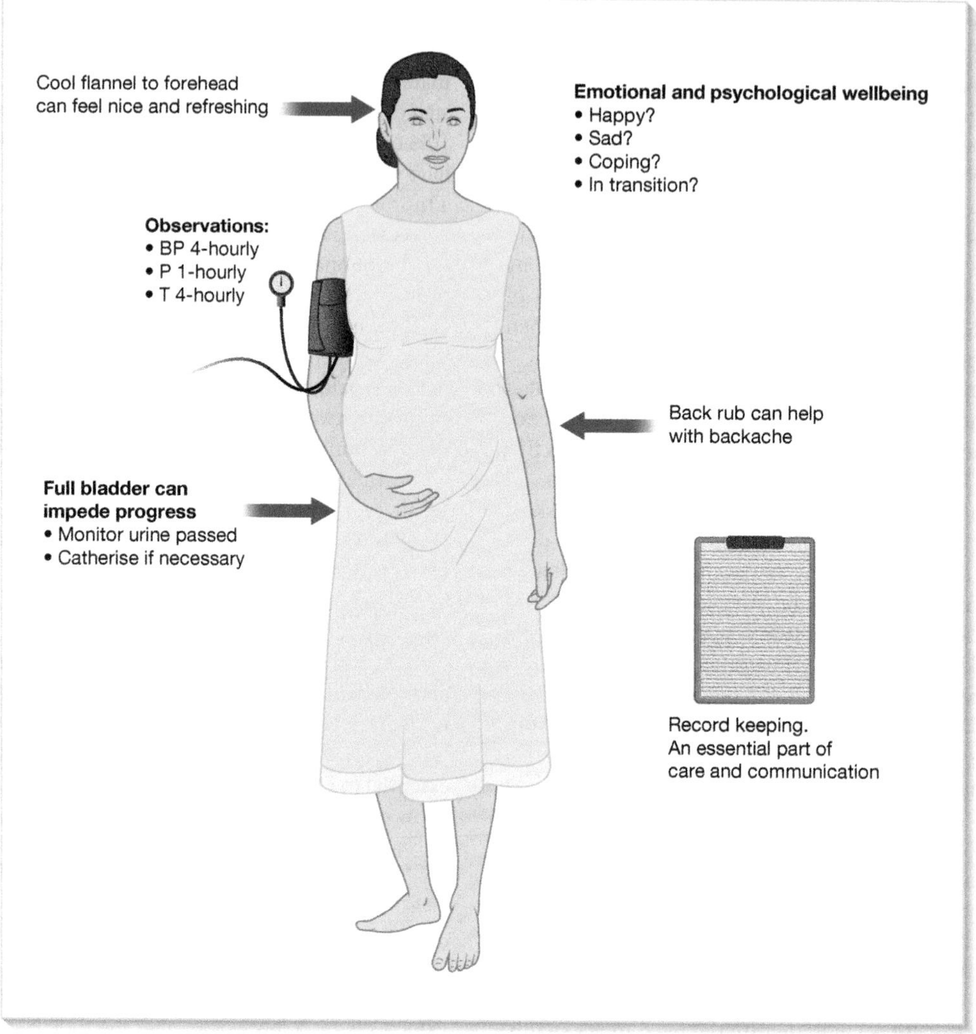

Cool flannel to forehead
can feel nice and refreshing

Emotional and psychological wellbeing
• Happy?
• Sad?
• Coping?
• In transition?

Observations:
• BP 4-hourly
• P 1-hourly
• T 4-hourly

Back rub can help
with backache

**Full bladder can
impede progress**
• Monitor urine passed
• Catherise if necessary

Record keeping.
An essential part of
care and communication

Key point

Always collate all information to look at the complete picture, not one
isolated factor. This is essential for comprehensive evaluation, risk
assessment and care planning.

Midwifery Skills at a Glance, First Edition. Edited by Patricia Lindsay, Carmel Bagness and Ian Peate.
© 2018 John Wiley & Sons, Ltd. Published 2018 by John Wiley & Sons, Ltd.

Overall assessment of the woman in labour requires a comprehensive overview of all the information gained from varying individual assessments so as to make a safe and appropriate plan of care. Other relevant chapters include:

- Positions in labour and birth (Chapter 27)
- Abdominal examinations in labour (Chapter 25)
- Vaginal examination in labour (Chapter 26)
- Supporting and caring for women in labour (Chapter 28) and
- Assessing fetal wellbeing in pregnancy and labour (Chapter 33).

This chapter will look at observations, bladder care in labour and documentation.

Intrapartum guidelines have a great emphasis on holistic care of the woman and fetus in labour as a unique biological unit and ensuring that one area is not focussed on at the detriment of others. Woman-led and woman-focussed care is at the heart of the guidelines. Effective communication is essential and so all findings should be communicated clearly and the woman's questions answered. This is equally important in the latent stage of labour when communication may be by telephone and a decision is made whether to come in or stay at home. It is recommended that expectations of what early labour is like are managed antenatally.

When the woman is in established labour the midwife must undertake regular observations as part of the risk assessment undertaken to ensure that the woman is receiving appropriate care in the correct setting (Figure 24.1). Observations in labour include temperature (T), pulse (P) and blood pressure (BP) and respirations (R).

Oxygen saturations (SaO_2) may be required if there is any need for facial O_2 to be given or if the woman has become unwell, such as if she has developed pre-eclampsia and/or pulmonary oedema.

On admission, a baseline T, P, R, BP will be recorded. Thereafter, routine observations are recorded on a partogram and consist of the following maternal observations (see Chapter 34 Monitoring the fetal heart in pregnancy and labour)

- First stage of labour:
  - P hourly
  - T, BP 4 hourly
  - Half hourly contractions
  - Frequency of passing urine (test for ketones)
- Second stage of labour:
  - BP, P hourly
  - T 4 hourly
  - Half hourly contractions
  - Frequency of passing urine (test for ketones).

The partogram allows for all elements to be documented together so as to see any trends that are emerging. The T, P, BP, R (if required) are recorded alongside fetal heart rate, contraction frequency and strength, cervical dilatation, descent of presenting part, liquor, any oxytocic drugs used, passing urine and fluid balance. There is normally a section to note any risk factors present and there is an action line that should guide the midwife and obstetrician in identifying any dystocia or deviations from the norm and take appropriate action.

In particular, the maternal pulse should be compared with the fetal heart rate and be part of the hourly 'fresh eyes' assessment to ensure the rates can be differentiated as there have been instances where maternal pulse has been wrongly recorded as the fetal heart rate.

A study examining the use of the partogram found that its use did improve the quality of delivery of care and allowed for logical and effective interventions. However, a systematic review of the effect of the partogram use on the outcomes for women in spontaneous labour at term found that there were no significant differences in outcomes between women who had a partogram in labour and those who did not. Nevertheless, it is standard practice to document all observations and assessments on the partogram in the UK and this is recommended by *NICE intrapartum guidelines* (NICE 2014).

Record keeping is an essential component in the care of the woman and communication between caregivers and midwives must record all care given and discussions. As well as the partogram the midwife will have a labour care pathway and continuation notes to write any extra information that is relevant. This can include other physiological events such as defecation or vomiting as these may also indicate maternal wellbeing / stage of labour.

The midwife should ensure the woman is encouraged to empty her bladder frequently as a full bladder can interfere with descent of the presenting part and increase the risk of postpartum haemorrhage if present after delivery. The woman may have altered/reduced sensation of the need to pass urine, particularly if she has an epidural. It is important to monitor fluid balance as if the woman has intravenous fluids running she may have a full bladder without taking in oral fluids and the urine output should be measured. This is also to identify if the bladder has incompletely emptied in which case a catheter may need to be passed (see Chapter 32).

An essential part of assessment in labour is to identify any deviations from the norm and escalate appropriately to the senior midwife obstetrician. It may be that the woman needs to transfer from midwifery-led to obstetric-led care. If this involves transfer from a birth centre or a midwifery led unit to the main delivery suite then the midwife should ensure the woman and her partner have all the necessary information and are aware of the reasons for transfer and exactly how and when this will happen. Regular observations include the woman's emotional and psychological wellbeing to ensure the midwife has a holistic assessment.

Risk assessment should be carried out throughout labour as the woman may develop complications. The observations discussed alongside the assessments detailed in the other chapters mentioned would enable the midwife to comprehensively risk assess and plan care accordingly.

Service user's view

'The midwife really made me feel less nervous and more able to cope when she explained what she was checking my pulse for. She explained the partogram to me when I asked, which made me feel I had more control over what was happening as I then had an idea of what it was all for.'

Verbal communication, service user, Berkshire

25 Abdominal examination in labour

Figure 25.1 Fetal presentations.

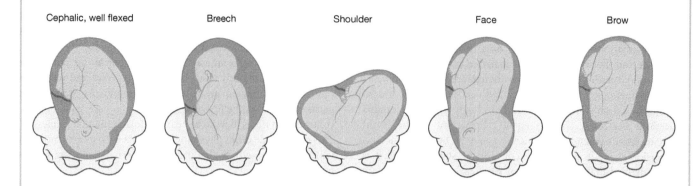

Cephalic, well flexed   Breech   Shoulder   Face   Brow

Figure 25.2 Pelvic palpation using two hands.

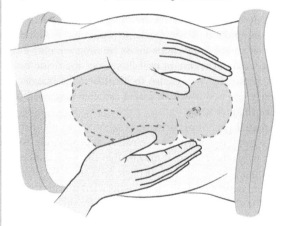

Box 25.1 Reasons for an abdominal examination in labour.

- To assess fetal size, lie, position, presentation, and engagement of the presenting part
- To assess descent and rotation of the presenting part
- To auscultate and monitor the fetal heart rate
- To assess the progress of labour before performing a vaginal examination
- To assess the position, presentation and fetal heart rate between the delivery of each baby in multiple births (such as after the birth of the first twin)

Figure 25.3 Engagement of the fetal head.

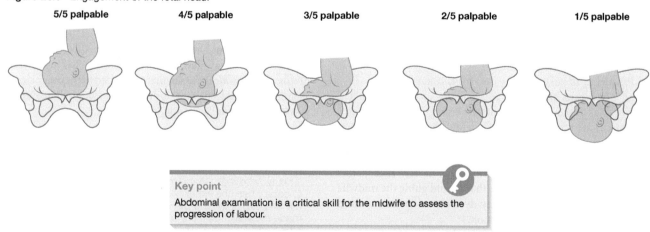

5/5 palpable   4/5 palpable   3/5 palpable   2/5 palpable   1/5 palpable

Key point

Abdominal examination is a critical skill for the midwife to assess the progression of labour.

Midwifery Skills at a Glance, First Edition. Edited by Patricia Lindsay, Carmel Bagness and Ian Peate.
© 2018 John Wiley & Sons, Ltd. Published 2018 by John Wiley & Sons, Ltd.

Labour can be an exciting, anxious, sensitive and very painful event. Therefore, it is important to approach and communicate with the woman in a sensitive, compassionate and caring manner. Prepare the woman for examination by gaining consent, maintaining her privacy and dignity and respecting any social and cultural needs. Document and communicate all findings to the woman.

Preparation

• Introduce yourself to the woman and her birth companion(s) and assess language needs.
• Obtain an initial history (ask how she is feeling). Ask about the length and frequency of contractions and any other pain she is experiencing.
• Ask about her baby's movements and any changes within the last 24 hours.
• Read the woman's maternity notes and review all antenatal screening results.
• Explain the procedure for carrying out an abdominal examination to the woman and gain informed consent. Also gain consent to have her birth companion(s) present during the examination, to maintain respect.
• Encourage the woman to empty her bladder, and then help her to adopt a semirecumbent position or left lateral position with a wedge to avoid aortocaval compression.
• Wash and dry your hands. Ask the woman to uncover her abdomen from the xiphisternum.

Box 25.1 outlines the reasons for an abdominal examination in labour.

The abdominal examination in labour follows the same principles as antenatal examination, but the emphasis will be in assessing progress during labour. To interpret and document the findings, it is important to know the anatomy and physiology of the pelvis and fetal skull for safe midwifery practice.

Throughout the examination, monitor the woman for signs of discomfort, abdominal pain and/or uterine contractions. Remember that stimulation of the fundus on palpation may stimulate a contraction.

Do not continue the examination during a contraction; this may cause discomfort to the woman and what can be felt will be limited. It is also important to let the woman know that the examination can be paused to minimise discomfort.

Observation

Note any visible fetal movements. Observe uterine shape, scars and uterine size:
• A supra pubic bulge may suggest the woman has a full bladder.
• A saucer-shaped dip over the umbilicus may indicate an occipitoposterior position; an unusually wide uterus may indicate a transverse lie.
• Observe the skin for presence of a linea nigra or striae gravidarum. Scars may indicate previous surgery, including appendicectomy, laparoscopy or uterine surgery such as previous caesarean section or myomectomy. Be alert to the signs and symptoms of uterine rupture, such as scar tenderness and persistent abdominal pain with or without abnormal uterine contractions and fetal heart rate.
• Observe changes in uterine contour during contractions.

Uterine size

• Assess whether the woman's fundal height correlates with gestational age in weeks (± 2 cm).
• If the fundal height seems large for gestational age, this may be due to multiple pregnancy, polyhydramnios or a macrosomic baby.
• If the fundal height measurement seems small for gestational age, this may be due to incorrect dates, intrauterine growth restriction or oligohydramnios.

Fundal palpation helps to establish fetal presentation (Figure 25.1). The buttocks felt in the fundus is indicative of cephalic presentation. A hard, round possibly ballotable head in the fundus may indicate a breech presentation. The frequency and intensity of the contractions can be assessed by gently resting a hand on the fundus.

Lateral palpation helps to determine fetal lie and position. The lie is normally longitudinal. An oblique or transverse may be due to placenta praevia, multiple pregnancy or uterine fibroids. With a transverse lie or oblique lie, there is a risk of umbilical prolapse if the membranes rupture. Lateral palpation helps assess the fetal size, attitude and tone. Uterine tone and amniotic fluid volume may also be assessed.

Pelvic palpation is used to confirm and assess presentation, attitude (whether flexed, deflexed or extended) and engagement of the presenting part. This is best done using a two-handed technique (Figure 25.2) and must be carried out gently, between contractions. Ask the woman to take a deep breath in, then let it out slowly. As she breathes out and the abdominal wall relaxes, follow it down with the fingers until the presenting part can be felt. Asking the woman to raise her knees slightly might also be helpful. In a normal vertex presentation, the head is flexed and the sinciput will be palpated at a higher level than the occiput.

A fetus with a deflexed head (military position) has a wider leading diameter. Where the fetal head is extended a brow or face presentation could be found. Brow presentation may cause obstructed labour, as the leading diameter may be too wide to pass through the pelvis.

Engagement of the presenting part is assessed to determine the woman's progress in labour. Engagement refers to how much of the presenting part (usually the head) has descended into the pelvis. It is calculated in fifths (Figure 25.3). An unengaged head in a nulliparous woman at term may indicate a malpresentation. For a multiparous woman, it is not uncommon for engagement of the presenting part to occur during labour.

Auscultation is carried out following abdominal palpation to detect and assess the fetal heart rate. The fetal heart is auscultated for 1 minute and recorded.

After the abdominal examination

• Cover the woman's exposed abdomen and help her into a comfortable position. Then wash and dry your hands.
• Discuss the findings with the woman.
• Fetal presentation, position and descent may be confirmed on vaginal examination, if necessary.
• Abnormal findings, for example malpresentation, must be referred to an obstetrician.
• Document the findings in the woman's notes. Some units use stamps or stickers in the woman's notes to summarise the findings on abdominal and vaginal examination.

26 Vaginal examinations in labour

Figure 26.1 Some positions identified at vaginal examination.

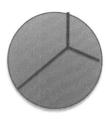

Left occipito-anterior

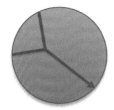

Right occipito-anterior

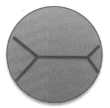

Right occipito-lateral

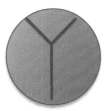

Direct occipito-anterior – well flexed head

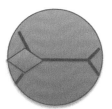

Left occipito-lateral – deflexed head

Figure 26.2 Station of the fetal head in relation to the ischial spines.
Source: Care in the first stage of labour. In *Mayes' Midwifery*, 14th edition. Macdonald S and Magill-Cuerden J (eds) (2010). Reproduced with permission of Elsevier.

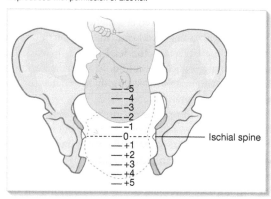

Ischial spine

Box 26.1 NICE guidance (2014) on vaginal examination (VE) in labour. Source: Adapted from NICE (2014).

Initial assessment:	If it is uncertain whether labour is established, it may be useful but not always necessary
	Offer VE if established labour is suspected
First stage:	Offer VE 4 hourly, if there is concern about progress or in response to the woman's wishes
	Offer VE 4 hours after starting oxytocin in labour
Second stage:	Offer VE hourly in active second stage
Diagnosing delay:	Cervical dilatation of less than 2 cm in 4 hours. For second and subsequent pregnancies, also look for a slowing of progress. Take into consideration the descent and rotation of the fetal head as well as the strength, duration and frequency of contractions

Box 26.2 Indications for vaginal examination (VE) in labour.

- To confirm the onset of labour
- To confirm the presentation and position of the fetus
- To ascertain whether the presenting part is engaged if there is doubt from abdominal palpation
- To assess the progress of labour
- To assess the progress of labour prior to administration of analgesia
- To rupture the membranes artificially
- To apply a fetal scalp electrode
- To exclude cord prolapse in the presence of ruptured membranes and an ill fitting presenting part
- To confirm the onset of the second stage of labour

Box 26.3 Contraindications to performing vaginal examinations in labour.

- Consent has not been obtained from the woman
- There is active bleeding
- There is a known placenta praevia
- Preterm labour is suspected
- There is suspected prelabour rupture of membranes

Key point

Vaginal examinations are invasive and can be distressing for the woman. Ensure that there is a clear indication to perform an examination, and that you will gain information that will aid your decision making in her care.

Midwifery Skills at a Glance, First Edition. Edited by Patricia Lindsay, Carmel Bagness and Ian Peate.
© 2018 John Wiley & Sons, Ltd. Published 2018 by John Wiley & Sons, Ltd.

Vaginal examinations (VEs) form part of the care of women in labour, being a means to assess the progress of labour. However, the procedure is highly invasive, and can be distressing and/or painful for many women. Midwives must consider this when initially discussing and gaining consent for a VE to be performed. Some women may be anxious about the whole childbirth experience, of which VEs may form a part, but others may have survived sexual abuse previously or have had female genital mutilation performed. In some cases, it may be impossible to perform a vaginal examination.

When used in conjunction with a holistic view of the woman and her labour, abdominal palpations and documented on the partogram, VEs help to provide a picture of the progression of labour to that point in time. However, they do not give any indication as to future progress, or the time of birth. They can provide an early warning of when labour is slowing (Box 26.1), which may be an indication of labour dystocia, but care should be taken to ensure that this is not over-diagnosed, thus leading to unnecessary interventions such as artificial rupture of membranes, the use of oxytocin to augment labour, or instrumental and caesarean births.

The indications and contraindications for VEs are given in Boxes 26.2 and 26.3. Consideration should be taken of the number of VEs performed during labour, due to the potential for ascending infections, especially when the membranes have ruptured.

Prior to undertaking a VE, a full explanation for the examination should be given, as well as what the examination entails, to the woman and her birthing partners. At all times, the midwife should ensure that privacy and dignity are maintained during the examination. This may involve asking birthing partners to wait outside, or to stand at the head of the bed, according to the woman's wishes, and leaving her covered until ready to perform the examination. The woman should also be asked to empty her bladder to aid her comfort during the examination.

VEs should always be performed using an aseptic non-touch technique, including routine hand washing and the use of sterile gloves. The use of vaginal examination packs varies, as does routine cleaning of the vulval area prior to the examination. NICE recommend the use of warm tap water for cleaning, but some maternity services will recommend the use of antiseptic lotions and local procedures should be adhered to.

Ask the woman to remove underwear and any sanitary pads, offering assistance if needed, then to lie semi recumbent, to avoid aortocaval compression, keeping covered as long as possible to maintain her dignity. Wash hands, put on an apron, and open the packs, including a sachet of single use lubricating gel.

An abdominal palpation should be performed to ascertain the position of the fetus, and to correlate the engagement of the fetal head abdominally with the vaginal descent. The fetal heart should be auscultated at this time. Where there is found to be descent vaginally with none or very little abdominally, this may be due to moulding and be a further indication of labour dystocia.

Wash hands again before putting on sterile gloves. The woman is asked to lift the cover, and position herself with her knees flexed and parted, and her heels together. The genital area is cleaned with either warm tap water or antiseptic lotion, from front to back, using a 'clean hand, dirty hand' technique, where the wet swab is passed from the hand to remain clean for the examination to the 'dirty' hand for cleaning, each swab being discarded after one wipe.

Inform the woman that she will feel touching her labia, and that it may feel uncomfortable. Using the lubricating gel, lubricate the first two fingers of the 'clean' hand, then gently part the labia with the 'dirty' hand. Initially, inspect the labia for signs of genital warts, vulval varicosities, scaring from previous perineal trauma or female genital mutilation. Note any vaginal loss, observing for a 'show', liquor, fresh vaginal bleeding or offensive discharge which may indicate infection.

When there is no uterine contraction, insert the two lubricated fingers into the vagina, slowly moving downwards and backwards until the cervix and/or presenting part is located. The vagina itself should feel warm and moist. A dry, hot vagina may indicate an obstructed labour. Gently feel around the cervix, assessing the consistency, the position, effacement, dilatation and the application to the presenting part. In early labour, dilatation can be assessed by parting the fingers. In the later part of the first stage, it is easier to feel around the rim of the remaining cervix. Continue to gently feel, note the presence or absence of membranes, then the presenting part, its position (Figure 26.1), the level of the presenting part in relation to the ischial spines to indicate descent (Figure 26.2), and the degree of flexion. The ischial spines are not easily palpated, so this measurement can be subjective.

As with all findings on vaginal examination, progress may be more readily assessed if repeated examinations are performed by the same person. The presence of caput and moulding should also be assessed.

Once the necessary information has been acquired, the fingers are gently withdrawn, the fetal heart auscultated and the woman made comfortable.

During the examination, if the woman feels pain, then either pause or stop the procedure.

A full explanation of the findings should be given to the woman and her birthing partners, with details of how the findings may impact the plan of care for her labour. All findings should be documented in the notes and on the partogram according to local policy.

Service user's view

'The midwife who performed my first vaginal examination made every effort to help me relax. She recognised that I was a little nervous, gave clear instructions, spoke to my partner and did not rush me or the examination. She performed the exam once I was relaxed and kept me informed throughout, comfortable afterwards and reassured me.'

Verbal communication, service user, Brentford

27 Positions in labour and birth

Figure 27.1 Standing or leaning against a wall or door. This position is good for swaying or rocking. Alternatively the woman can lean on her partner. Stairs can be used to mobilise and may be useful when labour has slowed.

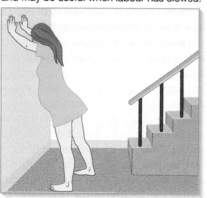

Figure 27.2 Sitting upright on a birthing ball. Like many of these positions if continuous fetal monitoring is required, this can be accommodated.

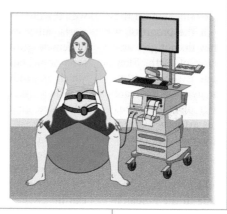

Figure 27.3 Supported squatting position. A partner can either stand or sit in a chair behind to provide support and safety for the woman.

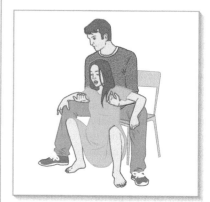

Figure 27.4 Kneeling while resting on a ball or beanbag. If on the floor, provide extra cushioning for her knees. If on a bed, the headboard can be held onto for extra support.

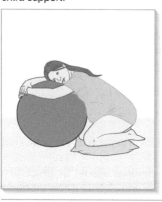

Figure 27.5 A sling or a rope maybe be available to hold onto or lean over. This maintains an upright position while offering support.

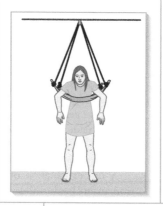

Figure 27.6 Immersion in water can provide comfort during labour and different positions can be explored when in a bath or pool, including leaning on the side of the pool for support in a kneeling position.

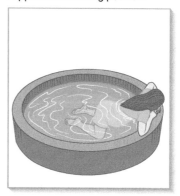

Figure 27.7 Resting on a chair. This position is useful if she wishes to have her back massaged.

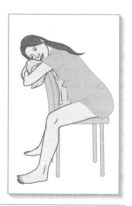

Figure 27.8 Supported kneeling. This can be on a bed, with a support person either side or on the floor with extra support for her knees.

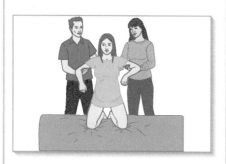

Figure 27.9 Lateral or side – laying position. A woman may use this to rest or when her mobility is reduced. Avoid a supine position, a wedge may be required to avoid rolling onto her back.

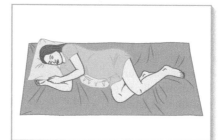

Figure 27.10 Sitting up on a bed or a mat on the floor with a bean bag for support. If using this position during pushing, be careful she does not slip down into a supine position.

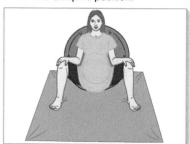

Key point

Review the birth environment and equipment to ensure it allows for free movement and changing of maternal position throughout labour. Listen to the woman and work in partnership to find a position that she finds most comfortable. Encourage mobility and upright positions, while considering the clinical circumstances.

Midwifery Skills at a Glance, First Edition. Edited by Patricia Lindsay, Carmel Bagness and Ian Peate.
© 2018 John Wiley & Sons, Ltd. Published 2018 by John Wiley & Sons, Ltd.

A high proportion of women still give birth in a semirecumbent position, often reinforced by media presentations, leading it to be considered normal. It is still common for women to labour on a bed, although there is no evidence to support any advantage. Midwives have a responsibility to share information about the advantages and disadvantages of different positions for labour and birth to facilitate an informed choice while providing women-centred care.

The RCM, RCOG and NICE encourage women to adopt whichever position they find comfortable during labour, encouraging mobility and upright positions and discouraging lying supine or semisupine. Upright positions include walking, sitting, kneeling, squatting, all fours, rocking and leaning against a wall/door/sling, and recumbent include supine, semirecumbent, lateral or side-laying. Positions in labour should also be considered when using a birthing pool (Figures 27.1–27.10).

The physiological advantages of remaining upright include the benefit of gravity helping the fetus to descend through the birth canal, improved application of the presenting part to the cervix and an increase in the effectiveness and efficiency of contractions. There is also a reduced risk of aortal-caval compression (the weight of the uterus can compress major blood vessels while in a supine position) that in turn may reduce fetal oxygenation.

An upright or 'sacrum free' position (where the pelvis is not resting on anything) also maximises the diameters of the pelvic outlet. By providing an environment whereby a woman feels in control and well supported there is a potential to enhance beta-endorphins and reduce maternal anxiety, both important and fundamental to promoting normal childbirth.

Remaining upright and mobile during labour not only increases maternal satisfaction but also reduces pain and the need for analgesics and epidural analgesia, shortens the length of labour, and reduces the incidence of episiotomy, assisted delivery and caesarean section. Fetal oxygenation is improved with fewer incidences of abnormal fetal heart rate patterns. Maximum effect is achieved by adopting an upright position throughout labour and birth.

During the second stage of labour the advantages continue with standing, squatting, kneeling and all fours enhancing the fetal ejection reflex making bearing down easier. Kneeling and all fours are the most protective of an intact perineum, while sitting, squatting and using a birth stool the greatest incidence of perineal trauma. If a recumbent position is used in the second stage, a lateral position is preferable. If a woman chooses a semirecumbent position when pushing, it is important to ensure she does not slip down the bed and become supine.

A potential negative consequence is the reported increase in estimated blood loss. However, it has been suggested that this may be due to more efficient collection and measurement of visible blood loss following birthing in an upright position.

Adopting different positions may help with a delay or difficulty in labour. For example, an all fours position may help with a premature urge to push or an oedematous cervix. While walking the stairs or lifting one knee higher than the other can help when labour has slowed or help correct asynclitism.

There is no one optimum position for birth; women will have differing needs and preferences. Midwives need to demonstrate, encourage and support women in exploring different positions. A woman's perception of her birth experience can be enhanced if information is shared as to the advantages and the practices that may affect her ability to mobilise, enabling her to make her own decisions.

Where possible, women should be given an opportunity to practice positions antenatally, preferably where they are choosing to birth. Antenatal education increases the likelihood of trying different positions and remaining mobile.

Midwives need to consider the environment, including reviewing the space available and whether any furniture needs to be moved (including the bed – women are more likely to stay on the bed if it is in a dominant central position) and source equipment (for example birth balls, stool, mats, beanbags) to facilitate positional changes. If an examination is undertaken on a bed the woman should be encouraged to move again once this has been completed.

Privacy is important; women may feel exposed when trying different positions. The woman's dignity must be maintained so she is not inhibited and has confidence in moving around and changing position.

There may be elements that restrict women from mobilising or exploring different positions (for example continuous fetal monitoring, intravenous infusions, narcotics or epidural anaesthesia). Sensitivity and adaptations may also be required if a woman has a disability that restricts movement and position change. In these circumstances the midwife should still assist the woman to be as mobile as possible. Changing position is vital when mobility is reduced to avoid the formation of pressure ulcers. If a woman wishes to lie in a supine position a wedge should be placed under her right side.

Upright positions can be tiring and there may be times that a woman wishes to rest and lay down. She should not be disturbed but encouraged to move and mobilise once ready. Kneeling over a ball or bed head can be a good position to rest in, it provides freedom of movement and ease of adjustment. Placing something under the woman's knees may be required.

Squatting can be a difficult position for some women and they may find this uncomfortable or not feel safe. They may choose to be supported if wishing to squat.

Midwives need to feel confident and competent in supporting women in different positions. Through experience and exposure, this may enhance midwives' willingness to do so. Asking midwives to document the different positions a woman has adopted in labour may also actively encourage them to support mobility and position changes in the future.

Service user's view.

'I was really lucky as my midwife helped me to try out different positions when I was in labour, I tried the birthing ball and when Charlie was actually born I was in an all-fours position, something I hadn't really thought about or even knew you could do. It really helped with my backache and I ended up with no stitches.'

Verbal communication, service user, London

28 Supporting and caring for women in labour

Figure 28.1 All aspects for care should be based on making the woman the centre of care.

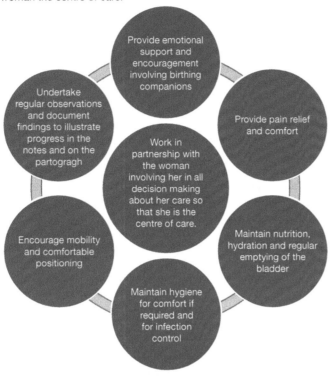

- Provide emotional support and encouragement involving birthing companions
- Undertake regular observations and document findings to illustrate progress in the notes and on the partograph
- Work in partnership with the woman involving her in all decision making about her care so that she is the centre of care.
- Provide pain relief and comfort
- Encourage mobility and comfortable positioning
- Maintain nutrition, hydration and regular emptying of the bladder
- Maintain hygiene for comfort if required and for infection control

Figure 28.2 Regular observation to be documented in established labour.
Source: National Institute of Health and Care Excellence (NICE) (2014).

- Four-hourly measurement of temperature and blood pressure
- Hourly pulse
- Half hourly palpation of the frequency, strength and duration of contractions
- A full abdominal palpation prior to any vaginal examination to confirm presentation, lie and descent
- A vaginal examination every 4 hours (if necessary to make decisions)
- Intermittent fetal monitoring with a Pinard stethoscope or doppler ultrasound for 1 minute, every 15 minutes after contractions and after vaginal examinations
- Continuous fetal monitoring if risk of intervention increases

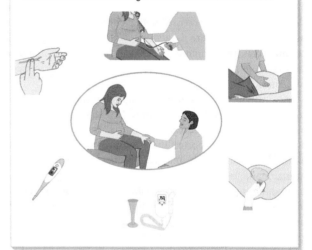

Box 28.1 Observation for transition between the first and second stage indicating impending birth.

 What the midwife may see:
- An apparent loss of control, intolerance, inability to cope
- Uncontrollable shaking
- The woman bears down with expulsive contractions
- A fresh 'show'
- Dilatation or gaping of the anus
- The anal cleft line (the purple line)
- A dome shaped curve in the lower back (Rhombus of Michaelis)
- A bulging and thinning perineum with contractions
- Gaping of the vagina with contractions
- Rupture of membrane if these had remained intact during labour

 What the midwife may feel:
- Less frequent but stronger contractions on palpation

What the midwife may hear:
- Deceleration of fetal heart rate with rapid recovery with each contraction due to vagal nerve stimulation
- The woman expressing the need to bear down with pressure on her rectum
- The woman expressing her feelings of inability to cope
- The woman expressing feeling nauseous (and may vomit)
- The woman grunts and become more vocal with contractions
- The woman expressing feelings of increased pressure on her rectum

 What the midwife may smell:
- The distinctive odour of fresh amniotic fluid with rupture of amniotic membranes
- Fecal matter as the presenting part depresses the rectum and causes expulsion of its content

Key point

What is paramount in the support and care provided in labour is that an effective partnership, built on effective communication and mutual trust, is established with the woman so that she is consistently informed and involved in decision making about her care and progress. She should feel able to express and discuss her desires and hopes for the experience she perceives will formulate an ideal labour. The midwife has to demonstrate that she has listened to and is responsive to the woman's needs, be an advocate by acting in her best interest, supporting her as far as possible to adhere to her birth plan for the best labour experience and safest outcome for the dyad.

Midwifery Skills at a Glance, First Edition. Edited by Patricia Lindsay, Carmel Bagness and Ian Peate.
© 2018 John Wiley & Sons, Ltd. Published 2018 by John Wiley & Sons, Ltd.

The first sign of discomfort building into regular and increasingly painful contractions elicits a mixture of emotions, ranging from anxiety to excitement about the impending birth. Wherever a woman chooses to give birth, the aim is to ensure that she receives one-to-one care that is individually adapted to her needs, and provided by a confident and competent midwife. The midwife needs to show commitment to respecting and addressing the emotional, psychological and physical requirements of the woman, ensuring she is comfortable throughout while providing the encouragement and support that is necessary to safely birth her baby.

Care will vary at the different stages of labour but is usually based on evidence such as the National Institute for Health and Care Excellence guidelines. However, what is paramount is that an effective partnership with the woman is established, built on successful communication and mutual trust. From the initial meeting the woman must be consistently informed and involved in decision making about her care and progress (Figure 28.1).

First stage of labour

The midwife is expected to utilise a variety of practical and interpersonal skills with effective verbal and non-verbal communication being paramount. Information should be presented in a manner that is easy for the woman to understand. Observation of how she responds to the discussion and further targeted questioning is important so that the midwife is aware of any additional actions that may be required, thereby enabling genuine involvement in all aspects of decision-making. The midwife needs to observe the woman's body language and facial expressions as labour progresses, and incorporate experience, intuitive skills, up-to-date evidenced knowledge and understanding of normal physiology to provide care, particularly during the transition period between first and second stage of labour.

Emotional support and encouragement

To enhance emotional support, additional help from a birthing partner is important. The woman should be the focus, surrounded by individuals who are compassionate and caring towards her needs. This can reduce the feeling of isolation as well as fear and anxiety that may accompany the experience of labouring in a new environment. These are all measures that increase the likelihood of a shorter labour, with less need for pain relief and an increased probability of spontaneous birth.

Nutrition and hydration

Not all women feel the need to eat or drink during labour but if the woman wants to, she can be encouraged to drink energy providing isotonic drinks instead of water or a light diet can be encouraged as the risk of gastric aspiration and Mendelson's syndrome is reduced due to the availability of epidurals and spinal analgesia. Eating, however, should be avoided if an opioid has been administered or risks of interventions during labour develop. Though not given routinely, H_2 receptor antagonists ought to also be accessible to reduce the acidity of the stomach content.

Hygiene for comfort and infection prevention and control

Feeling fresh and keeping clean may be difficult for the woman at this time, but if desired, a warm bath or shower could be offered and could have the added effect of reducing pain. Alternatively, assistance with tepid sponging may be welcomed and provide

opportunity for family involvement with her care. Keeping within universal infection prevention and control precautions remain vital.

Pain relief

The woman must be encouraged to make an informed choice about her method of pain relief (Chapters 78 and 79).

Mobility and comfortable positioning

Where possible, the woman should be encouraged to remain mobile and be supported to adopt comfortable optimal positions that promote progression in labour (Chapter 27). This should also reduce the chances of developing decubitus ulcers (pressure sores) from prolonged immobility.

Bladder care

Urine retention and bladder distention can cause long-term bladder damage, while a full bladder affects descent of the presenting part and delays labour. The woman should be encouraged to urinate frequently, but if she has difficulty passing urine, then an in-and-out catheter may be required with an indwelling catheter being introduced if the procedure is required more than once. Once the birth has occurred, she should be monitored and encouraged to void within 6 hours of delivery, informing the midwife when this has occurred so it can be documented.

Observation and documentation

Her vital signs, the wellbeing of the fetus and progress of labour must be monitored and documented regularly in the notes and on the partograph (Figure 28.2).

Second stage of labour

Using the same principles of care, the midwife now needs to observe for signs of transition between first to second stage and impending birth (Box 28.1). As this stage comes to an end, with the crowning of the presenting part of the baby, the midwife facilitates the birth of the baby into a safe and warm environment; in many cases culminating with skin-to-skin contact between the baby and new mother. The assistance of a second midwife to attend to the baby maybe required.

Third stage of labour

With the birth of the baby, the midwife continues to attend to the woman's comfort. Depending on her risk of postpartum haemorrhage and the woman's wishes, the midwife is required to await physiological delivery of the placenta or actively manage the third stage. With recommended delayed cord clamping, observations for signs of separation (contracted uterus, fresh bleed with lengthening of the cord), this stage is completed with delivery of the placenta and control of bleeding. The midwife needs to remain vigilant for evidence of excessive bleeding, which may need to be acted upon to prevent a postpartum haemorrhage.

Service user's view

'My midwife was wonderful. I felt that she listened to what my husband and I wanted. We had never met her before but it didn't matter. She was really supportive and very professional. We couldn't have done it without her. Now we have our beautiful little girl.'

First time mother, 6 hours after the birth of her baby, London

29 Supporting and caring for the partner

Figure 29.1 Becoming a father, creating a family.
Source: Photos reproduced with kind permission of the parents.

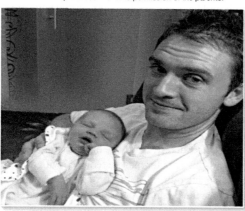

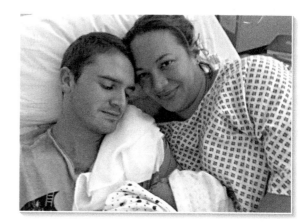

Box 29.1 Key points in care of the partner.

- Ask the partner what they wish to be called and use it when addressing them
- Discuss with both how involved they would like to be
- Any help requested must be meaningful so that the partner feels engaged with the care
- Communicate and explain
- Make sure physical needs are met: where to get food or drinks, where the toilet is
- If there is an emergency, make sure information is clear and timely

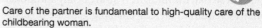

Key point

Care of the partner is fundamental to high-quality care of the childbearing woman.

Midwifery Skills at a Glance, First Edition. Edited by Patricia Lindsay, Carmel Bagness and Ian Peate.
© 2018 John Wiley & Sons, Ltd. Published 2018 by John Wiley & Sons, Ltd.

The beginning of pregnancy is the start of a lifelong journey. It may be the beginning of a new family (Figure 29.1), or the prospective addition of a new member to an established family. Naturally, most of the attention is focused on the woman as the chief custodian of the health of the developing child. Caring for childbearing women is the role the midwife is privileged to perform. However, caring for the partner is also essential as he or she is likely to be the main support for the woman on their shared transition to parenthood. Close involvement of the partner has social and psychological benefits for the woman, the partner and the infant. Sensitive midwifery care and support for the partner can be enabling and life-enhancing.

Antenatal and postnatal care

Antenatal care has traditionally focussed on the care of the woman; partners often find it difficult to attend as clinics are held during the day and taking time off work can be difficult. Even when the partner does attend there may be a feeling of exclusion:

'...she said hallo to my wife and turned her back on me...'

In some areas antenatal classes are held for partners only, led by male antenatal educators, such as DaddyNatal, which also offers online and print resources.

Similarly, some partners feel ignored during the postnatal period

'They don't actually sort of involve you as a couple anywhere along the line... I felt very left out...'

Normal birth

Most partners now expect to take an active role during pregnancy and labour, and to have their role accepted by staff. Many find they experience a mixture of emotions from being overwhelmed, to feeling vulnerable, to intense joy. For many partners this is an experience of growth and maturation as the new responsibilities become apparent:

'I have always tried to be confident... but now I have to be even more confident. Now I have to grow like an oak. Put out even bigger and stronger arms and... embrace this and...take care of this little mite...'

Ledenfors and Berterö 2016.

Other family types

Midwives need to be aware that the partner in a same-sex couple has an equal need for sensitive support. Lesbian partners may feel an equal need to be acknowledged as a parent:

'For me to be alone with the baby... without the other parent for a few minutes... was very important. I got to take responsibility for her for a little while. Then I felt recognised, I felt that she was my baby too.'

Dahl and Malterud 2015.

Emergencies

If an emergency arises it is common practice to ask the partner to leave. This may be in part to protect him/her from unpleasant or frightening sights and sounds. It may also be to enable staff to manage the woman's care without having to attend to the partner's needs as well. However, this may not be helpful:

Jerry was present at Kitty's caesarean, carried out as labour had not progressed. When she bled, he was asked to leave and was told that he could have their baby with him. He declined:

'[I was] not feeling mentally strong enough to have the baby because I was just panicking too much about Kitty'. The operation took 5 hours. While 'the information flow stopped completely,'

Jerry's need for information increased:

'Within half an hour [of leaving] I was wanting to find out. Some of the nurses and the midwives ... it was almost as though they were irritated by an anxious relative....'

Snowdon et al. 2012.

The role of partners in this situation shifts from participant to bystander. That this occurs at a point when their partner needs them most may be very traumatic.

The responsibilities and social and psychological changes precipitated by parenthood may provoke mood changes. Anxiety and depression may affect new fathers, with as many as 10% of men experiencing postnatal depression. Many do not receive the support they need and may feel ashamed of their feelings. Midwives should be prepared to discuss this in the antenatal period so that men who need support feel able to ask for it. Midwives should also be able to advise the partner of sources of help and support.

Partners want to be included but this has to be authentic. The points in Box 29.2 may be helpful reminders when caring for partners. They may also be helpful when attending to the needs of grandparents.

Service user's view
'These men felt forgotten.'

Snowdon et al. 2012

30 Care of the perineum in labour including episiotomy and suturing

Figure 30.1 Application of warm compress to the perineum during the head crowning.

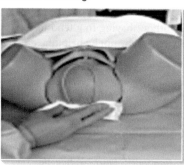

Figure 30.2 Infiltration of the perineum with lidocaine 1% prior to episiotomy.

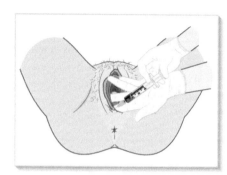

Figure 30.3 Right mediolaterial episiotomy.

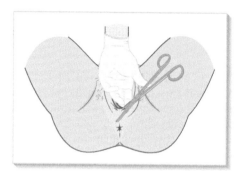

Figure 30.4 The first knot is secured approximately 1 cm above the apex of the wound.

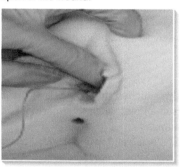

Figure 30.5 Continuous non-lock technique in the vagina mucosa.

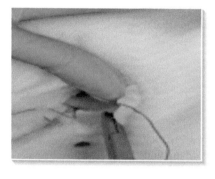

Figure 30.6 Introduce the needle into the perineal muscle from the posterior fourchette.

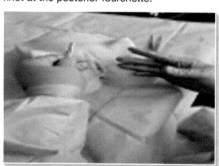

Figure 30.7 Continuous non-lock technique to the perineal muscle.

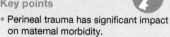

Figure 30.8 Subcuticular technique to the skin.

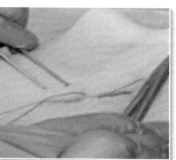

Figure 30.9 Finishing with the Aberdeen knot at the posterior fourchette.

Key points

- Perineal trauma has significant impact on maternal morbidity.
- Midwives need to be skilled in perineal trauma assessment and repair in order to minimise postpartum morbidity.
- Women need to be informed about methods of preventing perineal trauma, to enable them to make informed decisions.

Box 30.1 Classifications of perineal tears. Source: Adapted from RCOG (2015).

- **Intact perineum** No tears or lacerations involved
- **First-degree tear** Involves only the skin and/or mucosa
- **Second-degree tear** Involves skin and perineal muscles
- **Third-degree tear** Involve skin, perineal muscle and the anal sphincter
  - 3a: Less than 50% of external anal sphincter [EAS] thickness torn
  - 3b: More than 50% of EAS thickness torn
  - 3c: Both EAS and internal anal sphincter torn
- **Fourth-degree tear** Involves skin, perineal muscle, the anal sphincter, anal sphincter complex and anorectal mucosa

Midwifery Skills at a Glance, First Edition. Edited by Patricia Lindsay, Carmel Bagness and Ian Peate.
© 2018 John Wiley & Sons, Ltd. Published 2018 by John Wiley & Sons, Ltd.

In the UK, it is estimated that 85% of women will experience some degree of perineal trauma during vaginal delivery. This may be caused by spontaneous or surgical incision (episiotomy). Some women who experience perineal trauma will suffer from complications such as persistent pain, wound breakdown, wound infection, poor anatomical alignment, dyspareunia, urinary and faecal incontinence during the postnatal period. It is therefore important to explore what action could be taken by midwives during labour to minimise postpartum morbidity. It is crucial that every midwife is skilled in perineal trauma assessment and repair.

Perineal care in labour

There are different approaches employed by midwives to minimise the risk of perineal trauma. Providing continuous support, communicating effectively and working in partnership with women during labour can prevent perineal trauma.

Kneeling, upright and all fours position during the second stage of labour have been found to increase the chances of intact perineum, although there is no evidence to suggest that these positions prevent labia tears. The lateral position has also been associated with lower rates of perineal trauma and pain postnatally. Sitting, squatting and birth stools are known to have the highest incident of perineal trauma.

There is conflicting evidence when it comes to perineal protection. The hands-on or hands poised (HOOPS) trial was the first study that compared the hands-on versus hands-poised approach during the second stage. The study found no difference in perineal trauma between the two groups. Since then, researchers have either reported significantly higher incidence of perineal laceration with the hands-on technique or argued that the hands-on approaches could be beneficial in minimising the rate and degree of perineal injuries.

Supporting the perineum with the thumb and index finger has been found to be effective in reducing the tension of the perineal tissue, and subsequently preventing trauma. Similarly, application of warm compresses (Figure 30.1) and slow delivery of the head during the second stage is known to reduce perineal trauma. Both hands-on and hands-poised approaches can be used to facilitate spontaneous birth. It is important that midwives inform women about methods of preventing perineal trauma, to enable them to make informed decisions. Box 30.1 provides the classifications of perineal tears.

Episiotomy

Episiotomy is the surgical incision of the perineum during childbirth to enlarge the birth canal. The main types are the midline and mediolateral incision. The latter is most commonly used in the UK. The incision begins at the posterior fourchette and is made at an angle of 45–60 degrees, avoiding damage to the Bartholin's gland.

Indications for episiotomy are:
- Suspected fetal compromise
- Instrumental birth
- Shoulder dystocia (assess if episiotomy is needed)
- Breech delivery (assess if episiotomy is needed).

Before performing episiotomy:
- Seek consent and document.
- Use an aseptic technique to avoid introducing infection.
- Insert two fingers between the fetal head and perineum to protect fetal tissues.
- Infiltrate along the mediolateral line with lidocaine 1% (Figure 30.2).
- Avoid damage to Bartholin's duct and gland.
- Allow the perineum to thin before the incision, to reduce the risk of bleeding.

When and how to perform the incision (Figure 30.3):
- Best after infiltration
- Perineum should be thin and 3–4 cm long
- During a contraction
- Cut between the two fingers to protect the baby's head.

The continuous suturing technique is associated with less short-term pain. This is a three-stage technique using absorbable suture material, for example 2-0 Vicryl Rapide™. The first knot is secured approximately 1 cm above the apex of the wound (Figure 30.4). The vaginal wound is sutured up to the posterior fourchette (Figure 30.5). The needle is then introduced into the perineal wound to suture the perineal muscle (Figures 30.6 and 30.7). The skin is repaired using subcuticular technique (Figure 30.8), finishing with the Aberdeen knot at the posterior fourchette (Figure 30.9). The National Institute for Health and Care Excellence recommends this method.

Preparing for suturing:
- Ensure privacy and dignity
- Explain the procedure and seek consent
- Offer inhalational analgesia if the woman has no working epidural.

Systematic examination:
- Wash hands, wear a gown and sterile gloves prior to the assessment to minimise the risk of infection.
- Check with the woman to ensure that local or regional analgesia is effective.
- Carry out a visual assessment of structures involved in the trauma.
- Identify the apex before suturing is commenced.
- Perform vaginal and rectal examination before the repair to establish full extent of the injury. This should be carried out for all women who have had vaginal delivery, even those with intact perineum, to rule out anal sphincter injury and button-hole tear. Change gloves afterwards.
- Assess the amount of blood loss throughout.
- Swabs, instruments and needles should be checked and signed by two people.
- Ensure that the tissues are correctly aligned anatomically throughout the procedure.
- Avoid the routine use of a tampon, as women who have no regional analgesia may find it uncomfortable. If the use of the tampon is required, remember to secure the tail with an artery forceps.
- Perform rectal examination after repair, to ensure that no sutures have been inserted into the rectum.
- Rectal non-steroidal anti-inflammatory drug (Diclofenac suppository) should be offered routinely unless contraindicated.
- Document in records.
- Draw a diagram illustrating the extent of the trauma.

The aftercare discussion should include:
- Perineal hygiene
- Dietary advice
- Pelvic floor exercise.

Service user's view

'I think people need to know that birth isn't this pretty picture. It isn't the Home and Away birth of three pushes and you're out.'

Verbal communication, service user, Berkshire

31 Examination of the placenta and membranes

Figure 31.1 Maternal surface of placenta showing cotyledons and sulci. Amnion visible.

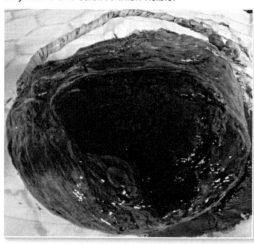

Figure 31.2 Fetal surface showing a centrally inserted umbilical cord and blood vessels radiating outwards.

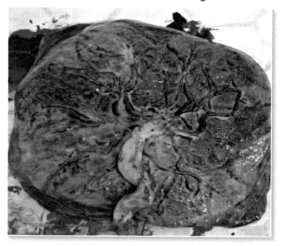

Figure 31.3 Umbilical cord with typical twisted appearance, Wharton's jelly, two arteries and a vein.

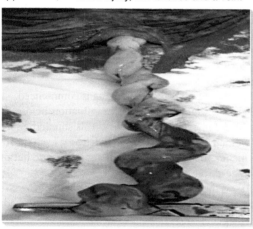

Figure 31.4 Umbilical cord with umbilical vein and two umbilical arteries.

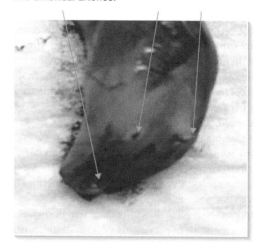

Figure 31.5 Separation of chorion (left) and amnion (right).

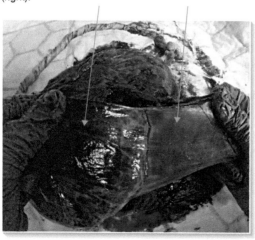

Figure 31.6 Placenta with a large succenturiate lobe and blood vessels.

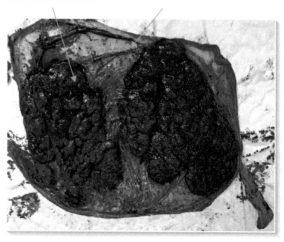

Source: All images courtesy of Sara Phillips and Christine Bell, Maternity Unit, Royal Berkshire Hospital, Reading.

Midwifery Skills at a Glance, First Edition. Edited by Patricia Lindsay, Carmel Bagness and Ian Peate.
© 2018 John Wiley & Sons, Ltd. Published 2018 by John Wiley & Sons, Ltd.

The placenta and membranes are examined shortly after birth to ascertain completeness. Retained placental tissue or membranes may lead to postpartum haemorrhage (PPH) or uterine infection. Information may be gained about the intrauterine environment and the wellbeing of the baby.

The **term placenta** is round or oval, deep red/maroon in colour, 20–22 cm in diameter and 2–3 cm at the centre and thinner at the edge. There are two surfaces – maternal (Figure 31.1) and fetal (Figure 31.2) – and two membranes.

The fetal surface lies closest to the fetus. The umbilical cord is usually inserted centrally or slightly off centre; a lateral 'Battledore' insertion may occur. Blood vessels radiate to the edge of the placenta (Figure 31.2).

The maternal surface has 15–20 cotyledons separated by grooves/sulci. Each cotyledon has its own blood supply (Figure 31.1).

Umbilical cord: This approximately 50 cm or more in length, and contains two arteries and a vein suspended in Wharton's jelly (Figures 31.3 and 31.4). A thin cord may be associated with intrauterine growth restriction and a thicker cord with diabetes, macrosomia or hydrops fetalis.

Membranes: The chorion is the outer, opaque, friable membrane that lines the uterus and extends to the edge of the placenta. The amnion is the smooth, stronger, inner, translucent membrane that covers the umbilical cord (Figure 31.5).

Preparation for examination

Ensure the mother's condition is stable, that she is comfortable, has a contracted uterus and is not bleeding excessively. Explain the rationale for the examination. Be prepared for parents to observe and to facilitate any wishes for disposal of the placenta, for example taking the placenta home or wrapping the placenta with the baby if a Lotus birth.

To prevent any transmission of a blood-borne infection, non-sterile gloves and an apron should be worn. Hands should be washed before and after the examination. Examine the placenta in good light, on a flat surface that is protected to contain blood spillage. A syringe and needle may be needed to sample cord blood.

Examination

When examining the placenta and membranes be systematic and use your senses to observe, feel and smell.

Place the placenta on a flat surface, fetal surface uppermost (Figure 31.2). Note the size, shape, colour and smell. A placenta has little odour, but if infection is present it may smell offensive. Look to see if there are any additional/Succenturiate lobes visible in the membranes. Note fatty deposits, infarctions (localised tissue death), or grey, gritty calcification (lime salt deposits). Although of interest, these are not of clinical significance

Examine the umbilical cord, observe the insertion point, note the length, any true knots or formation of thrombi.

Inspect the cut end of the cord to determine if two arteries and a vein are present, (Figure 31.4). A missing artery may signify increased risk of anomalies such as renal agenesis and will require paediatric referral for the baby.

Lift the placenta by the cord, the membranes can be observed and the hole seen where the baby has passed through the membranes. Note any vessels or placental tissue in the membranes. Turn the placenta over to examine the maternal surface (Figure 31.1).

Check both membranes are present by separating the amnion from the chorion (Figure 31.5).

Examine the maternal surface, ensure all the cotyledons are present, fit together, without gaps and with a uniform edge. Reposition any broken cotyledons and observe for completeness.

Spread out the membranes to look for blood vessels leading into the membranes that may suggest a succenturiate lobe (Figure 31.6) is retained in the membranes. If retained in the uterus, this may lead to PPH or sepsis. Again, note any greyness, grittiness, infarctions or fatty deposits.

Take cord blood samples for blood gas analysis if the baby is born by caesarean section or has a low Apgar score. Samples for blood group and Rhesus factor will be taken if the mother has a Rhesus-negative blood group.

Where maternal sepsis is suspected or confirmed, for example chorioamnionitis or prolonged membrane rupture, cord samples will be taken for blood culture. Swabs from the fetal and maternal surfaces are also required.

Follow local policies for further investigations and tests that are needed if the baby has an abnormality, or has died.

Dispose of the placenta as per local policy, or if the mother wishes to take the placenta home place this in a sealed container. If the mother has a lotus birth where the cord is uncut, the placenta may be washed and wrapped in a soft cloth and placed with the baby. The mother may be advised that separation of the baby from the placenta is likely to take several days. Any indications of infection such as an offensive smell should be discussed with the midwife.

Record your findings in the maternal notes, reporting any abnormalities to the obstetrician. Retain any incomplete placenta/membranes for further examination. Student midwives should have their examination of the placenta observed by their mentor and all records require counter signing.

Inform the mother of the results of the examination. If the placenta or membranes appear incomplete, she should be advised regarding lochial blood loss, passing clots and signs of sepsis. The mother should be advised to seek early professional advice from a midwife or doctor if she is symptomatic. The maternal notes should clearly state if the placenta or membranes are incomplete to alert other healthcare professionals that PPH or sepsis may arise postnatally.

If the mother has delivered at home and there are significant concerns about retained placental tissue, transfer to obstetric care should be considered.

Service user's view

'I was fascinated to see my son's placenta; I was amazed that such a small thing could be a complete life support system for my child.'

Lynn, service user, London

32 Urinary catheterisation

Figure 32.1 Diagram of female external genitalia and catheterisation.

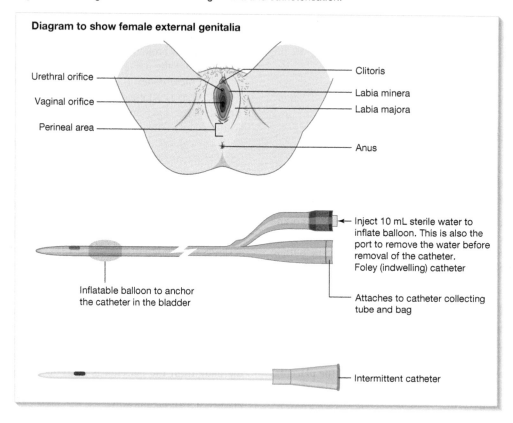

Diagram to show female external genitalia

- Urethral orifice
- Vaginal orifice
- Perineal area
- Clitoris
- Labia minera
- Labia majora
- Anus

Inject 10 mL sterile water to inflate balloon. This is also the port to remove the water before removal of the catheter.
Foley (indwelling) catheter

Inflatable balloon to anchor the catheter in the bladder

Attaches to catheter collecting tube and bag

Intermittent catheter

Box 32.1   Indication for catheterisation.

Catheterisation is required for a number of reasons during labour, birth and the postnatal period.
- Prior to a caesarean section or any other abdominal surgery to minimise damage to the bladder and improve visualisation during the procedure
- Prior to forceps or ventouse delivery
- If a woman is unable to micturate during labour perhaps due to epidural anaesthesia
- During the third stage of labour as a full bladder will impede normal uterine activity
- To fill the bladder, if the umbilical cord has prolapsed
- Women who are critically ill and need precise fluid balance, for example following a major obstetric haemorrhage or pre-eclampsia
- If urinary retention (an inability to pass urine) is diagnosed at any stage

Key point

Urinary catheterisation should be avoided if possible as it can cause pain, infection and/or trauma.

Box 32.2   The urinary bladder.

The bladder is a hollow muscular organ situated in the anterior of the pelvis and when full can displace the uterus and may lead to labour dystocia and poor uterine activity and can also prevent involution of the uterus in the postnatal period. The action of progesterone on the smooth muscle of the urinary tract during pregnancy can predispose pregnant women to urinary tract infections.

Box 32.3   Equipment required.

- Sterile Foley catheter
- 10 mL sterile water
- 10 mL sterile syringe and drawing up needle
- Sterile drainage bag and stand
- Sterile gloves
- Sterile catheter pack
- Anaesthetic gel
- Cleansing solution and a disposable sheet

Midwifery Skills at a Glance, First Edition. Edited by Patricia Lindsay, Carmel Bagness and Ian Peate.
© 2018 John Wiley & Sons, Ltd. Published 2018 by John Wiley & Sons, Ltd.

Urinary catheterisation is increasingly used in a number of women during labour, preoperatively and in the postnatal period. During the physiological process of labour, bladder care is a fundamental part of midwifery care, with the National Institute for Health and Care Excellence making recommendations on the frequency for passing urine from admission through labour, birth and postnatal period.

Knowledge of the anatomy and physiology of the urinary tract is vital in being able to make considered clinical decisions when caring for pregnant women who require urinary catheterisation (Figure 32.1).

Urinary catheterisation drains urine using a small hollow tube (catheter), which is inserted into the bladder, most commonly via the urethra, using an aseptic technique. Catheters are made from a variety of materials Including plastic, silicone, PTFE (Teflon) and latex. Due consideration should be given when choosing the type of catheter where a patient has a latex allergy. The catheter may be left in situ secured in the bladder by a small balloon on the tube inflated with sterile saline, which drains urine continuously into a collection bag (indwelling or Foley catheter) or inserted and immediately removed once the urine has drained (intermittent). Catheterisation is a relatively straightforward procedure; however, it does carry some risk. Boxes 32.1 and 32.2 outlines indication for catheterisation.

Complications

Urinary catheterisation should be avoided if possible as it can cause pain, infection and/or trauma. Pain can be caused by the introduction of the catheter into the urethra. The urethra is lined by transitional epithelium cells, which are not lubricated and are also very sensitive. By using a sterile lubricant, such as 6 mL lidocaine 2% gel, tissue damage can be minimised but this will also give an anaesthetised effect to the urethra, helping to manage any pain or discomfort. Infection is often caused by poor aseptic technique where micro-organisms are introduced as the catheter is inserted, from the hands of the practitioner or from the flora of the perineum. Where catheterisation is prolonged, the risk of infection increases; therefore an assessment of need must be made regularly.

Procedure

Midwives should consider the risks of using a catheter alongside the benefits and always discuss with the woman prior to the procedure. They must also ensure that the woman's identity has been checked and that informed consent has been given for any procedure. The midwife needs to gather all the equipment required for the procedure (Box 32.3).

The midwife may need to assist the woman into a semirecumbent position, helping her to remove any underwear or sanitary towels, with her knees bent, hips flexed, ankles together and feet resting on the bed.

An aseptic technique must be used throughout the procedure, prepare the equipment by opening the packs on to a clean trolley that can be taken to the bedside. The midwife must ensure that hands are washed and sterile gloves are used to minimise the risk of introducing infection. The disposable sheet should be placed under the woman's buttocks helping to maintain an aseptic field.

Separate the labia and clean the vulva using the dominant hand, from front to back starting with the labia majora and then the labia minora using each swab once only.

Locate the urethral orifice and insert the anaesthetic gel and allow it to take effect for 3–5 minutes before inserting the catheter. Remove gloves, wash and dry hands thoroughly and put on a second pair of sterile gloves.

Using a gauze swab to separate the labia, introduce the tip of the catheter into the urethra passing it slowly in an upward and backward direction until urine is visualised.

If there is any difficulty in passing the catheter or the woman is in pain, the procedure should be stopped.

If catheterisation is erroneously placed into the vagina and not the urethra, the catheter must be discarded and a new sterile one used.

Once urine is seen the catheter can be advanced further and the balloon inflated by slowly injecting the sterile water from the syringe into the valve. If there is any pain this could indicate that the balloon is misplaced in the urethra and not in the bladder. The catheter needs to be attached to the drainage bag and this is then attached securely to the bedside.

Clear the area, correctly dispose of any equipment and remove gloves and wash hands.

The procedure for intermittent catheterisation is the same except the catheter is single-use and is removed once urine is drained.

Removal of the catheter should be considered according to the woman's clinical condition. Gather together a disposable receiver, 10 mL syringe, non-sterile gloves, disposable sheet and cleansing solution. Place the disposable sheet under the woman's buttocks, wash hands and put on gloves. Deflate the balloon by withdrawing the water into the syringe. Ask the women to inhale and remove the catheter smoothly and quickly as she exhales and place it into the receiver. Cleanse the perineum as per local protocols.

The woman's urinary function and output must be monitored according to local protocols following removal of a catheter. The woman should be given information to ensure she is aware of the need to void within the first 6 hours, that her output should equal her input, possible signs of urinary retention, increase oral fluids and to be aware of urethral irritability or trauma from the catheterisation.

The midwife should document the procedure with the indications, any complications and details of all the equipment and drugs used.

Service user's view

'The midwife was well prepared and explained the benefits and all the risks to me prior to the procedure, which made me feel included in the decision making process and in control of my care.'

Verbal communication, service user, Berkshire

33 Assessing fetal wellbeing in pregnancy and labour

Figure 33.2 Identifying the fundus.
Source: Perinatal Institute, Birmingham, UK. Reproduced with permission of the Perinatal Institute.

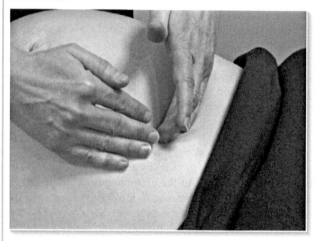

Figure 33.3 Measuring fundal height.
Source: Perinatal Institute, Birmingham, UK. Reproduced with permission of the Perinatal Institute.

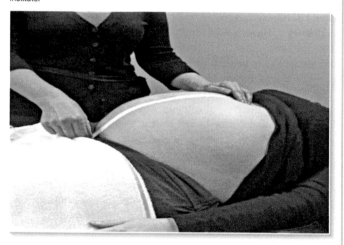

Figure 33.4 Listening with a Pinard stethoscope.

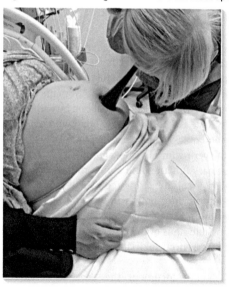

Box 33.1 Antenatal screening and diagnostic tests.

Women are offered a range of screening and diagnostic tests during their pregnancies which will give an indication of fetal wellbeing. These include:
- Serum screening for chromosomal abnormalities as part of the Combined Test or Triple Test
- Chorionic villus sampling or amniocentesis to obtain samples for cytogenetic testing for chromosomal abnormalities
- Blood tests for antibodies (anti-D, anti-C, anti-K)
- Blood tests for infectious diseases such as HIV, hepatitis B and syphilis

Key point

Always ask permission from the woman before any examination, including abdominal palpation.

The aim of assessing fetal wellbeing in pregnancy and labour is to achieve the birth of a healthy baby. This is can be done by confirming normal fetal growth and development, but also early detection of deviations from the norm so timely intervention can take place.

Assessment can be accomplished in a number of ways, including antenatal screening and diagnostic testing (Box 33.1), measuring fetal growth, ultrasound scanning and monitoring fetal movements. Assessing maternal wellbeing also provides vital clues, as poor maternal health may negatively impact on the fetus.

Ultrasound scan

All pregnant women are offered an ultrasound scan (USS) at 10 to 13 weeks to:
- Assess fetal viability
- Date the pregnancy
- Undertake nuchal translucency screening for chromosomal abnormalities.

A further scan is offered at 18–20^{+6} weeks to detect fetal structural abnormalities. Third trimester scans are not routinely

Midwifery Skills at a Glance, First Edition. Edited by Patricia Lindsay, Carmel Bagness and Ian Peate.
© 2018 John Wiley & Sons, Ltd. Published 2018 by John Wiley & Sons, Ltd.

offered although there is some research suggesting they have a place in detection of intrauterine growth restriction (IUGR).

Further USS will be offered if indicated:
- To accurately assess the position of the fetus
- For suspected IUGR
- Women at high risk of IUGR.

If symphysis fundal height (SFH) measurement is likely to be inaccurate, such as with high BMI (e.g. a BMI over 35) or multiple pregnancies, women may be referred for serial assessment of fetal size. Women who have risk factors for IUGR should be offered routine umbilical artery Doppler scans from 26 to 28 weeks of pregnancy.

Fetal movements

Women should be encouraged to monitor fetal movements (FM) and should report if their number reduces or the pattern changes. Whilst perception of FM will vary, most women can identify when the frequency reduces significantly.

For reduced fetal movements (RFM) under 28 weeks' gestation the fetal heart (FH) should be auscultated with a hand-held Doppler. If the FH is heard, reassure the woman. There is no evidence supporting the use of cardiotocograph monitoring (CTG) or USS in the absence of other clinical indications.

After 28 weeks' gestation women should be advised to lie on their left side and focus on FM for 2 hours. If they do not feel 10 or more movements in 2 hours, they should contact maternity services.

Women with significantly reduced or absence of FM should contact maternity services immediately and be monitored using a CTG to exclude fetal compromise. Women with recurrent RFM should be reviewed and undergo further investigations such as USS to assess growth and liquor volume.

Abdominal examination and palpation is fundamental to assessing fetal wellbeing. See Chapter 25.

Assessing fetal growth is a key means of assessing fetal wellbeing. From 24 weeks' gestation the SFH should be measured at every appointment and plotted on a growth chart (Figure 33.1, which can be found in the Appendices at the end of the book). The RCOG recommends the use of customised growth charts. If the SFH measures below the 10th centile on one occasion, or slow or static growth is demonstrated on serial measurements, the woman should be referred for USS assessment.

Measuring the fundal height

- Ensure privacy.
- Position the woman in a supine position with her legs extended.
- Wash hands.
- Palpate the abdomen to locate the fundus (Figure 33.2).
- Use a single patient use tape measure with the centimetres on the underside to reduce the risk of bias
- Secure the tape at the fundus with one hand. Keeping the tape in contact with the skin, measure along the longitudinal axis of the fetus to the upper border of the symphysis pubis without correcting to the abdominal midline (Figure 33.3).
- Measure only once.

- Wash hands.
- Document the distance in centimetres on a customised growth chart.

Liquor volume

During abdominal palpation abnormalities of liquor volume may be suspected. Polyhydramnios, too much liquor, may be suspected if the uterus appears larger than expected, looks tight and shiny and feels tense to palpate. A fluid 'thrill' may be seen if the abdomen is tapped.

Oligohydramnios, too little liquor, may be suspected when the uterus feels small and compact. The fetal parts may be easily palpated. Both polyhydramnios and oligohydramnios can be confirmed by USS.

Auscultation of the fetal heart

A pinard or fetal stethoscope should be used for the initial assessment to confirm that the sounds are the FH as the maternal pulse may be picked up by electronic methods and mistaken for the FH. The maternal pulse should be palpated simultaneously to establish a difference in rates to further confirm it is the FH being auscultated (Figure 33.4).

Fetal wellbeing in labour

A key indicator of fetal wellbeing is maternal wellbeing. If the mother is unwell this is likely to impact on the fetus. The midwife should assess maternal wellbeing, including observations of vital signs and urinalysis.

Women should be asked about FM at the first point of contact during labour. Women reporting reduced FM should be monitored using electronic fetal monitoring (EFM) throughout labour. FM during labour is an indication of a healthy fetus. FM should be anticipated following stimulation such as a vaginal examination, and the absence of such may indicate fetal compromise.

The FH should normally be auscultated every 15 minutes in the first stage of labour and every 5 minutes or after every contraction in the second stage for women. Auscultation should take place after a contraction for 1 minute and the rate should be counted and recorded.

Liquor colour and smell

Liquor is usually clear and has an inoffensive smell. A change in colour from clear to green/brown may indicate the liquor is contaminated with meconium. This may be a sign of fetal distress. Whilst a pinkish tinge may be normal, any significant blood staining may be a sign of haemorrhage. An offensive smell is indicative of infection.

Service user's view

'I found it reassuring that they measured the baby and I could see that it was growing on the chart in my book.'

Charlotte, primigravida, Manchester

34 Monitoring the fetal heart in pregnancy and labour

Figure 34.1 Using a Pinard stethoscope.

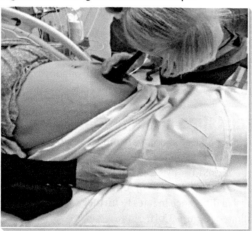

Figure 34.2 Using a hand-held fetal doppler.

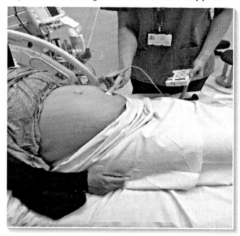

Figure 34.3 CTG monitoring.

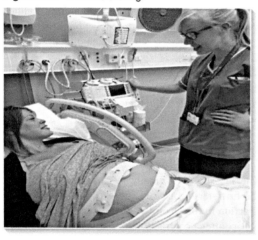

Figure 34.4 Fetal scalp electrodes.

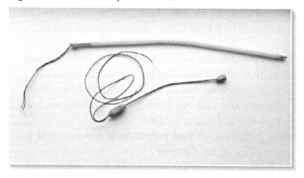

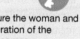

Key point

Listening to the fetal heart rate can only reassure the woman and midwife of the wellbeing of the fetus for the duration of the auscultation and is not a predictor of good outcomes.

Figure 34.5 Position of electrode on fetal skull.

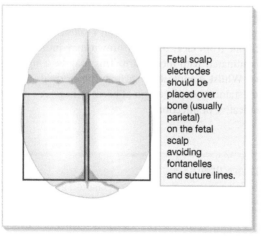

Fetal scalp electrodes should be placed over bone (usually parietal) on the fetal scalp avoiding fontanelles and suture lines.

Midwifery Skills at a Glance, First Edition. Edited by Patricia Lindsay, Carmel Bagness and Ian Peate.
© 2018 John Wiley & Sons, Ltd. Published 2018 by John Wiley & Sons, Ltd.

It is the role of the midwife to provide appropriate care during pregnancy and labour, which promotes normal birth and detects complications in mother and/or fetus. Maternal consent is required for any procedure.

Auscultation of the fetal heart

Best practice for auscultation is to listen with a Pinard stethoscope (Figure 34.1), although a hand-held fetal Doppler may also be used (Figure 34.2). Abdominal examination (see Chapter 25) is used to identify the best location on the maternal abdomen to hear the fetal heart (FH), which is over the fetal shoulder.

Intermittent auscultation is when the FH is listened to for short periods of at least 1 minute. This is a suitable method during pregnancy and throughout low-risk labours. When listening to the FH the midwife should record the following:
- Rate – should be counted for a full minute and recorded as a single number.
- Variability – the differences that occur within the heart rate and should be heard during the course of auscultation.
- Accelerations – whether or not rises in the heart rate are heard.
- Decelerations – whether or not decreases in the heart rate are heard. Any decelerations should be noted and continuous monitoring commenced immediately.

Maternal pulse should be palpated simultaneously and recorded.

During pregnancy

During pregnancy there is no evidence to support regular auscultation of the FH as the 'snapshot' of wellbeing. Therefore, the midwife should not routinely auscultate during antenatal examinations but can do so if requested by the woman. Instead care should be taken to ensure that women are aware of the importance of fetal movement as an indicator of a healthy fetus.

First stage of labour

Auscultation should be performed at the first contact when the woman is in labour and at every assessment thereafter, with maternal pulse recorded to differentiate between the two.

During the first stage of established labours (from 4 cm dilatation to commencement of pushing) the FH should be auscultated every 15 minutes. The midwife should listen for at least 1 minute immediately following a contraction taking note of the features above, with any deviations from normal noted, recorded and acted upon, continuous monitoring commenced and a member of the obstetric team informed.

Second stage of labour

During the active second stage of labour (from commencement of pushing until the birth of the baby) the FH should be auscultated every 5 minutes or after every contraction. Again this should be immediately after a contraction for a minimum of 1 minute.

Electronic fetal monitoring

In cases where the pregnancy/labour is affected by complications or medical complexities, continuous monitoring of the FH may be indicated. Electronic fetal monitoring is carried out using a cardiotocograph (CTG) machine. This provides the midwife with a continuous record on paper of the FH rate as well as an indication of uterine activity.

The CTG transducer should be placed on the maternal abdomen where the FH has been heard with a Pinard stethoscope and is held in place with an elasticated belt. The toco (which is a pressure sensor to identify uterine activity) is then placed at the highest point of the fundus and held in place with a second belt (Fig. 34.3). It is important that the uterus is in a resting phase (soft) when this is applied and that the percentage reading on the machine is low, <10. If this is not the case there is a button on the machine that will reset the reading to zero.

Antenatally the woman may be given a button to press to record fetal movements felt, if this function is available on the machine. Some machines record this automatically through the transducer. Following commencement of the CTG recording the midwife should record the following details on the trace:
- Date and time
- Woman's name and hospital number
- Gestation
- Indication for CTG
- Maternal pulse
- Midwife's name and signature at completion of monitoring.

The following is an example of indications for CTG monitoring in pregnancy and/or continuous monitoring in labour (this is not exhaustive).
- **Pregnancy:**
  Maternal: abdominal trauma, prolonged rupture of membranes
  Fetal: reduced fetal movements, deceleration on intermittent auscultation.
- **Labour:**
  Maternal: suspected sepsis or chorioamnionitis, tachycardia (>120 bpm) on two occasions 20 minutes apart, severe hypertension, obstetric emergency (e.g. haemorrhage, cord prolapse, seizure), oxytocin use, fresh vaginal bleeding, delay in first or second stage
  Fetal: significant meconium liquor, abnormal presentation (including cord presentation), suspected growth restriction, fetal heart rate <110 bpm or >160 bpm, deceleration on intermittent auscultation, oliogohydramnios or polyhydramnios.

Interpretation

NICE guidelines set out the parameters used in most of the UK by which the FH should be assessed for normality. This should be done hourly, unless otherwise indicated by previous assessments in which case every 30 minutes is more appropriate.

Fetal scalp electrode

If the FH cannot be monitored adequately by abdominal transducer, a fetal scalp electrode (FSE) may be considered (Figure 34.4). An FSE is a clip or screw-like device, which is attached to the fetal scalp, with consent of the woman, during a vaginal examination. There is direct contact, giving rise to a more consistently recorded CTG. The FSE is normally applied over one of the parietal bones (Figure 34.5). They should only be used with extreme caution where there is maternal infection or malpresentation.

Service user's view

'I found being able to hear my baby's heartbeat all of the time reassuring, especially as the doctors said there may be a problem. However, I hadn't quite realised the impact of being strapped to a monitor; it meant I was tied to the bed, ended up with an epidural and assisted delivery and this all had an effect on my physical recovery, psychological state following birth and the relationship I formed with my daughter. With my son, I was determined not to go down that road again!'

Service user, Essex

The Apgar score

Table 35.1 APGAR scoring.

	Apgar scoring	2	1	0	1 minute	5 minutes	10 minutes
A	Appearance (Colour)	Pink all over	Pink (but hands and feet are bluish)	Pale or bluish-grey			
P	Pulse (heart rate)	Heart rate above 100 beats per minute	Heart rate below 100 beats per minute	Absent heart rate			
G	Grimace (reflexes)	Cries, sneezes, coughs or turns away with stimulation	Facial movements (grimace) only with stimulation	No response to stimulation			
A	Activities (muscle tone)	Well flexed arms and legs with active movements	Arms and legs flexed with little movements	'Floppy' tone with no movement			
R	Respiration (rate and effort)	Good cry, breathing is spontaneous	Weak cry, irregular/ laboured breathing	Not breathing			
				Total Score			

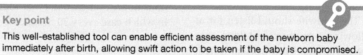

Key point

This well-established tool can enable efficient assessment of the newborn baby immediately after birth, allowing swift action to be taken if the baby is compromised.

Midwifery Skills at a Glance, First Edition. Edited by Patricia Lindsay, Carmel Bagness and Ian Peate.
© 2018 John Wiley & Sons, Ltd. Published 2018 by John Wiley & Sons, Ltd.

Assessment at birth

The birth of a baby is an exciting time for the parents and the family. For many people, the moment of birth is full of emotions and anxiety, including concerns about the baby's condition. The process of birth (other than by elective caesarean section) can be a hypoxic experience for the baby, because significant respiratory exchange at the placenta is prevented for a duration of 60–65 seconds during an average contraction. Most babies tolerate this well, but the few that do not may require help to establish normal breathing following birth.

At delivery, the midwife's initial concern, amongst other things, is usually about the baby's ability to adapt to the outside world, such as the physiological changes in the heart function and the initiation of respiration. The midwife uses the Apgar scoring system to assess the condition of the baby at birth in the first instance, and then follow up with a full physical examination to confirm normality and to detect any deviation from the norm.

The Apgar score

This system helps to rate a baby's colour, heart rate, reflexes, muscle tone, and respiration with a total score from 0 to 10 (maximum score of 2 for each of the 5 components assessed). Thus, the Apgar score quantifies the clinical signs of the neonate such as cyanosis or pallor, bradycardia, depressed reflex response to stimulation, hypotonia, and apnoea or gasping respirations. Although the Apgar score was named after Virginia Apgar, it is often referred to as an acronym for: Appearance, Pulse, Grimace, Activity, and Respiration.

The Apgar score is used by health professionals to assess the condition of the baby at 1 and 5 minutes of birth, and at 10 minutes if the score remains low (i.e. 6 or below). This helps to quickly identify those babies who may require additional cardiorespiratory support at birth. The Apgar score is based on a score of 0 to 10. The higher the score, the better the baby's condition at birth. A score of 7 or above is considered normal, which indicates that the baby is in good health with good adaptation to extra-uterine life. A score of 10 is very rarely given as almost all neonates lose 1 point for having bluish hands and feet, which is normal at birth. Any score below 7 is considered low and is an indication that the baby may require attention from the neonatal team. The lower the score, the more help the baby is likely to need to adjust to extrauterine life. A low Apgar score may arise from a difficult delivery or a caesarean section birth, for example fluid in the baby's airway/lungs. Although a baby with a low Apgar score may need help with breathing and/or physical stimulation to get the heart beating at a healthy rate (i.e. 100 beats per minute or more), it is not necessarily indicative of intrapartum asphyxia. Most of the time, a low score at 1 minute will improve to near normal by 5 minutes with minimal intervention.

It is important to recognise the limitations of the Apgar score. The scoring system is an expression of the baby's physiological condition at one point in time (i.e. at birth), which includes subjective components. Factors such as maternal medication, congenital malformation, gestational age and trauma can influence the Apgar score. The score alone cannot be considered to be evidence of, or a consequence of, asphyxia, nor does it predict individual neonatal mortality or neurological outcome, therefore should not be used for that purpose. Although a 1-minute Apgar score of 0–3 does not necessary predict any individual baby's outcome, a 5-minute score of 0–3 clearly correlates with neonatal mortality and morbidity such as cerebral palsy. However, large population studies have uniformly reported that most babies with low Apgar scores do not always develop cerebral palsy. Therefore, it should be noted that a lower Apgar score does not mean a child will have serious or long-term health problems. The score is not designed to predict the future health of the child.

Using the Apgar scoring chart (Table 35.1) as an assessment aid, the midwife will be able to arrive at a total score quickly when assessing the baby at birth. For example, a baby born in good condition with the maximum score of 2 each for well flexed arms and legs, heart rate of 110 beats per minute, strong cry (i.e. breathing spontaneously), but with bluish hands and feet (scoring 1) and facial grimace with stimulation only (scoring 1) at 1 minute will have a score of 8. If the baby quickly progress to having sneezes and turns/pulls away with stimulation by 5 minute, the score will go up to 9, with hands and feet remaining slightly bluish.

However, a baby is born in poor condition with 'floppy' tone (score 0), facial grimace only (score 1), heart rate of 80 per minute (score 1), looking pale (score 0) and not breathing (score 0) will have an Apgar of just 2 and will require immediate life support and the neonatal team should be summoned urgently. The midwife should then commence neonatal resuscitation whilst awaiting the neonatal team to arrive. Communicating with the parents is vitally important to enhance the parents' understanding of their baby's health status at this time.

The Apgar score provides an easy and convenient way of conveying the condition of the baby following birth. The midwife is required to understand the significance of the score and its use in assessing the neonate at birth and explain this to the parents. The score and the result of any intervention should be clearly and correctly documented in the maternal/ neonatal notes as well as the baby's personal child health record (PCHR).

36 The midwife's examination of the baby at birth including identification of the neonate

Figure 36.1 Newborn examination.

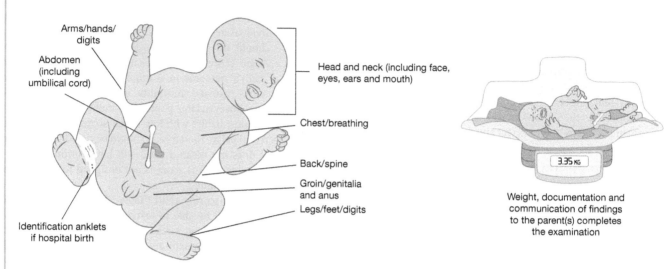

- Arms/hands/digits
- Abdomen (including umbilical cord)
- Head and neck (including face, eyes, ears and mouth)
- Chest/breathing
- Back/spine
- Groin/genitalia and anus
- Legs/feet/digits
- Identification anklets if hospital birth

3.35 KG

Weight, documentation and communication of findings to the parent(s) completes the examination

Table 36.1 Key issues to consider prior to the examination.

History	Consider antenatal, medical and intrapartum
Birth outcome	Mode of birth (normal, instrumental/operative)
Informed consent	Parent(s) received relevant information to make informed decision and provide consent
Room temperature	Babies lose heat through evaporation, conduction, convection and radiation. Every effort should be taken to ensure an optimal thermoneutral environment
Time allowed for parent–baby relationship	Time should be allowed for parent–baby interactions, skin-to-skin contact and initiation of breastfeeding
Proximity of baby to parent(s) at the time of the examination	Ensuring safety and taking precautions to prevent infection, every effort should be taken to ensure baby and parents are in close proximity. This allows for health education, explanation and an opportunity to answer questions posed

Box 36.1 Identification (ID) of the newborn. Source: Adapted from National Patient Safety Agency (2008). *Identification of neonates.* http://www.nrls.npsa.nhs.uk/EasySiteWeb/getresource.axd?AssetID=60202&type=full&servicetype=Attachment (accessed February 2017).

ID labels/anklets information
TWIN/TRIPLET I/II/III (if applicable)
Mother's surname   Baby's gender boy/girl   Baby's date and time of birth
Baby's NHS Number (or in line with local policy)

Checking ID labels/anklets
Following birth, ALL ID labels MUST be checked with the mother and her birth partner (or member of staff where necessary) before being applied. During hospitalisation they must be checked daily by the midwife as part of the routine daily examination of the baby.

If an ID label/anklet becomes detached from the baby:
Produce and apply a new ID label.
If *both* ID label/anklets are lost: inform midwife in charge of the shift; check every other baby's wristbands on the ward before ID labels are replaced; follow local NHS Trust policy/risk management procedures and complete an incident form.

Key point
The examination of the newborn should be carried out in a timely manner as soon as practicable after birth, in the presence of the parent(s), with a full explanation throughout the procedure.

Midwifery Skills at a Glance, First Edition. Edited by Patricia Lindsay, Carmel Bagness and Ian Peate.
© 2018 John Wiley & Sons, Ltd. Published 2018 by John Wiley & Sons, Ltd.

The initial examination of the newborn by the midwife at birth is essential, as the transition from intrauterine life to extrauterine existence becomes a reality. It sets the parameter for care and provides a baseline to inform the subsequent detailed newborn and infant physical examination (NIPE) (Lomax 2015). It also provides an opportunity for health education for the parent(s).

The baby transitions from a warm, calm and fluid environment, one that is life sustaining, to one that is drier and harsher, where physiological adaptations must be made quickly in order to adjust satisfactorily to the demands of extrauterine life. Colour, tone, breathing and heart rate are vital signs when assessing wellbeing. A midwife's understanding of this process of adjustment and change are factored into the systematic physical examination of the baby at birth.

Prior to the examination, informed consent from the parent(s) must be obtained, including rationale. The room should be at an ambient temperature, supporting a thermoneutral environment, to minimise heat loss throughout the assessment, as outlined in Table 36.1.

The **initial assessment** commences with inspection or observation using the **Apgar score** (Chapter 35). The midwife employs a systematic 'top to toe' approach when performing the examination.

Examination of the skin should be done at the moment of birth and forms a core part of the continuing assessment of the neonate. Apart from the skin colour (e.g. obvious perfusion, pallor or cyanosis), the midwife is also observing for signs of underlying infection (may be apparent if liquor was offensive in odour at birth), lesions, birthmarks, signs of bruising and presence/absence of **vernix, lanugo** or meconium staining.

The temperature of the baby should be checked in line with local policy and documented.

Head and neck (including face, eyes, ears and mouth): Starting from the head, the scalp is examined for any bruising or swelling (e.g. **caput succedaneum**). Any moulding, elongation of the head, asymmetry/abnormal shape, characteristic facies such as Down syndrome and size of sutures and fontanelles are noted and referred to a paediatrician as required. The head circumference is measured to establish a baseline parameter. The midwife then assesses the neck for any signs of swelling, asymmetry or extra skin folds.

Ears: Note position and any preauricular skin tags or malformation.

Eyes: Note any asymmetry, presence/absence of eye(s), any epicanthic skin folds and any obvious corneal opacities.

Nostrils: Observe breathing and note any nasal flaring or evidence of choanal atresia.

Mouth: Externally, the condition of the lips is assessed to exclude any congenital malformations such as cleft lip as well as the angle of the chin to note any chin recession. The midwife inspects the inside of the mouth noting any anomalies such as any abnormal tongue protrusion, ankyloglossia, any defects such as cleft palate or the presence of teeth at birth.

Chest/breathing: Respiratory rate is observed to detect any early signs of abnormality such as tachypnoea, sternal recession, grunting noise or high-pitched cry. Any obvious chest mass should be noted and communicated to the parent(s) and paediatrician.

Abdomen (including umbilical cord): check to ensure the umbilical cord is securely clamped. Detailed examination of the placenta at birth will reveal presence/absence of umbilical vessels. The midwife will also inspect for any signs of swelling of the abdomen or herniation.

Arms/hands/digits: Check movement and note muscle tone. The arms are also checked for any irregularity, absence or asymmetry. The digits of each hand are examined to confirm normality and exclude anomalies, for example extra or fewer digits.

Groins/genitalia and anus: The groin area is inspected to exclude any unexpected masses. Inspection of the genitalia usually confirms gender. The position of the urethra is noted in male babies. Patency of the anus is checked. The passage of meconium or urine at birth should be noted and must be included as part of contemporaneous record keeping.

Legs/feet/digits: These are checked for any irregularity, absence or asymmetry and also extra or fewer digits.

Back/spine: The curvature of the spine is noted as well as any lesions, swelling, bruising and dimpling at the base of the spine.

Weight: The baby must be weighed, the birth weight checked by the parent(s) and recorded.

Figure 36.1 summarises this examination.

Identification of newborns

The National Patient Safety Agency (2008) uses the term 'wristband' to address both wristbands and any other form of identity band, for example anklets. Their guidance for identification of the newborn relates to the hospital setting only, as detailed in Box 36.1.

Documentation/communication

Following the examination, all findings, including any deviation from normal, must be communicated to the parent(s) and documented in the records (paper-based and electronic).

Service user's view

'Postnatal care should be led by the woman's own midwife, who should help her to develop the element of her postnatal personalised care plan, and provide care alongside others, including: Perform the new-born examination.'

NHS England 2016

37 Appearance and characteristics of the well term neonate

Figure 37.1 Neonatal primitive reflexes (left to right): Moro (startle) reflex, rooting reflex, palmar grasp reflex and stepping reflex.

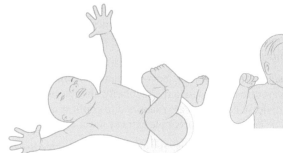
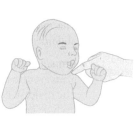
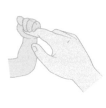
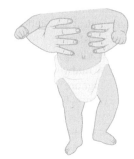

Figure 37.2 Minor abnormalities noted in the first few days of life.
Source: *Neonatology at a Glance*, Third Edition. Edited by Tom Lissauer, Avroy A. Fanaroff, Lawrence Miall and Jonathan Fanarof. © 2016 John Wiley & Sons, Ltd. Reproduced with permission of John Wiley & Sons.

Distortion of the shape of the head from delivery (molding)
Caput succedaneum, cephalhematoma Chignon after vacuum extraction

Traumatic cyanosis – skin discoloration and petechiae over the head and neck or presenting part from cord around the baby's neck or from a face or brow presentation. The tongue is pink

Peripheral cyanosis of the hands and feet (acrocyanosis). Present in most newborn infants on the first day

Lanugo: fine, downy hair, starts to shed at 32–36 weeks' gestation

Vernix: greasy, yellow-white coating present at birth, a mixture of desquamating cells and sebum which protects fetus from maceration *in utero*

Cracking and peeling of skin, particularly over hands and feet. Most pronounced in post-term infants. This scaling and desquamation is physiological

Swollen eyelids but no discharge from the eye

Subconjunctival haemorrhages – from delivery

Small white cysts along the mid-line of the palate (Epstein pearls). Cysts of the gums (epulis) or floor of the mouth (ranula)

Breast enlargement may occur in newborn infants of either sex. A small amount of milk may be discharged

Umbilical hernia – more common in Black infants, usually resolves within 2–3 years

Vaginal discharge – small white discharge or withdrawal bleed in girls. A prolapse of a ring of vaginal mucosa may be present

Positional talipes Feet adopt *in utero* position. If marked, parents can be shown passive exercises by physical therapist

Key point
Accurate assessment of health and development at birth is essential to provide safe care.

Appearance

A term baby is one born between 37 and 42 weeks' gestation. The dermis is well formed and the skin is usually smooth, with adequate subcutaneous fat and good muscle tone. The skin is generally well perfused although transient mild blueness of the feet and hands is normal at birth. The skin should be free from blemishes. Injuries such as cuts, bruises, marks from forceps blades or ventouse cups must be recorded. Movements, including chest wall movement, are symmetrical. Asymmetrical limb movement may indicate skeletal, muscle or nerve damage. The infant will be vigorous and the cry lusty, not weak or high-pitched.

Physiology

The average weight at birth is 3.5 kg, with a normal range of 2.7–4.6 kg. The average length is 50 cm and the average occipitofrontal head circumference is 35 cm. The heart rate is between 110 and 160 beats/minute. The respiratory rate is 30–50 breaths/minute. Respiration is noiseless; respiratory 'grunting' must be investigated at once. The average systolic blood pressure is 75–100 mg/Hg, and the circulating blood volume is 85–90 mL/kg. The normal body temperature range is from 36.5 to 37.4°C (axillary).

Reflexes

Appropriate neurological development is indicated by the presence of primitive or primary reflexes. Some, such as the sucking reflex, are essential to survival. These reflexes can be elicited in the healthy term infant and should disappear with increasing maturity. Their absence in the neonate is suggestive of depression of the central nervous system. Similarly, persistence of primitive reflexes beyond infancy may be a sign of central nervous system pathology.

Reflexes that can be elicited in the neonatal period include (Figure 37.1):
- Sucking reflex
- Rooting reflex
- Moro (startle) reflex
- Palmar grasp reflex
- Plantar grasp reflex
- Stepping reflex
- Placing reflex
- Asymmetric tonic neck reflex.

Feeding

Breastfeeding is the optimal method of infant nutrition and provides all the fluid and nutrient requirements for the infant. It also encourages proximity to the mother thus helping maintain body temperature and normal heart and respiratory rate. Some babies will not be breast fed, either from maternal choice or from necessity. For these babies safe, suitable breast milk substitutes are available. See Chapters 43 and 44 for further information on infant feeding.

Elimination

The infant will usually pass urine and meconium within 24 hours of birth. Once milk feeding starts the stools change from dark green meconium to brownish (changing stools) then to yellow, usually at around 5 days of life. Urinary output is usually approximately 100–200 mL/kg/day by 7 days of life. However, as the renal cortex is relatively immature at birth the neonate has limited ability to concentrate urine and conserve water or electrolytes. A dehydrated infant will therefore still produce an adequate volume of urine. Urate crystals appear as a brick-red deposit in the nappy and are usually harmless.

Minor abnormalities

Some variations in appearance of the newborn are considered normal (Figure 37.2). These include:
- Head shape: moulding and caput succedaneum should resolve quickly. Sutures and fontanelles are palpable. Cephalhaematomas are not usually evident at birth.
- Skin: white spots (milia) may appear on the face, naevi such as 'stork bites' and 'port wine stains' may be visible. Blue/grey patches ('Mongolian' spots) may be seen, commonly on the back or buttocks of Black, Asian or mixed heritage infants. The skin of a postdates infant may be dry and may crack. Blueness of the hands and feet should disappear within 48 hours. The appearance of jaundice within hours of birth is not normal. Vernix may be present in skin folds and a little lanugo may still be seen, although this has usually disappeared by 40 weeks.
- Mouth: teeth are occasionally present. The presence of tongue-tie may be seen.
- Limbs: positional talipes may be present.
- Genitalia: in female babies a white vaginal discharge may be seen and pseudomenstruation may occur. In male babies the testes should be descended.
- Trunk: transient breast enlargement may be seen in babies of either sex. There may be an umbilical hernia.

Service user's view

'Many women emphasised that it was important for health professionals to listen to what they were saying.'

Healthtalk 2016

38 Overall daily assessment of the term neonate including vital signs and bladder and bowel function

Box 38.1 Aims of daily assessment of the term neonate.

- Answer parents questions about their baby's health/ promotion
- Provide reassurances that all is well with their baby
- Monitor or refer promptly to the appropriate professionals when deviation from the normal is identified including any child protection concerns. Deviations are classified as non-urgent, urgent or emergency which act as a guide to how promptly these concerns should be dealt with

Box 38.2 Good practice points.

Introduce self to parents
Explain the rationale for the assessment
Obtain consent
Read through notes
Ask if any parental concerns
Wash hands
Undress baby
Talk to parents as assessment is undertaken
Explain findings
Redress baby
Thank parents
Wash hands
Document in notes
Monitor/report any abnormalities

Box 38.3 Top-to-toe check list.

Assess overall appearance
Head
Eyes
Nose
Mouth
Trunk
Skin
Arms and hands
Breasts
Abdomen
Umbilical cord
Genitalia
Buttocks
Spine
Legs and feet
Weigh if required

Box 38.4 Vital signs.

Temperature
Axillary (into the armpit) temperature
36.4–37.2° C

Heart
120–160 BPM
The heart rate may vary from 100 BPM during sleep to 180 BPM when crying

Respirations
30–40 breaths/minute, but not exceeding 60, shallow and irregular, with periods of apnoea (temporary cessation of breathing) for 10–15 seconds

Figure 38.1 Bladder function: (a) urates and (b) pseudomenstruation.
Source: Reproduced with permission of NCT (www.nct.org.uk).

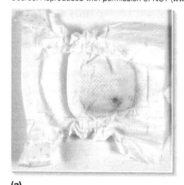
(a)

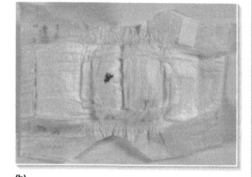
(b)

Figure 38.2 Bowel function.
Source: Reproduced with permission of NCT (www.nct.org.uk).

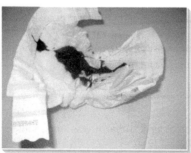
(a) Days 1–2 meconium

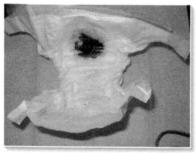
(b) Days 3–4 changing stool

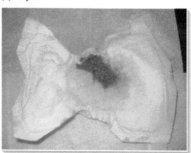
(c) Days 5–6 Changing colour, no more meconium

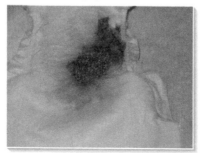
(d) Day 7 milk stool

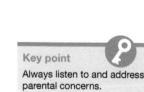
Key point
Always listen to and address parental concerns.

Midwifery Skills at a Glance, First Edition. Edited by Patricia Lindsay, Carmel Bagness and Ian Peate.
© 2018 John Wiley & Sons, Ltd. Published 2018 by John Wiley & Sons, Ltd.

For most term neonates adapting to extrauterine life is a normal physiological event. But in order to thrive and develop, they depends on others to provide their basic needs, and to be vigilant on their behalf for any changes to wellbeing.

The overall daily assessment of the term neonate, including vital signs, bladder and bowel function, acts as an important screening tool to ensure wellbeing is maintained. This assessment is a continuation in a modified format and not a replica of the examination of the newborn check. Box 38.1 outlines the aims of the assessment.

Effective communication is vital for the parents to understand the findings and know who to contact for support. An aid to this is the individualised postnatal care plan (IPCP), which should be reviewed and updated at each visit.

At every visit the midwife should ensure consent is obtained, including the rationale for the assessment. The examination should be undertaken in a warm, private well-lit room with one or both parents present and findings clearly explained in words that the parents can understand.

Before the assessment read the IPCP. The original birth examination should be used as a comparison in case any visible marks or bruising are found, to ensure that no physical abuse has occurred. Midwives have a duty to report concerns about the vulnerability or abuse of the baby.

Box 38.2 summarises best practice when completing the assessment. A systematic approach is required in order to complete the assessment satisfactorily and to prevent any omissions occurring (Box 38.3). Before checking the baby, it is important to ask the parents if they have any concerns.

The baby needs to be considered holistically, commencing with overall appearance: tone, movement, posture, sleepiness and rousability. The head can then be checked, particular attention is paid to the fontanelles, which if sunken is a sign of dehydration. The eyes of the baby should be clear, and checked for signs of infection. As most babies are obligatory or preferential nose-breathers the nostrils should be checked for signs of dry secretions that could interfere with the baby's ability to breathe properly.

An ideal time to mention infant feeding is when checking the baby's mouth, as it can be incorporated to queries about possible thrush or tongue-tie. Infant feeding is an integral part of the health promotion activity during the assessment (see Chapters 43 and 44).

The baby can then be undressed and the trunk, arms and hands exposed. If there are any concerns that the baby is unwell perform a set of observations:

- Respirations observing pattern, rate and depth
- Heart rate can then be listened to
- Axillary temperature reading is always performed last as the thermometer will need to be held in place, and might upset the baby and thus can impact on the normal reference ranges for these vital signs (Box 38.4).

Both sexes may present with transient breast engorgement due to a withdrawal of maternal oestrogens and the parents need to be reassured that this will resolve.

The baby's abdomen should look and feel soft and rounded. The umbilical cord should be checked for signs of infection.

At this point the baby can have its upper body redressed whilst the bottom half is exposed.

The contents of the nappy can be a source for much discussion as checking bladder and bowel function is an indicator that the baby is feeding normally and that the body systems are functioning normally. Parents need to be reassured regarding the frequency and contents of wet and dirty nappies.

The assessment of bladder function can be challenging especially as the bladder capacity in the neonatal period is around 10 mL. Another contributory factor is that urine output can be difficult to monitor due to the absorbency of disposable nappies.

Parents can be reassured by getting them to put a piece of tissue paper inside the nappy. Parents also need to be informed that a build-up of urates can cause pink crystals to appear which may be mistaken for blood in both sexes. Moreover, female neonates may develop pseudomenstruation due to a withdrawal of maternal oestrogens (Figure 38.1b).

The stool pattern is dependent on the method of feeding. Parents can be reassured that their baby's stool pattern is normal by discussing how the first stool, meconium, a greenish black colour, changes, and that within 2–3 days, breastfed babies stools turn yellow. If formula fed the stools may vary from yellow, brown or greenish in colour. From day 4 and in the first weeks, the baby will pass at least two stools a day which should be similar in size to a £2 coin. (Examples of contents are provided in Figure 38.2).

The check ends with an inspection of the buttocks, spine, legs and feet. A blue or blue/grey discoloration of the skin over the buttocks, back and legs may be due to a pigmented birth mark known as Mongolian blue spots.

Local guidelines may apply and the baby undressed completely and weighed. However, it is recognised that healthy babies can lose weight in the first week of life. The baby can then be dressed.

It is important to thank the parents and explain the findings. If any abnormalities were found they must be acted upon and either monitored or a referral made to the appropriate healthcare professional.

Finally, remind the parents that if they have any concerns before the next visit who they can contact. All the findings should be documented in the neonate's child health record book.

Service user's view

'I have always enjoyed the community midwife postnatal home visits. It's nice to share those special days with my baby under the care of midwives who have supported me through my pregnancy.'

Verbal communication, service user, fourth baby, Swindon

39 Newborn and infant physical examination

Figure 39.1 Auscultatory sites.
Source: Photograph reproduced with kind permission of the parents.

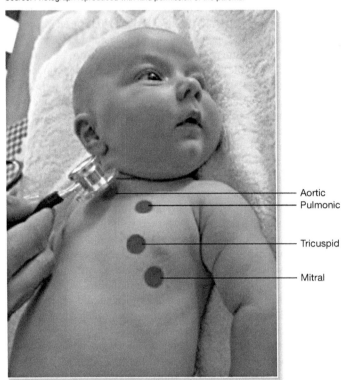

- Aortic
- Pulmonic
- Tricuspid
- Mitral

Figure 39.2 Ortolani's test.
Source: Photograph reproduced with kind permission of the parents.

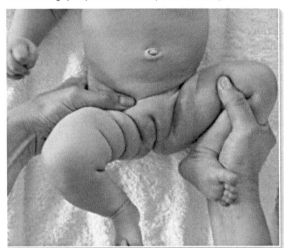

Key point

NIPE is a holistic examination that is ideally undertaken by the midwife who delivered the baby as part of postnatal care. It should be carried out with the parent(s), explaining the process as the midwife proceeds methodically though the examination.

Midwifery Skills at a Glance, First Edition. Edited by Patricia Lindsay, Carmel Bagness and Ian Peate.
© 2018 John Wiley & Sons, Ltd. Published 2018 by John Wiley & Sons, Ltd.

The Newborn and Infant Physical Examination (NIPE) is part of Public Health England's National Screening Programme, who provide national standards for the newborn examination that is offered to parents within the first 72 hours of birth. Part of this requires gaining informed consent prior to the examination and ensuring detailed records are completed afterwards to ensure appropriate referral and action is taken.

The aim is to detect deviations from the normal that may lead to long-term morbidity or even neonatal/infant death. Currently, midwives who have undertaken additional training can do this examination. NIPE is now also part of undergraduate midwifery education.

NIPE is a holistic examination that is ideally undertaken by the midwife who delivered the baby as part of postnatal care. The midwife will have insight into the maternal, neonatal and family history. The examination includes taking a comprehensive medical, family, and social history as well as gaining information regarding the antenatal, intrapartum and early postnatal periods. Some services run NIPE clinics and the midwife must be vigilant in taking a thorough history, particularly if they have not met the family before.

Midwives are not required to diagnose specific abnormalities but to recognise deviations from the normal and refer appropriately. A further examination will be performed by the General Practitioner at 6–8 weeks of age, enabling a second opportunity to screen for deviations from the normal.

Four key areas are screened as part of the NIPE standards:

Eyes: Observe the position of the eyes, that they are open and symmetrical. This examination is performed using an ophthalmoscope to visualise the red reflex as well as to detect conditions such as congenital cataracts and retinoblastoma. The maternal history is important when looking for congenital conditions or infections that may affect the development of the eyes.

Heart and chest (Figure 39.1): Make sure that the neonate is awake and calm and observe colour and tone and whether he/she is moving all limbs symmetrically and without difficulty.

Observe closely for circumoral cyanosis and count the respirations. There should be equal inspiration and expiration and rise and fall of the chest, no sternal recession or grunting. Observe for signs of nasal flaring as this may indicate a cardiac problem. Place the pad of one finger on the sternum and gently press down until the skin turns white. Remove the finger and note when the pink colour returns. This is the capillary refill time and should be approximately 2–3 seconds. Longer than this may indicate a problem, particularly if there are also other symptoms, and should be investigated by a paediatrician. Place a hand gently over the chest so that fingertips fall just below the left nipple to find the point of maximum impulse or apex beat. A sensation may be felt here that is commonly likened to a cat purring. This is 'thrill' and indicates a murmur or turbulent blood flow. Place the side of the hand on the sternum to feel for a 'heaves' where the heart may push the hand upwards very slightly with each impulse. This may indicate the presence of an enlarged right ventricle.

Using a paediatric stethoscope, listen for one minute in each of the four areas of the heart, the mitral, tricuspid, aortic and pulmonic. Also palpate the right brachial pulse when in the mitral area to ensure that they are equal in rate, rhythm and volume.

Part of the cardiac examination involves checking to see if both the left and right femoral pulses are present. If one or both are absent, this may indicate a cardiac anomaly. Place both index fingers in the inguinal canal below the inguinal notch and palpate for the femoral pulses. Once found, compare the left femoral with the right brachial pulse, found in the antecubital fossa. They should all be equal in rate, rhythm and volume. This gives an indication that the fetus has made the adaptation to extrauterine life.

It is also good practice to perform pre- and postductal oxygen saturations on all neonates as some cardiac conditions are not picked up by listening to the heart itself. Once the neonatal heart has made the adaptations to extrauterine life, the oxygen levels before the blood flows into the heart (preductal) and after it flows out of the heart to the body (postductal) should be similar. Fluctuations in oxygen levels may provide an early indication of heart anomalies.

Hips: The hip examination is key to screening for any abnormalities that may be present or develop and, as a result, is now called developmental dysplasia of the hip (DDH). The midwife should be vigilant in this examination to ensure any concerns are identified early to avoid long-term problems, pain, impaired mobility and possibly complex multiple surgeries.

NIPE guidelines recommend that all neonates are screened using the Ortolani and Barlow manoeuvres. The Ortolani manoeuvre (Figure 39.2) aims to detect if the hip is already dislocated, and the Barlow manoeuvre to detect if the hip is dislocatable. If an audible clunk is heard this is a positive result.

If an abnormality is detected, the baby should be referred for an ultrasound scan (USS) within 2 weeks of age and followed up by a paediatric orthopaedic surgeon. Treatments for a positive diagnosis include a Pavlik harness, spica cast or surgery. NIPE recommend an USS for neonates with first degree family history and those that have been breech presentation after 36 weeks, irrespective of mode of delivery.

Testes: The scrotum should be symmetrical, uniform in colour and covered in rugae. The penis should be 2–3 cm long. Any groin or scrotal swelling may indicate a hernia or hydrocele. Note the raphe, a line that runs from the tip of the penis, through the scrotum down to the anus. Observe that there is a patent urethral meatus at the tip of the penis. Occasionally, it can be found further down along the raphe, this is called hypospadias.

Bilateral undescended testes should be reviewed by a paediatrician within 24 hours to rule out metabolic and intersex conditions. Unilateral undescended testis should be reviewed by the GP at the 6–8 week check.

40 The term, preterm and growth-restricted baby

Figure 40.1 Term baby.
Source: *Neonatology at a Glance*, Third Edition. Edited by Tom Lissauer, Avroy A. Fanaroff, Lawrence Miall and Jonathan Fanaroff. © 2016 John Wiley & Sons, Ltd. Reproduced with permission of John Wiley & Sons.

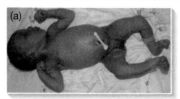
(a)

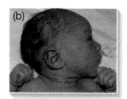
(b)

Figure 40.2 Preterm baby.
Source: *Neonatology at a Glance*, Third Edition. Edited by Tom Lissauer, Avroy A. Fanaroff, Lawrence Miall and Jonathan Fanaroff. © 2016 John Wiley & Sons, Ltd. Reproduced with permission of John Wiley & Sons.

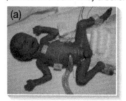
(a)

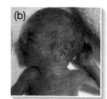
(b)

Figure 40.3 Growth-restricted baby.

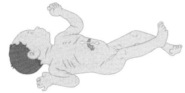

Table 40.1 Maturational changes in appearance, posture and development with age.
Source: *Neonatology at a Glance*, Third Edition. Edited by Tom Lissauer, Avroy A. Fanaroff, Lawrence Miall and Jonathan Fanaroff. © 2016 John Wiley & Sons, Ltd. Reproduced with permission of John Wiley & Sons.

Gestation	23–25 weeks	29–31 weeks	37–42 weeks (term)
Birthweight (50th centile)	At 24 weeks – Female: 620 g; Male: 700 g	At 30 weeks – Female: 1.4 kg; Male: 1.5 kg	At 40 weeks – Female: 3.4 kg; Male: 3.55 kg
Skin	Very thin, gelatinous. Dark red all over body	Medium thickness. Pink	Thick skin with cracking on hands and feet. Pale pink: pink all over ears, lips, palms and soles
Ears	Pinna soft, no recoil	Cartilage to edge of pinna in places, recoils readily	Firm pinna cartilage to edge of pinna, recoils immediately
Breast	No breast tissue palpable	One or both breast nodules 0.5–1.0 cm	One or both nodules >1.0 cm
Genitalia	Male: scrotum smooth, testes impalpable. Female: prominent clitoris. Labia majora widely separated, labia minora protruding	Male: scrotum – few rugae, testes – in inguinal canal. Female: labia minora and clitoris partially covered	Male: scrotum – rugae, testes in scrotum. Female: labia minora and clitoris covered
Posture	Extended, jerky, uncoordinated	Some flexion of legs	Flexed, smooth limb movements
Vision	Eyelids may be fused or partially open. Absent or infrequent eye movements	Pupils react to light	Looks at faces. Follows faces, curvy lines and light/dark contrast in all directions
Hearing	Startles to loud noise		Turns head and eyes to sound. Prefers speech and mother's voice
Breathing	Needs respiratory support. Apnoea common	Sometimes needs respiratory support. Apnoea common	Need for respiratory support uncommon. Apnoea rare
Sucking and swallowing	No coordinated sucking	Coordinated at 32–34 weeks' gestation	
Feeding	Usually need PN (parenteral nutrition)	Gavage (nasogastric) feeds. Sometimes need PN (parenteral nutrition)	At term, cries when hungry. Takes full feeds on demand. Coordinates breathing, sucking and swallowing
Taste		Reacts to bitter taste	Differentiates between sweet, sour, bitter. Prefers sweet
Interaction	Seldom available for interaction. Easily overloaded by sensory stimulation		Makes eye contact and alert wakefulness
Cry	Very faint		Loud
Sleep/wake cycle	Intermediate sleep state		Clearly defined sleeping and waking states

> 🔑 **Key point**
> Accurate assessment of gestational age is an important skill. Babies have different care needs and health challenges depending on gestation and weight at birth.

Assessment of gestational age

Most babies are born at term and are healthy (Figure 40.1). However, low birthweight (LBW) babies, that is <2.5 kg at birth, comprised 7% of livebirths in 2014 (ONS 2015). Babies weighing <1.5 kg at birth are classed as very low birthweight and babies <1 kg as extremely low birthweight.

Babies may be LBW because they are born preterm, because they are constitutionally small or because intrauterine growth has not followed the expected trajectory (growth restriction). The baby may at increased risk of perinatal morbidity or mortality. Accurate assessment of gestational age is essential to ensure appropriate care. A useful assessment tool is the Ballard Score (Lissauer *et al.* 2016).

Preterm babies

A preterm baby is one born alive before 37 weeks' gestation (Figure 40.2). Worldwide, prematurity is the leading cause of death before the age of 5 years. Subclassifications include very preterm (i.e. 28–32 weeks' gestation) and extremely preterm: (<28 weeks' gestation). A baby may be delivered preterm deliberately (elective preterm birth) if it is medically indicated. Examples of such situations are higher-order multiple pregnancies, or maternal or fetal disease where continuation of the pregnancy would be risky for the health of mother or fetus. However, the majority of preterm labours are idiopathic (spontaneous.)

Risk factors for spontaneous preterm birth include:

- Maternal infection
- Uterine malformations
- Multiple pregnancy
- Maternal substance misuse
- Domestic abuse.

Characteristics of the preterm baby

The appearance and characteristics are dependent on the gestation at birth. The skin is thin and at very early gestations the dermis is almost gelatinous, eyelids fused and fat stores absent. Nails are small and soft and lanugo may be seen on the skin. Body systems such as the respiratory and gastrointestinal systems are immature and do not function well. The muscle tone is poor and the infant lies with limbs extended. Table 40.1 shows maturational stages at different gestations.

Problems of the preterm baby are:

- Birth asphyxia and birth trauma
- Respiratory problems/chronic lung disease
- Feeding/nutritional difficulties
- Poor thermoregulation
- Susceptibility to infection
- Intraventricular haemorrhage
- Jaundice.

Small for gestational age babies

The definition of small for gestational age (SGA) is an estimated fetal weight (EFW) or abdominal circumference (AC) below the 10th centile; severe SGA is an EFW or AC below the 3rd centile. The fetus may be constitutionally ('normally') small, with growth appropriate for maternal ethnicity or size (RCOG 2013) or the cause may be pathological. SGA is not synonymous with intrauterine growth restriction (IUGR). Growth restriction implies the presence of pathology that is interfering with the fetal growth potential (Figure 40.3). Pathologies may be non-placenta mediated such as fetal anomalies or infection, or placenta-mediated such as maternal disease that may affect transplacental transfer of nutrients.

Risk factors for IUGR include:

- Previous SGA baby, stillbirth or pre-eclampsia
- Maternal substance misuse
- TORCH infections (toxoplasmosis, other – syphilis, parvovirus, varicella-zoster, rubella, cytomegalovirus, herpes)
- Maternal disease such as pre-existing diabetes, renal disease or chronic hypertension
- Repeated antepartum haemorrhage
- Chromosomal anomalies.

Characteristics of the IUGR baby

Constitutionally small babies will show gestationally appropriate development and appearance. Growth-restricted babies usually have a head circumference appropriate for gestational age. However, fat stores are poor or absent and there is poor skeletal muscle mass. The skin is often dry, meconium stained and appears loose, with skin folds. Nails may be long and hair abundant. The abdomen may be scaphoid, AC reduced, and ribs visible. The umbilical cord may be thin and meconium stained. The baby often has a wizened, malnourished appearance.

Problems of a growth-restricted fetus are:

- Birth asphyxia
- Meconium aspiration
- Hypoglycaemia
- Polycythaemia
- Jaundice
- Poor thermoregulation
- Pulmonary haemorrhages
- Necrotising enterocolitis.

Service user's view

'Having a premature baby is something you don't expect to happen to you.'

NHS Choices. 'My son was born at 25 weeks.' Available at: http://www.nhs.uk/conditions/pregnancy-and-baby/pages/premature-baby-mum.aspx

41 Providing daily hygiene for the neonate including changing a nappy

Box 41.1 How to clean the baby's eyes, ears, mouth, face, neck and hands.

- Wash hands before and after procedure so as not to spread infection
- Position the baby on its back on the changing mat
- Partially undress the baby covering with a towel if exposed
- Keep the nappy on until ready for the nappy change
- Notice any unusual features – sticky eyes, rashes, excoriations and jaundice
- Dip a single cotton wool ball in the warm water
- Wash each of the baby's eyes inward to outward in a single wipe before disposing so as to minimise any infection transfer
- Wash the external rim of each of the baby's ears avoiding the inner canal using a single wipe to minimise any infection transfer. Never use cotton buds as they can damage delicate structures.
- Continue to wash the baby's face, mouth, chin, neck and hands as above and do not over vigorously try to wash away vernix or lanugo
- Gently dry the baby

Box 41.2 How to clean the nappy area.

- Wash and dry hands
- Undo the vest and roll up underneath the baby's back
- Gently lift the baby's body by raising the ankles in an upward direction
- Loosen the nappy tapes on disposable or terry towel clips
- Wash genitals and buttocks using water soaked cotton wool balls/wipes
- Girls – front to back single wipe
- Boys – keep penis covered as they may urinate
- Notice any skin conditions, which may be caused by infrequent hygiene, infections such as thrush, sensitivity to washing products or creams
- Notice excretion – meconium, transitional stools and urine outputs
- New born babies may need changing 10–12 times a day and this decreases in frequency as they grow older
- Replace dirty nappy with a new one by lifting baby up by the ankles
- Discard dirty equipment and nappy into a secure disposal receptacle
- Carefully dry skin folds
- Apply barrier cream as manufacturer instructions
- Secure the nappy tapes or terry towel fasteners
- Discuss the follow up for conditions requiring additional treatment or medication
- Wash hands and dispose of waste appropriately, using policy and procedure
- Document

Figure 41.1 Changing a nappy.

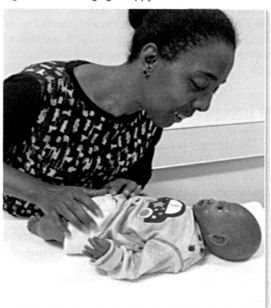

Box 41.3 How to clean the umbilical cord.

- Cleanse with cotton wool balls dipped in water
- Observe for periumbilical redness, stickiness or offensive smell
- Keep cord clean and dry by exposing to the air
- Avoid chafing on nappy
- Antiseptics not routinely advised
- Wash hands before and after cord care

Key point

Midwives play an important role in empowering parents to be confident in baby care during the postnatal period. Care contacts are opportunities for assessment, discussion and clarification and should aim to support lasting confidence and fulfilment in the transition towards mother and parenthood.

Professional standards and best practice clinical guidelines outline the professional responsibilities for those involved in promoting safe, evidence-based and effective care for mothers, babies and their families following birth. Interactions that empower parents to discuss and clarify information on baby hygiene and how to change a baby's nappy are valued opportunities to build parental confidence. A focus on individualised care enables midwives to identify what is important to mothers and parents. Initial care interactions involving discussions and demonstrations on daily neonatal care can be used to consolidate antenatal discussions and to clarify parents' concerns on neonatal health and development, common health issues, screening choices, care pathways and what to do if they are worried.

Person-centred approaches to maternal and neonatal care pathways are useful partnership reference points to enable healthcare professionals to assess, plan, implement and evaluate appropriate care with parents and to ensure routines are responsive and sensitive to each baby's circumstance. Although NICE (2006) advocates both parents should be encouraged to participate in care so as to learn about their baby's needs and capabilities, this might not always be possible and healthcare professionals should be sensitive to women's social circumstances.

In facilitating support on daily hygiene and nappy changing it is important to use communication styles and methods that are appropriate and effective in meeting a range of individualised learning preferences and situations. Facilitation strategies may include demonstration, information giving talks, client or group-led question and answer discussions, sign posting to resources such as *NHS Choice* leaflets, web links, films, peer and support networks. These strategies can be tailor made to strengthen a positive experience of parenting and used to 'mix and match' care opportunities to make sure they are timed and relevant to individual parent's needs, expectations and confidence levels.

Handovers and documentation of care plans at every stage of the antenatal, intrapartum and postnatal maternity journey are important professional responsibilities to ensure continuity and care partnership are helpful and relevant to parents either in the hospital or home setting. For example, demonstrating daily neonatal hygiene routines immediately postbirth when the mother may still be in pain and adjusting to early motherhood may not be an optimal time. It may be more sensitive to discuss practicalities of nappy changing and daily hygiene later in the postnatal period alongside infant feeding information and support. Healthcare professionals should be mindful not to overwhelm parents and joint discussion as the when the best time is to discuss baby care is an important consideration in ensuring receptivity in assimilating information.

Where possible, try to promote a peaceful, unhurried and uninterrupted ambience to baby care so that parents are enabled to enjoy the wonder and emotional involvement of getting to know their baby. As acknowledged by authors investigating care for preterm infants, tender touching and caressing behaviour by parents to their babies can play an important role in supporting positive parental experiences and could encourage future confidence in baby holding, touching and calming.

General information to discuss with parents

It is important to prepare equipment and plan actions so as to prevent any injury to either themselves or to the baby. Consideration should include safety awareness to minimise any risks and to ensure that babies are never left unattended or in precarious or hazardous environments. In addition, both temporary and permanent baby changing facilities should aim to protect carers from back and musculature strain.

Equipment and environment

Hands must be washed and dried before and after any care given. All care must be documented. Ensure the environment is warm and free from draughts – around 24°C or 75°F. Ensure all equipment is within easy reach. Equipment includes:

- A safely positioned changing mat or a flat towel-covered surface
- Cotton wool balls for eyes, ears, mouth and hands (wipes for buttocks only)
- Bowl of warm water comfortable to touch around 37°C
- Barrier cream for buttocks
- Disposal bag or bin
- Replacement clothes.

Nappy changing (Figure 41.1) offers parents, siblings and family and friends with potentially rewarding opportunities to get to know the new baby. Benefits of understanding new born behaviour and early relationships and drawing attention to the baby's individuality and behavioural cues may be helpful. This can include discussion of reflexes and sleep/feeding cycles in conjunction to discussing the impact of carers touching, holding, visual and vocal patterns. Parents are generally eager to plan a daily hygiene routine when the baby is contently awake and healthcare professionals can discuss issues such as why, when, where, how to undertake cleaning the face, neck, hands and bottom. Advice in the *Birth to Five* booklet (Public Health Agency 2016) indicates that babies do not need a bath every day and a 'top and tail' daily hygiene routine, as outlined in Boxes 41.1, 41.2 and 41.3, is recommended.

42 **Bathing the newborn**

Box 42.1 Environment and equipment.

N.B. hands must be washed and dried before and after any care given. All care must be documented
- Make sure the environment is warm and free from draughts – around 24°C or 75°F
- Decide what bathing facilities to use and prepare either a plastic baby bath, sink, regular bath (not shower) rubber stabilising mats, sponges and supports
- Many parents are keen to bath share and discussion should focus on water temperature, ways to minimise infection and handling transfer risks
- Consider safety and moving and handling issues – prevent spillages, slipping and back strain
- Make sure all equipment is within easy reach
- Cotton wool balls
- Water should be sufficient but if cleansers are preferred make sure they are suitable for newborn skin to avoid allergic reactions
- Towels, clean nappy and clothes

Key point

In designing responsive and flexible care, healthcare professionals should sensitively balance health messages around safety and infection control with strategies to increase feelings of parental confidence and achievement.

Box 42.2 How to bath the baby.

- Wash hands before and after procedure so as not to spread infection
- Follow the 'Top and Tail' approach outlined in Chapter 41
- Fill bath to a level that covers the bay's shoulders and does not overfill the bath
- Add cold water first before hot water top ups
- Perform the 'elbow' test
- Enjoy communicating with the baby
- Take off the baby's clothes
- Dispose of the nappy and wipe nappy area skin clean before lifting into the bath
- Support the baby by sliding one arm to support the head and neck and gently hold the arm
- Support the baby's bottom with the other hand whilst lifting the baby into the bath
- Maintain the upper body support
- Use the free hand to wash the front and back of the baby remembering that babies can be wriggly and slippery
- Gently lift the baby up and out of the bath
- Pat dry with a soft towel and wrap to make the baby feel secure and warm
- Only use mild moisturising lotions as indicated by manufacturer's instruction if the skin is dry.
- Be observant for allergic reactions
- Put on nappy and clothes
- Cuddle and coo to baby

Figure 42.1 Bathing the baby.

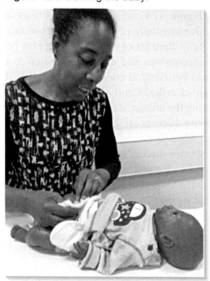
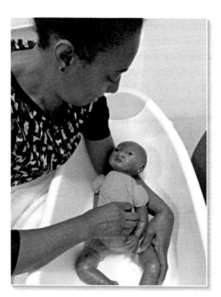
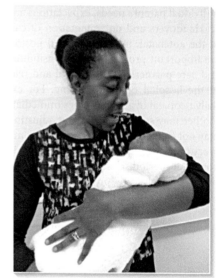

Midwifery Skills at a Glance, First Edition. Edited by Patricia Lindsay, Carmel Bagness and Ian Peate.
© 2018 John Wiley & Sons, Ltd. Published 2018 by John Wiley & Sons, Ltd.

This chapter overviews care in relation to bathing a baby, exploring evidence-based care in providing baby baths for the neonate as well as a step by step approach to care.

The emphasis on evidence-based practice has led to significant changes in newborn baby bathing recommendations. Whereas 20 years ago bathing babies immediately after birth was common, current recommendations advocate bathing should be delayed until more than 24 hours after birth due to the significant risks of hypothermia. This is of major importance for low birth weight and premature babies. Opportunities to promote informed parental decisions about baby bathing that are compliant with professional principles outlined in the Code arise at various points along the neonatal care pathway. Bathing can be discussed at the initial newborn check, during the 72-hour examination that forms the United Kingdom (UK) National Screening Programme and as part of ongoing postnatal care. There are many useful leaflets and web-based resources that the healthcare professional can signpost parents to.

In order to promote individualised care around bathing, the baby's parents should be invited to talk about what is important to them and to share concerns that might relate to their antenatal and/or perinatal clinical history. As identified by the Care Quality Commission Maternity Services Survey (CQC 2015), there are further opportunities to review the information that is given to mothers about baby care and consideration should be given to factors such as parity, previous experience, continuity of care and carer. Baby bathing demonstrations and discussions, whether done as part of antenatal or postnatal care, are opportunities for parents to share emotional experiences about adjusting to parenthood and can include acknowledgement of love, joy, pride, anxiety and/or insecurities.

Bathing a baby provides an opportunity to examine the baby's skin and assess for possible infection vulnerabilities caused by chafing, soreness or breakdown in integrity. Initially, term babies are often covered in a layer of creamy lanugo, which provides a protective function in the adaptation to the extra uterine environment in the first 24 hours. Lanugo may be very noticeable in preterm babies and less so in postmature babies, who often have dry and cracked skin and postnatal bathing should consider the implications of bathing as part of a general assessment and care planning. Careful observation will detect any potential adverse skin conditions, which range from minor transient changes to more serious conditions that may carry risks of infection and discomfort.

Many parents express concerns around baby bathing and it is an aspect of care that can get overlooked in the priorities of hospital and community postnatal activities. Parents often ask questions about the frequency, location and method of baths and the following questions might be useful in routinely initiating discussions with parents caring for low-risk babies.

When and how often?

The decision as to how often to bath a baby is a personal preference. WHO (2013) recommendations advocate that the baby is not bathed within the first 24 hours but recognise that if earlier bathing is the cultural norm that it is not done until 6 hours following birth. For some parents establishing a daily bath is a rewarding routine to be done alongside regular 'top and tail' cleanses (see Chapter 41) whereas for others once or twice a week is more acceptable. Many parents are eager for support the first time they do a bath and talking through ways to establish daily routines that accommodate personal responsibilities and choices are valued. Planning bath time to avoid interruptions often promotes an atmosphere of relaxation and enjoyment, and discussions could include the involvement of others, such as partners and siblings, and cover ways of establishing regular sleep and play routines around feeding. The benefits of skin-to-skin contact on neonatal development and wellbeing has been acknowledged in healthcare literature and bath time may be a good opportunity to enjoy skin-to-skin cuddles. Boxes 42.1 and 42.2 indicate the key points in bathing the newborn. Figure 42.1 illustrates the care.

43 Breastfeeding

Box 43.1 Impact of feeding choice.

Babies fed with breastmilk substitutes face increased risks of:
- Intestinal infections
- Respiratory and ear infections
- Necrotising enterocolitis in preterm babies
- Allergy-related conditions
- Type 1 and type 2 diabetes
- Obesity
- Childhood leukaemia
- Suboptimal bonding
- Sudden infant death

Breastfed children may experience better:
- Neurological development
- Cardiovascular health

Successful breastfeeding reduces the mother's risk of:
- Breast cancer
- Ovarian cancer
- Postnatal depression
- Osteoporosis and bone fractures

See BFI Website at http://www.unicef.org.uk/BabyFriendly/ for evidence

Box 43.2 Benefits of skin-to-skin contact.

Benefits of skin-to-skin contact for baby:
- Lowers blood cortisol (stress hormone)
- Stabilises heart and respiratory rates
- Stabilises body temperature
- Raises infant oxytocin and endorphin levels
- Stimulates breast-seeking behaviours and optimises feeding reflexes
- Increases breastfeeding at 6 weeks

Benefits for the mother:
- Lowers blood cortisol and promotes relaxation
- Raises blood oxytocin levels which initiate the let-down reflex, promote bonding and stimulate instinctual mothering behaviours

Figure 43.1 Different positions for holding the baby.

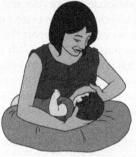
Cross Cradle Hold

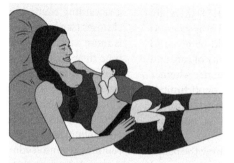
Laidback

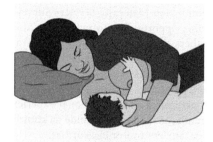
Side-lying

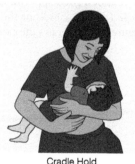
Cradle Hold

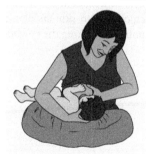
Rugby Ball

Key points

- Breastfeeding optimises the infant's immediate and long-term wellbeing, facilitates a loving mother-baby relationship and enhances maternal health.
- Skin-to-skin contact immediately after birth enables both mother and baby to follow their instincts and get breastfeeding off to a great start.
- Enabling the mother to help her baby achieve a good latch is essential for effective milk transfer and an enjoyable breastfeeding experience.
- Encouraging the mother to hold and watch her baby will help her be sensitive to her baby's needs and respond early to cues for feeding and comfort, so optimising her hormonal responses and milk supply.
- Praise, encouragement and skilled support help women keep going through early concerns and become confident breastfeeding mothers.

Box 43.3 Confirming effective feeding.

Signs of effective feeding include
- Mother feeds baby frequently in response to feeding cues
- Mother relaxed and in well-supported position
- Baby held close, in line, with head free and nose to nipple
- Baby takes a mouthful of breast tissue not just the nipple
- Baby has rounded cheeks and their chin is close to the breast
- Lips are opened wide - lower lip is curled outwards
- More areola visible above the upper lip than below the lower lip
- Rapid sucking initially, then settles to a slower deeper suck
- Swallows seen every few sucks and audible after day 3
- Infant stays attached and relaxed at the breast
- Mother feels a deep tugging but no pain after first few seconds
- Signs of high oxytocin (after-pains, breast tingling, milk leaking)
- Baby ends the feed themselves
- Nipple not misshapen, inflamed or cracked
- Breasts fill between feeds and feel softer afterwards (after day 3)
- Many wet nappies and two or more dirty nappies each day
- Baby gaining weight (regains birth weight by 10-14 days)

Box 43.4 CHINS Acronym.

Many NHS Trusts use the acronym CHINS to help staff remember what results in a good position for breastfeeding:

Close

Head-free

In-line

Nose-to-nipple

Sustainable

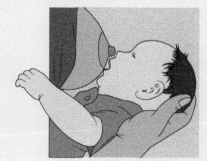

Breastfeeding is the physiological norm for human babies, and has nurtured their growth and development for 200 000 years. The effects of feeding babies with modified cows' milk are still coming to light (Box 43.1), but breastfeeding provides optimal nutrition, primes the immune system, stimulates neurological development, facilitates a loving mother–baby relationship and enhances maternal health.

Despite social pressures to bottlefeed, many women choose breastfeeding but some struggle due to lack of skilled support and stop sooner than they wanted. Midwives are key to helping women achieve their breastfeeding goals.

First feed

During labour, ask the women how she would like to welcome her baby and explain the benefits of skin-to-skin contact (Box 43.2). With her consent, place the newborn on her chest, where it can be assessed and dried. Let the baby rest; covered with a dry towel and hat. Observe them frequently to maintain safety. If undisturbed and un-medicated (no opiates in labour), babies will crawl and attach at the breast using a series of instinctive behaviours. This is best facilitated with the mother in a laidback position as gravity holds the baby against the mother's body, enabling them to move and suckle. Encourage the mother to follow her instincts to help her baby.

Laidback feeding is most restful but some women prefer an upright position. This can be more difficult for the baby as gravity pulls them away from the nipple. Figure 43.1 shows different ways she can hold her baby. Help the woman get comfortable with her back and shoulders supported. She should hold the baby very close to her body ensuing the baby's arms are not between them. The baby's head should be free to tilt back. The baby's ear, shoulder and hip should be in line, not twisting to reach the nipple. Finally the baby's nose should be level with the nipple so when the baby tilts its head back to open its mouth wide, the nipple is in the right place. The mother can express a little milk and brush the nipple against the baby's lips to stimulate the rooting reflex. If she is holding her breast, her fingers should be well behind the nipple. When the baby opens its mouth wide, she should swiftly bring them closer (with the nipple directed towards the roof of the mouth) so the baby can draw in a good amount of the pigmented areola as well as the nipple.

Give verbal guidance and demonstrate using a doll. Avoid holding the woman's breast – this can be disempowering compared with achieving a successful latch for herself. If a woman wants more practical help, offer to put your hands over hers to guide her as she helps her baby. Once the baby is well latched, encourage the woman to relax. The baby should remain in skin-to-skin contact until after this first feed. Encourage the mother to ask for help with the next feed.

Responsive feeding

Feeding should be part of a sensitive reciprocal relationship. Keep mother and baby together, encourage the woman to notice early feeding cues (e.g. stirring, lip-licking, rooting) and to hold, watch and feed her baby frequently. These behaviours raise maternal oxytocin levels, triggering the milk ejection reflex (driving milk down the ducts to the nipple) and facilitating bonding by enhancing mothering behaviours. Infant oxytocin levels are also raised and stimulate brain development. The more she watches her baby the sooner the mother will understand their needs. She should offer the breast in response to any early cues for feeding or comfort, well before the baby get distressed as they cannot feed when crying. Each feed triggers the pituitary gland to release prolactin. This hormone stimulates the lactocytes in the breast to secrete more milk – so frequent feeding will establish a good milk supply.

Assessing breastfeeding

Ask the mother how she feels feeding is going and listen carefully to any concerns she has. Consider her wellbeing as pain, anaemia or infection can affect her ability to cope with feeding. Ask about the baby's feeding pattern and nappy contents. Infrequent wet and dirty nappies or a slow change from meconium suggest insufficient milk transfer. Examine the baby to confirm wellbeing or detect signs of poor feeding such jaundice. Most newborns lose weight initially as they pass meconium and excrete (as urine) the excess fluid they were born with. Whilst a loss of up to 10% of birthweight is considered acceptable, a baby who has lost 7–10% should be carefully assessed and the mother supported to increase milk transfer. Greater weight loss requires an infant feeding specialist or medical practitioner referral.

Observe a breastfeed to give the mother positive feedback about her skills or if you have concerns about her feeding experience or the baby's wellbeing. Box 43.3 indicates signs of effective feeding. If the woman is experiencing nipple pain, suggest alternative ways of holding and latching the baby, based on the CHINS acronym (Box 43.4). If you or the mother are concerned about milk intake, encourage her to enjoy periods of skin-to-skin contact, feed more frequently, including at night (more prolactin is released at night), offer both breasts every feed, and stimulate the baby to keep suckling. Also offer additional visits from a breastfeeding support worker.

Praise and encouragement help women keep going through early difficulties. Breastfeeding can take a few weeks to get established but becomes a lovely relaxed experience as the mother's confidence grows.

Service user's view

'The midwife helped me have skin-to-skin time immediately after he was born. It was amazing that my baby, with just a little help, knew how to find my nipple and start to feed even though he wasn't even an hour old… I carried on feeding in a laidback position as it was so relaxing for both of us.'

Roz, a first-time mother, Manchester

44 Formula feeding

Figure 44.1 How to make up a formula feed.

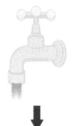
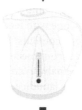

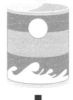
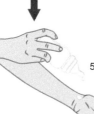

1. Wash hands and work surfaces with hot soapy water

2. Use freshly boiled water

3. Fill a sterilised bottle with the correct amount of water

4. Add the required amount of formula, levelling off the scoop with a knife. Replace teat and cap and shake to mix

5. Test temperature of milk on inside of wrist

Box 44.1 Equipment.

Equipment required for safe formula feeding
- Bottles with removable teats and teat covers
- Bottle brush and teat brush
- Sterilising equipment (may be a steam steriliser, microwave or cold-water steriliser)
- Formula milk powder (or cartons of sterile readymade formula milk)

Sterilising feeding equipment
- Wash hands well with hot soapy water
- Wash and rinse bottles and teats. Use hot soapy water and clean bottle/teat brushes
- Rinse clean equipment with cold running water
- Place equipment in the steriliser
- Always follow the manufacturer's instructions for any type of steriliser as there are many different types
- Only remove equipment from the steriliser when you wish to use it
- Clean and disinfect any work surfaces on which you will prepare the bottle
- If a bottle will not be used immediately, ensure that both the teat and teat cover are in place so that the sterility of the teat and inside of the bottle is maintained
- Dishwashers are not safe to use as sterilisers as they do not reach the high temperatures required to sterilise equipment. Bottles, teats and brushes may be cleaned in a dishwasher, but they will not be sterile

Figure 44.2 Responsive feeding.

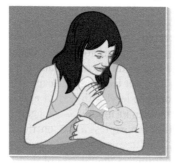

Responsive feeding is an important way to encourage secure attachment in infants. Parents should be encouraged to hold the baby close, sing or talk to their baby, and maintain skin-to-skin cantact whenever possible.

Box 44.2 Top tips.

1. Do not use mineral or other bottled water as this may be harmful to an infant
2. Always add water and formula in the amount recommended by the manufacturer in accordance with the baby's age
3. Never add anything else to a bottle, e.g. rice, rusk, flavoured powders

Key point

Parents who choose to formula feed their babies – either exclusively or alongside breastfeeding – should be given clear, non-judgemental, evidence-based advice about preparation of formula feeds in order to limit the risks to babies.

Midwifery Skills at a Glance, First Edition. Edited by Patricia Lindsay, Carmel Bagness and Ian Peate.
© 2018 John Wiley & Sons, Ltd. Published 2018 by John Wiley & Sons, Ltd.

Breastmilk is the optimum source of nutrition for babies under 1 year and mothers should be supported and encouraged wherever possible to breastfeed or give expressed breastmilk. However, despite relatively high levels of breastfeeding initiation, rates of exclusive breastfeeding in the UK decline significantly from 6 weeks postbirth, with less than 1% of babies exclusively breastfed at 6 months. It is essential that midwives are able to give clear, supportive evidence-based advice to those parents who make the decision to give their baby formula milk.

Constituents of first infant formula milk

Most infant formulas are derived from cows' milk that has been dehydrated and treated to make it suitable for very young infants. This is usually then fortified with a variety of vitamins, minerals and other ingredients in an attempt to mimic the constituents of breastmilk. A small percentage of babies may be allergic to the proteins in cows'-milk formula and may require soya-based milk available on prescription. Some formulas are made with goats' milk but these should not be given to babies with cows'-milk allergy.

Advice for parents regarding types of formula milks

Under the terms of the WHO International Code of Marketing of Breastmilk Substitutes, advertising and promotion of formula milk is strictly controlled.

Parents should be reassured that, except in cases of diagnosed cows'-milk-protein allergy, all first infant formulas will be suitable for babies under 6 months old and there is no evidence to support the suggestion that any one brand is 'better' than another. Furthermore, there is no evidence to suggest that after the age of 6 months babies require those milks marketed as 'follow-on' or 'growing-up' milks. Parents should be advised that there is no need to move on from first infant formulas until the age of 1, when ordinary cows' milk may be introduced.

Sterilisation and preparation of formula milk

Sterilisation of all equipment is essential and parents should be taught how to sterilise bottles and prepare feeds, even when using readymade formula (Figure 44.1; Boxes 44.1 and 44.2). Busy and tired parents may be tempted to make up an entire day's formula feeds at one time, storing them in the fridge to heat up as needed. However, this significantly increases the risk of bacteria breeding in the milk and so they should be advised to make up each individual feed as required.

How to give a formula feed

Babies should be kept sitting as upright as possible for a bottle feed. Their body and head should be in line to enable easy sucking and swallowing, and their head should be well supported. Babies should never be left 'propped up' on a pillow or similar to feed, as this increases the chance of choking. To avoid the baby taking in air whilst feeding, the bottle should always be held at an angle that ensures the teat is full of milk. The baby may not wish to take the same amount of milk each time, or may be slower or faster to feed at different times; this is normal and parents are encouraged to be responsive to their baby's individual needs at every feed. Babies should never be forced to finish a bottle, and leftover milk should be discarded straight after the feed. Formula-fed infants may need breaks during feeds and may require gentle 'winding' during or after the feed.

Baby-led, responsive formula feeding

Evidence is clear that a strong maternal–infant bond in the first days and weeks of life can help to promote secure emotional attachment and brain development in the infant. This evidence has often been based on observations of breastfeeding mothers; however, parents who have chosen to formula feed should also be encouraged to regard feeds as an opportunity to develop this close attachment with their baby and learn to respond to their needs. Skin-to-skin contact whilst bottlefeeding should be promoted as a way to keep babies warm, secure and to help develop a loving connection through the increase in oxytocin levels in both mother and baby (Figure 44.2). Equally, parents should be encouraged to maintain eye contact whilst giving formula, stroking, cuddling and talking to their babies as they feed. The UNICEF Baby Friendly Initiative suggests that parents try to give the majority of feeds themselves in order to increase this connection during these important early months.

Making up a formula feed

- Feeds should be made up as required and not stored.
- Ensure that all equipment is correctly sterilised.
- Wash hands and work surfaces with hot soapy water.
- Boil fresh tap water in a clean kettle and allow to cool slightly (not more than 30 minutes cooling time). Do not use water that has already been boiled.
- Bottled, mineral or artificially softened water should not be used as it may contain levels of minerals that are unsuitable for an infant.
- Always follow the manufacturer's instructions when making up feeds to ensure the correct amount of water and powder for the age of the baby.
- Fill the bottle with the appropriate amount of slightly cooled boiled water.
- Add the required amount of formula as per manufacturer's instructions. Always level off the amount of formula in the powder scoop to avoid overfilling the scoop.
- *Never* add extra formula powder, sugar, cereals etc. to the feed.
- Replace the teat and cover and gently shake the bottle to ensure the powder is fully mixed with the water.
- Do not touch the teat.
- Ensure the feed is at an appropriate temperature. Cool the feed down by running under the cold tap if necessary. Never heat up a feed in a microwave as this can cause 'hot spots', scalding and burns.
- Test the temperature of the feed before giving to the baby. The easiest way is by dropping a little on the inside of the wrist. It should feel warm, not hot or cold.
- Discard any unused milk after feeding.

Service user's view

'I think it's really nice to be able to share that responsibility [bottle feeding] with your partner.'

Earle 2000

45 Other feeding methods

Figure 45.1 Cup feeding.

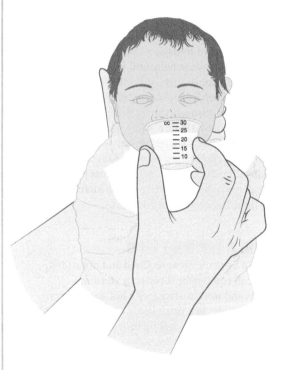

Figure 45.2 Syringe feeding.

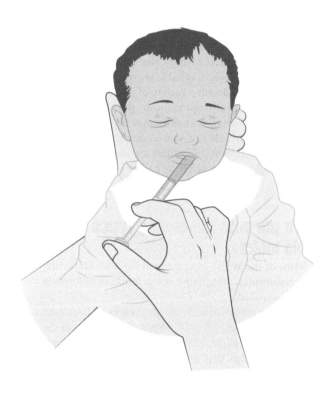

Figure 45.3 Tube feeding.

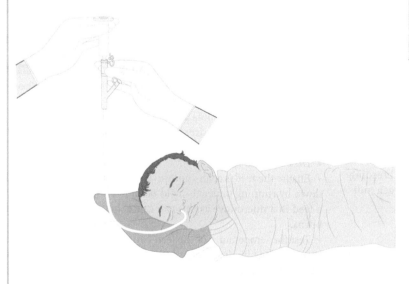

> **Key point**
>
> Infant feeding is an emotional experience for all parents. Midwives should be mindful of the emotional care needs of parents whose babies require support with feeding.

Midwifery Skills at a Glance, First Edition. Edited by Patricia Lindsay, Carmel Bagness and Ian Peate.
© 2018 John Wiley & Sons, Ltd. Published 2018 by John Wiley & Sons, Ltd.

For the newborn baby to survive and thrive it must make a successful transition to enteral feeding after birth. Most babies achieve this smoothly and continue to feed well, either at the breast or from a bottle. However, some need support to maintain adequate nutrition and hydration. These babies may be small and relatively weaker, such as preterm infants, or may have a congenital anomaly that makes feeding more difficult, such as an orofacial cleft. Midwives will need to work with parents to ensure the infant's nutritional needs are supported. The following are common strategies to provide additional milk for the baby and, if the mother is breast feeding, are preferable to using a bottle and teat. Breastfeeding mothers should be encouraged to give expressed breastmilk rather than formula.

Basic principles of cup and syringe feeding

- Use only when clinically indicated.
- Discuss with, obtain the consent of, and involve the parents.
- Wash hands before and after.
- Use sterile, single-use equipment.
- Discard unused milk.
- Document all supplementary feeds.
- Used in addition to, not instead of, breast feeds.
- After feeds remove bib and make baby comfortable.

Cup feeding

Used when additional feeds of 3–5 mL or more are required (Figure 45.1).
- Wrap baby in a blanket and place a bib under the chin.
- Hold baby in an upright position.
- Rest the edge of the cup on the baby's lower lip, tilted to allow milk to touch the lip.
- Allow baby to lap or drink the milk.
- Feed at the baby's pace.
- Do not move the cup until the baby has finished.
- The baby will indicate when it has had enough, usually by turning the head away.

Syringe feeding

Used when additional feeds of 3–5 mL or less are required (Figure 45.2).
- Wrap baby in a blanket and place a bib under the chin.
- Hold baby in an upright position.

- Place the nozzle of the syringe between the gum and the cheek.
- Syringe no more than 0.2 mL of milk into the mouth at a time.
- Allow baby to swallow the milk before delivering another bolus of 0.2 mL.
- Continue until feed has finished or baby rejects more feed.

Tube feeding

Babies who are unable to suck and swallow adequate amounts of milk may need supplementary feeding by nasogastric tube. This is only undertaken by staff who have been trained and demonstrated competence in the procedure. Parents will be trained to insert and feed by tube if the baby is discharged while still being tube fed. The tube must be inserted correctly and the position in the stomach confirmed. The position is confirmed before every feed or medicine is given, after any vomiting episode and at least once every shift. An incorrectly placed tube may lead to inadvertent instillation of milk into the airways, with possibly fatal consequences. Tube size is usually 6FG.

When inserting a nasogastric tube the type and size must be based on individual needs. It is essential that the midwife refer to local evidence-based policy and procedure in order to ensure the safety and comfort of the child. During insertion of the tube there will be a need for two people to pass the tube; one carrying out the procedure and the other supporting the baby and parent(s).

The type of tube passed, size, method used to secure the tube and the tube feeding regimen must be documented.

Feeds may be given as slow boluses from a syringe, with the flow rate controlled by gravity (raising or lowering the syringe; Figure 45.3). The tube is flushed with water before and after every use and should be removed as soon as it is no longer required.

Infants with orofacial clefts

Infants born with an orofacial cleft may need some assistance to feed. Many are able to breastfeed with appropriate assistance in the early days. For those who cannot, or whose mothers do not wish to, special teats are available.

Service user's view
'Feeding him went really well… I was just nervous he was going to choke on it or something.'

Stevens *et al.* 2014

46 Neonatal blood screening ('heel prick')

Figure 46.1 Equipment – lancets.

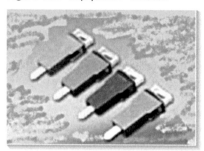

Figure 46.2 Recommended sampling area as indiated by shading.

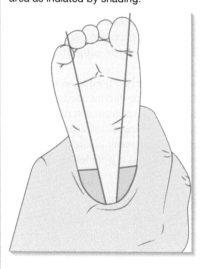

Figure 46.3 Screening card.

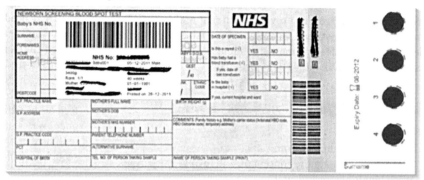

Box 46.1 Top tips for taking a blood spot sample.

- Check that the card has not expired
- Use the baby's NHS number barcoded label, affix this to all pages of the card
- Get parents to check the details and amend as necessary before starting to take the sample
- Cleanse the heel with tepid water, allow to dry
- Hold lancet device firmly against one of the two shaded areas of the heel (as shown)
- Fill each circle with a single drop of blood – check that it has soaked through to the back of the card
- Allow the blood spots to dry before placing in special glassine envelope
- Dispatch the card in the same day (or within 24 hours) using the barcoded prepaid envelope

Key point

The midwife should ensure that parents have the necessary information about the NBS screening and the importance of their babies being screened.

Midwifery Skills at a Glance, First Edition. Edited by Patricia Lindsay, Carmel Bagness and Ian Peate.
© 2018 John Wiley & Sons, Ltd. Published 2018 by John Wiley & Sons, Ltd.

The newborn blood spot (NBS) screening programme is recommended for all babies born in the UK. It should be done between days 5 to 8, but ideally on day 5 (counting day of birth as day 0). This aims to achieve early detection, referral and treatment for babies affected by any of the following conditions to improve their health, and prevent severe disability or even death.

Congenital hypothyroidism

The thyroid gland of the fetus starts functioning at about 20 weeks' gestation to produce thyroxine for general development. About 1 in 3000 babies born in the UK has congenital hypothyroidism (CHT) and lack the hormone thyroxine, which in turn affects their growth and can lead to learning disabilities. However, early detection and treatment with thyroxine allows them to develop normally.

It is important to remember that the routine day 5 test may not identify very preterm babies with this condition. Therefore, all babies born at less than 32 weeks' gestation are recommended to have a preterm repeat test at 28 days of age or on discharge home, whichever is the sooner, to ensure they are appropriately screened.

Sickle cell disease

Sickle cell disease (SCD) affects haemoglobin and the oxygen-carrying capacity of the red blood cells, hence it is also known as sickle cell anaemia. This is a serious inherited blood disorder in which the normal round flexible disc-like cells change to elongated sickle or crescent-moon shapes when deoxygenated and under stress, forming clusters and blockage, resulting in tissue hypoxia, causing pain and severe anaemia. Babies who have SCD will require specialist care throughout their lives. The incidence in the UK is about 1 in 2000 babies.

Cystic fibrosis

Cystic fibrosis (CF) is an inherited condition that affects the digestive system and the lungs. Babies with CF tend to gain weight slowly, are susceptible to chest infection and can become very ill. However, early treatment with a high-energy diet, medication, and physiotherapy can prolong and improve the quality of their lives. The incidence of CF in the UK is about 1 in 2500 babies.

Inherited metabolic diseases: Phenylketonuria

Phenylalanine is an amino acid found in milk and many protein foods. Babies with phenylketonuria (PKU) lack the enzyme phenylalanine hydroxylase (PAH) in their liver to metabolise and convert phenylalanine into tyrosine, which is essential for normal brain development. The incidence of PKU in the UK is 1 in 10 000 babies. However, treatment with special dietary supplement for those affected is very effective, and should commence as soon as diagnosis is confirmed because the brain appears to be most vulnerable during the first 18 months of life.

Medium-chain acyl-coA dehydrogenase deficiency

In MEDIUM-chain acyl-coA dehydrogenase deficiency (MCADD), fat is not being metabolised properly, which can give rise to complications such as seizures, respiratory distress and even coma or sudden death. However, most babies are asymptomatic at birth. Although MCADD is a lifelong condition, again, its management is relatively straightforward with special diet to allow those affected to lead a reasonable healthy, normal life. Incidence in the UK is around 1 in 10 000 babies.

Four other genetic and metabolic anomalies (maple syrup urine disease (MSUD), isovaleric acidaemia (IVA), glutaric aciduria type 1 (GA1) and homocystinuria (pyridoxine unresponsive) (HCU)) are also being tested for since 2015.

Communication and documentation

Before the test, the midwife must ensure that parents have the necessary information about the NBS screening and the importance of their babies being screened. They should be given time to consider their options beforehand, preferably with access to written information. Fully informed parental consent is required prior to the test. Although written consent is not necessary, parental consent must be recorded in both the maternity/neonatal notes and the NBS screening section of the personal child health record (PCHR).

Parents can opt out of having their babies screened for all or any of these conditions. However, they can only opt out of inherited metabolic diseases as a group and not by each condition. If a parent declines screening, this must be recorded in the maternity/neonatal notes and PCHR for each condition declined. The sample card should be marked showing each condition declined, and be sent to the NBS screening centre to communicate this.

Parents should be made aware that all normal results will be available on the child health database for their GP and health visitor to access by baby's 6-week check-up, unless otherwise notified of any issues before then. As this is a screening test, they should also be made aware of the likelihood of false-positive results, which may necessitate further tests.

Taking the NBS sample

The NBS sample is usually obtained by the midwife. It involves pricking the baby's heel (Figures 46.1 and 46.2) and collecting four drops of blood (five drops in Scotland) onto a specially designed blood spot screening card (Figure 46.3). The midwife should explain the test procedure and ensure informed parental consent is obtained.

The NBS sample card should be checked for damage and expiry date. The required details on the card should be completed before the blood spots are collected. Mother should be encouraged to hold baby (put to breast if breastfeeding) to provide baby comfort. The midwife should wash her hands, put on gloves and cleanse the baby's heel with tepid water (do not use alcohol) and allow to dry. Hold lancet device firmly against baby's heel for the puncture (Figure 46.1), and lower baby's foot to improve blood flow. Do not squeeze the baby's foot or allow the heel to touch the card. Fill each circle with a single drop of blood to soak through to the back of the card. Allow the blood to dry before placing the sample card into the glassine envelope provided and dispatch the sample on the same day (or within 24 hours). Always ensure the sample is taken correctly to avoid unnecessary repeat (Box 46.1).

Place a spot plaster on baby's heel after the test and advise parents regarding care of the puncture site and report any adverse effect such as bruising around the area.

47 Maternal venepuncture, including glucose tolerance testing

Box 47.1 Required equipment.

- Locally used vacuumed system with 21g needle
- Required specimen bottles
- Approved skin decontaminant
- Non-sterile gloves
- Apron
- Antiseptic handrub
- Sterile gauze
- Disposable tourniquet – if available/best practice
- Adhesive plaster (consider allergy)
- Specimen request form
- Portable sharps box

Figure 47.2 Inserting the needle bevel edge uppermost at a 10–30 degree angle.

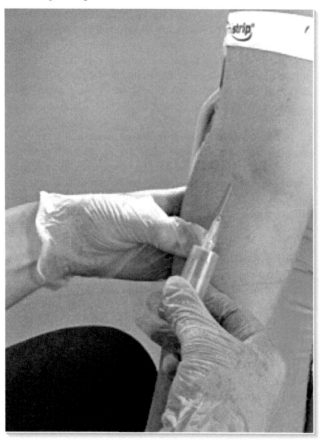

Figure 47.1 Accessory cephalic, median cubital and basilic veins.

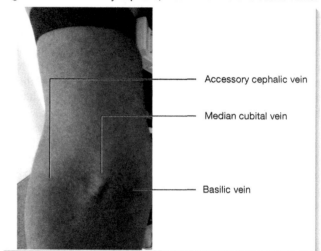

Accessory cephalic vein

Median cubital vein

Basilic vein

Box 47.2 Order of the draw. Source: Brooks (2014).

1. Sterile tubes e.g. blood culture
2. Coagulation tubes
3. Serum tubes
4. EDTA (ethylenediaminetetraacetic acid)
5. Glycolytic inhibitor
Specimen bottles inverted after filling for required amount of time

Box 47.3 Correct labelling of specimens.

Four points of identity on every sample as required by local policy
- First name
- Surname
- Date of birth
- Unique number (Hospital or NHS number)

Key point

Venepuncture should be carried out safely with competence, confidence and consideration of the woman at all times.

Venepuncture is the entering of a needle into a vein in order to obtain a specimen of blood. Venepuncture can also be used for the administration of a drug intravenously in an emergency situation. The physiological changes during pregnancy, for example increased blood supply and generalised warmth of the woman, promote vasodilatation and thus the veins are more visible. Therefore venepuncture performed on a pregnant woman is considered to be easier than at other times.

Indications for venepuncture

- Antenatal 'booking' bloods
- Assessment of full blood count and rhesus antibodies
- Fetal antenatal screening tests
- Ongoing monitoring of existing medical conditions, e.g. haemoglobinopathies, epilepsy, diabetes, pre-eclampsia
- Cross matching or 'group and save'.
  This list is not exhaustive.

Midwifery Skills at a Glance, First Edition. Edited by Patricia Lindsay, Carmel Bagness and Ian Peate.
© 2018 John Wiley & Sons, Ltd. Published 2018 by John Wiley & Sons, Ltd.

Midwives' role and responsibility

It is the midwife's role to provide comfort, privacy, dignity and respect at all times. This will help to ensure that the woman is able to give informed consent. Some women present with a phobia of needles that causes them great anxiety. The midwife should take time and provide support to improve the whole experience; this includes the use of coping strategies and 'pain relieving cream'. The woman's medical history should be considered as the cream can interact with some medications. Also, there is a time factor to consider as 1–5 hours are needed for the cream to work effectively.

Choosing the site and vein

The site normally used is in the antecubital fossa. Preference as to which arm needs to be discussed with the woman. The veins here are easily accessible and are the accessory cephalic, median cubital and basilic veins (Figure 47.1). Once a tourniquet is in place, assessment of the suitability of the vein can be made, considering size and mobility. Palpation will allow this assessment, ensuring that the vein is 'full and bouncy' with the consideration of valves (feels like a small nodule), arteries (pulse felt) and nerves. Although hitting a nerve is very rare, a knowledge of the position of the median and ulna nerves, plus ensuring the angle of needle insertion is within 10–30 degrees, will reduce the risk of occurrence.

Assessment of the condition of the skin should be made. There should be no bruising, scarring, infection or inflammation present. If present, another site must be found.

Procedure

- Wash your hands with soap and water and put on non-sterile gloves and apron to reduce the risk of healthcare-acquired infection.
- Clean a plastic receiver using locally approved wipes. Leave to dry. Take off gloves and then wash and dry hands thoroughly.
- Gather equipment (Box 47.1), ensuring it is in date and the packaging is intact.
- It is important to discuss the procedure with the woman and gain informed consent.
- Ensure that this is the correct woman for venepuncture by checking details and required samples on the blood form verbally with the woman and/or if relevant by patient ID band.
- Ensure the woman is in a comfortable and accessible position, with a good light source.
- Position the tourniquet approximately 5–7 cm above the antecubital fossa.
- Assess and palpate the vein for quality and accessibility for venepuncture. The woman may be asked to make a fist a couple of times to make the vein 'full and bouncy' and therefore more easily visible.
- Remember the site of entry and release tourniquet.
- Decontaminate your hands and put on non-sterile gloves.
- As micro-organisms can enter the body or circulatory system at the skin site, cleanse the skin with approved decontaminant for 30 seconds and allow to dry for 30 seconds.
- Assemble required equipment and reapply tourniquet.
- Do not repalpate the vein as this will contaminate the skin.

- With the aim of anchoring the vein, use your non-dominant hand to apply slight tension to the skin just below the entry site.
- With your dominant hand, insert the needle with the bevel edge uppermost at a 10–30 degree angle (Figure 47.2).
- Attach the specimen bottles with your non-dominant hand considering the 'order of the draw' (Box 47.2) to reduce the risk of cross-contamination of additives.
- Bottles are self-filling but if blood does not appear then gently 'adjust' the position of the needle. Consider the potential for causing bruising.
- When the required samples have been obtained, release the tourniquet and remove the needle and syringe. Dispose of these directly into the sharps box.
- Immediately apply pressure (or ask the woman to do this) with gauze or cotton wool ball to the puncture site. With her arm horizontal, retain the pressure for at least 1 minute.
- If no allergies identified, apply a plaster dressing when bleeding has subsided.
- Take off gloves and wash and dry your hands.
- Label the blood bottles and complete the request form (Box 47.3) while the woman is still present.
- Dispose of equipment correctly and reclean the receiver.
- Document and act on results as they become available.

Glucose tolerance test

Glycosuria of >2+ (= 30 mmol/L) on one occasion and >1+ (= 15 mmol/L) on two occasions warrants further investigation for possible onset of gestational diabetes. Women who have presented with risk factors and/or previous gestational diabetes require a 2-hour 75 mg oral glucose tolerance test (OGTT). Those with previous gestational diabetes are tested twice: once at booking and then 24–28 weeks' gestation. Those with risk factors are tested at 24–28 weeks' gestation (NICE 2015).

Preparation for an OGTT is:
- The woman must not eat for 8–12 hours before the OGTT; she is permitted to drink water only.
- Local policy and procedure must be followed.
- Consider omission of certain medications as these can affect the overall test result – discuss this with the multidisciplinary team.

At the time of the test, a fasting blood sugar is taken. Then 75 mg of glucose is drunk by the woman. Blood is taken at hourly intervals up to 2 hours or just one sample is taken at 2 hours (RCOG 2013).

A diagnosis of gestational diabetes is made if a woman presents with:
- A fasting plasma glucose level of 5.6 mmol/L or above; or
- A 2-hour plasma glucose level of 7.8 mmol/L or above.

If the test results indicate a diagnosis of gestational diabetes, the woman should be offered a joint diabetic and antenatal review within 1 week (NICE 2015).

Service user's view

'My blood was taken by a student midwife. She was excellent. I didn't let on I was a nurse and knew what to expect.'

Verbal communication, service user, Essex

48 Cord blood and neonatal capillary blood sampling

Box 48.1 Indication for obtaining cord blood sample.
Source: NICE (2014).

- Emergency caesarean section
- Forceps delivery
- Fetal blood sampling in labour
- Baby born in poor condition on the basis of abnormal heart rate, breathing or tone
- Babies of mothers who are rhesus negative or have unusual antibodies
- Cord blood bank collection

Figure 48.1 Technique for obtaining cord blood.

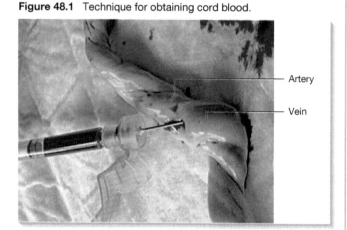

Artery

Vein

Figure 48.2 Labelling of samples.

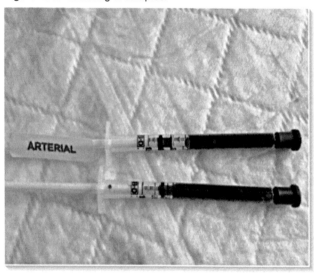

ARTERIAL

Figure 48.3 Equipment.

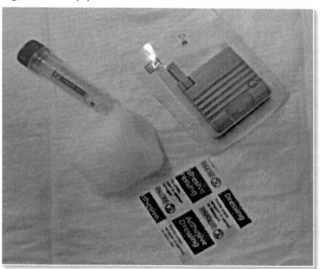

Figure 48.4 Recommended site for heel puncture.

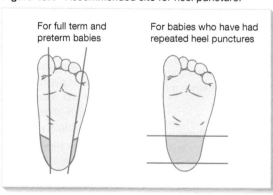

For full term and preterm babies

For babies who have had repeated heel punctures

Key point

Cord blood is rich in stem cells. The NHS national blood transfusion service collects, stores and supplies cord blood from voluntary contributions.

Midwifery Skills at a Glance, First Edition. Edited by Patricia Lindsay, Carmel Bagness and Ian Peate.
© 2018 John Wiley & Sons, Ltd. Published 2018 by John Wiley & Sons, Ltd.

Cord blood is a sample of blood taken at birth from a baby's umbilical cord. It is not a requirement to obtain cord blood routinely (NICE 2014) (Box 48.1). The umbilical cord consists of three closely adjacent blood vessels; two arteries, which carry deoxygenated blood from the fetus, and one vein, which carries oxygenated blood to the fetus (Figure 48.1). The single vein is usually the largest structure and hence easier to obtain a sample from. If only one sample is required then either the vein or artery may be used. Umbilical cord gas analysis will, however, require a sample from both the vein and artery.

Obtaining cord bloods for blood gas analysis

- Do not clamp the cord earlier than 1 minute following the birth unless there is concern about the baby's condition (NICE 2014). Samples need to be collected within 60 minutes of birth, having noted the time of cord clamping to ensure correct interpretation of results.
- Equipment: apron, sterile gloves, two heparinised syringes with needle, sharps box, labels to identify the sample to the baby and as arterial or venous.
- Wash hands. Don gloves, apron and eye protection. Refer to local infection control policies for further advice, particularly relating to maternal blood-born viruses.
- Double clamp the umbilical cord 10 cm apart. Clamp as close to the fetal end as possible to facilitate access to remaining cord in the event of repeat sampling.
- Identify an artery and vein within the umbilical cord.
- Insert the needle into the appropriate vessel at a 45 degree angle and withdraw the blood. Ensure the needle is well placed into the centre of the vessel to avoid contamination of blood with air (Figure 48.1). If air bubbles are seen in the sample, safely discard and repeat with a new syringe and needle.
- Withdraw the needle from the cord. Safely remove needle from syringe and discard in compliance with local policy.
- Place the bung on the end of the syringe. Gently agitate the syringe by rolling between thumb and forefinger to ensure that heparin is dispersed appropriately to prevent clotting of the sample. Label syringes (Figure 48.2).
- When samples are taken for umbilical cord gas the analysis should be performed within 30 minutes, as samples will deteriorate after this time.
- Inform doctors of the blood gas results and document findings appropriately.
- Discuss the findings with the parents.

Cord blood is rich in stem cells. The NHS national blood transfusion service collects, stores and supplies cord blood from voluntary contributions. Cord blood collected is then used to treat patients suffering from life-threatening diseases. Currently, some hospitals within the greater London area have subscribed to this service. For more information visit NHS Blood Transfusion at: http://www.nhsbt.nhs.uk/cordblood/about/

Neonatal capillary blood sampling

A heel puncture is a simple and convenient method of obtaining a blood sample from a baby. This technique is usually performed for tests including blood sugar monitoring, bilirubin levels, full blood count analysis and newborn blood spot screening. In the event that a capillary sample is required for newborn blood spot screening, it is essential that midwives adhere to current national guidance such as NHS newborn blood spot screening programme (Public Health England 2016). This will ensure that parents are provided with evidence-based information to enable them to give the required fully informed verbal consent. Puncturing the skin on the baby's heel is associated with increased pain. Mothers should therefore be encouraged to be involved in the procedure by providing skin-to-skin contact, breastfeeding or use of a pacifier as this is known to minimise discomfort, and make the baby feel secure (Uga *et al.* 2008). Health professionals need to recognise the real anxiety and stress that parents may experience before and during blood sampling from their baby.

Taking capillary sample

Procedure adapted from Public Health England (2016):
- Equipment – see Figure 48.3.
- Examine the baby's heel to identify an appropriate puncture site. Ensure that baby and mother (if she is present) are in a comfortable and secure position.
- Clean the heel with cotton wool/gauze soaked in tepid tap water. It is not necessary to warm the baby's foot first but it is useful to dress the baby warmly to facilitate a good blood flow.
- Wash hands and apply gloves.
- Hold the foot gently yet securely and puncture the heel using an automated device no deeper than 2 mm for a term baby. Use either the external or internal limits of the calcaneus (Figure 48.4). If repeated sampling is required then use an automated incision device of no more than 1 mm depth within the plantar area of the foot to reduce risk of trauma and infection.
- Allow the foot to hang to encourage blood to flow. Do not squeeze the foot.
- Collect the blood required into the capillary tube/blood bottle/screening card.
- When the sample is complete, wipe away excess blood with gauze/cotton wool and apply gentle pressure.
- Apply a hypoallergenic plaster if required and remind parents to remove 2 hours following the procedure.
- Remove gloves, wash hands and dispose of equipment according to local policy.
- Label samples immediately before leaving the bedside/cot-side/bedroom.
- Document the procedure according to local policy. Depending on rationale for sampling, inform doctors of result and discuss implications of findings with parents.

Service user's view

'It's hard being a parent having a little baby having blood taken. Trying to hold him still and keep him occupied was one of my fears… it was over before I even realised they had started… the thought about them hurting my baby was in my head but the relief that he wasn't traumatised and he was back to his smiley self made me feel at ease.'

Verbal communication, service user, Cambridge

49 # Venous cannulation of the woman

Figure 49.1 Key parts.

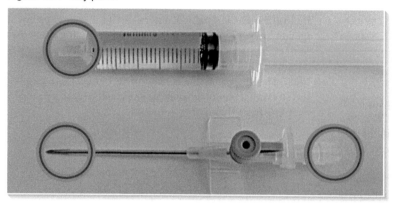

Figure 49.3 Equipment.

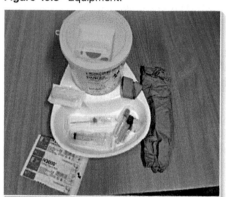

Figure 49.2 Suitable veins.

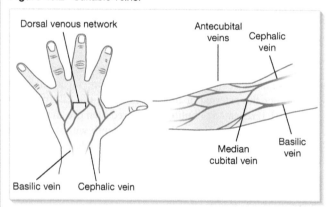

Dorsal venous network

Antecubital veins

Cephalic vein

Basilic vein

Median cubital vein

Basilic vein

Cephalic vein

Figure 49.4 Inserting the cannula.
Source: Reproduced with permission of Jamie Lindsay.

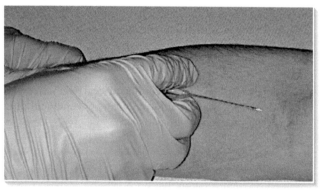

Key point

Any staff member attempting venous cannulation must have been assessed as competent to do so.

Table 49.1 VIP score.
Source: Weston D, Burgess A and Roberts S (2017). *Infection Prevention and Control At a Glance*. Reproduced with permission of John Wiley & Sons.

Appearance	Score	Stage
IV site appears healthy	0	No signs of phlebitis Action: OBSERVE CANNULA
One of the following signs is evident: • Slight pain near IV site or • Slight redness near IV site	1	Possibly first signs of phlebitis Action: OBSERVE CANNULA
Two of the following signs are evident: • Pain at IV site • Erythema/redness • Swelling	2	Early state of phlebitis Action: RESITE CANNULA
All of the following signs are evident: • Pain along path of cannula • Erythema/redness around site • Swelling	3	Medium state of phlebitis Action: RESITE CANNULA AND CONSIDER TREATMENT
All of the following signs are evident and extensive: • Pain along path of cannula • Erythema/redness around site • Swelling • Palpable venous cord	4	Advanced stage of phlebitis or start of thrombophlebitis Action: RESITE CANNULA AND CONSIDER TREATMENT
All of the following signs are evident and extensive: • Pain along path of cannula • Erythema/redness around site • Swelling • Palpable venous cord • Pyrexia	5	Advanced stage thrombophlebitis Action: INITIATE TREATMENT/RESITE CANNULA

Midwifery Skills at a Glance, First Edition. Edited by Patricia Lindsay, Carmel Bagness and Ian Peate.
© 2018 John Wiley & Sons, Ltd. Published 2018 by John Wiley & Sons, Ltd.

Venous cannulation (the introduction of a cannula into a vein) is one of the commonest procedures of inpatient care. Indications are:

- Administration of fluids
- Drug administration
- Administration of blood or blood products
- Prior to epidural analgesia
- In preparation for potential complications of complex situations such as multiple births
- Administration of drugs and fluids in an emergency.

Venous cannulation requires standard aseptic non-touch technique (ANTT) – key parts must not be touched (Figure 49.1).

Choice of cannula site is important. The veins of the forearm or hand of the non-dominant side should be considered first. Avoid:

- Any site with signs of infection, inflammation, bruising or scarring
- Impalpable veins
- Veins over points of flexion or bony prominences
- Veins close to an artery
- Veins that look or feel thrombosed
- Nerves in the lower arm.

The vein chosen should be long, straight and feel firm, rounded and slightly 'bouncy' to palpate. Commonly used veins are those in the dorsal venous network in the back of the hand and the cephalic, basilic and median cubital veins in the forearm (Figure 49.2). The size of the cannula should be sufficient to allow rapid administration of fluids, including blood, in an emergency. In maternity care this is usually 16 gauge (grey).

Prior to cannulating the woman:

- Identify the patient
- Explain and gain consent
- Check if allergic to any dressings/tapes used
- Wash the skin if visibly dirty
- Position the woman comfortably, with arm supported, and ensure privacy
- Wash hands, apply tourniquet and locate a suitable vein
- Loosen tourniquet; cleanse hands
- Assemble equipment
- Topical anaesthetic may be offered.

Equipment

See Figure 49.3.
Clean clinical procedure tray
Non-sterile gloves
Single use tourniquet
Skin cleansing agent (2% chlorhexidine gluconate in 70% isopropyl alcohol)
Ported cannula (correct size, 'safe' cannula if available)
Needle-free extension set (if used)
Sterile transparent cannula dressing
Blood tubes if required
Syringe and 0.9% saline for flush
Sharps container
Alcohol hand rub (if local policy requires)
Patient's notes including Visual Infusion Phlebitis Score (VIPS) chart.

Procedure

See Figure 49.4.
- Wash and dry hands; clean the clinical procedure tray.
- Collect equipment.
- Clean hands and apply non-sterile gloves.
- Assemble equipment, draw up flush solution and flush extension set if used.
- Clean the site for 30 seconds using locally approved disinfectant and allow to dry.

- Reapply tourniquet – do not repalpate vein.
- Using your non-dominant hand, anchor vein below the puncture site.
- Using ANTT, insert cannula at an angle of 15–30°, depending on depth of vein, bevel up – warn the patient just before insertion ('sharp scratch').
- Advance cannula until loss of resistance is felt and blood is seen in the flashback chamber.
- Lower the angle and advance plastic cannula slightly, while withdrawing needle, watching for second flashback in the cannula.
- *Never* reinsert the needle.
- Apply gentle pressure over insertion site, release tourniquet and remove needle completely, disposing of it in sharps' container.
- Take blood samples if required.
- Flush cannula and attach needle-free bung.
- Apply dressing according to local policy.
- Make patient comfortable, dispose of equipment and wash your hands.
- Document date and time of insertion, cannula site, gauge, batch number, name of person inserting, reason for insertion, number of attempts.
- Date the dressing.
- Observe for adverse reactions.
- Make two attempts to cannulate only.

Ongoing care

- Wash your hands before and after touching cannula site.
- Clean port and allow to dry for 30 seconds before administering drugs or fluids.
- Observe cannula site for signs of infection at least daily.
- Record VIP score at least daily (Table 49.1).
- Replace cannula after 72–96 hours.
- Observe dressing daily and replace after 7 days or if loose or contaminated.
- Remove when no longer required and before discharge.

Removal

- Confirm patient identity, explain procedure and gain consent.
- Assemble equipment: clean clinical procedure tray, non-sterile gloves, gauze or other dressing, tape, sharps container, patient's notes.
- Wash your hands before, don gloves.
- Check cannula site.
- Peel the dressing towards insertion site until completely loose.
- Withdraw cannula while simultaneously applying pressure with gauze dressing over the insertion site.
- Maintain pressure on puncture site until bleeding stops.
- Dispose of cannula in sharps container at once.
- Apply dressing.
- Remove gloves and wash hands.
- Document date of removal, reason for removal and name of person removing.
- Record VIP score at removal.

Potential complications

- Fainting
- Pain
- Haematoma formation
- Phlebitis
- Cellulitis/infection.

50 Urinalysis

Figure 50.1 Examples of sampling hubs from indwelling urinary catheters.

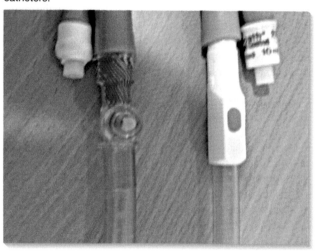

Box 50.1 Taking a mid-stream urine specimen (MSU).

- The woman may clean her labia of any excess vaginal secretions with water. This stage is debatable, as some studies have not demonstrated any benefit
- While holding the labia apart, she will then void the first part of the urine stream into the toilet, then catch the middle part in a (sterile) wide-mouthed container, finishing in the toilet.
- Consideration needs to be made of the contortions necessary to undertake this when heavily pregnant. Providing a sterile jug, the contents of which can then be transferred into a universal container, may be cost effective if it allows accurate diagnosis.

Box 50.2 Characteristics of urine.

Colour: straw-coloured.
Clarity: clear (if cloudy or containing debris may indicate infection or other disease)
Blood: considered an abnormal finding although often simply caused by contamination especially from a sample taken during early labour or postnatally. In a non-contaminated sample blood in the urine may indicate infection, renal system trauma or renal disease
Leucocytes (white blood cells): a high leucocyte presence is usually suggestive of infection.
Nitrates: present in some bacterial infections.
pH: reflects acid-base balance of the body. A normal reading is 5-6, above 7 may indicate infection.
Specific gravity: normal 1.010 (dilute) to 1.025 (concentrated). High concentrations can indicate dehydration, a common problem especially around labour and the early postnatal period.

Box 50.3 Infections.

Any urinary tract symptoms (frequency, pain on micturition, loin pain, malodourous smell, abnormal colour of urine) or vaginal infection symptoms (discharge, itching, suprapubic/loin pain) will prompt collection of a urine specimen to send to the laboratory to confirm/aid diagnosis.

Asymptomatic bacteriuria is routinely screened for in pregnancy (or as part of a septic screen) as it may lead to pyelonephritis, which is frequently associated with premature labour.

Chlamydia is usually asymptomatic, and may be diagnosed by urine screening or vaginal swab.

Group B streptococcus (GBS) can be found in urine, which is treated but is also commonly the beginning of a GBS pathway of intervention to prevent transmission to the baby at birth.

Box 50.4 Assessment for pre-eclampsia.

It is suggested that if significant (1+) protein is detected on dipstick, further investigations to quantify protein when pre-eclampsia is suspected are carried out. A 24-hour urine collection remains the gold standard for protein assessment (≥ 300 mg/24 hours is considered abnormal), however there are many errors possible in undertaking this collection, and the time until a result is available may be problematic. To carry out this test, the bladder should be emptied and time noted (start time), all urine collected in the next 24 hours and a 15-minute warning to pass the last specimen carried out. Other timed collections are possible (2-hour collection, 12-hour collection) but these are not common. More usually undertaken in current practice is a protein-creatinine ratio (PCR): a laboratory test on urine which can identify significant proteinuria (≥ 30mg/mmol). It is important to note that proteinuria may sometimes be the first (and only) sign before severe disease takes over.

Box 50.5 Depending on testing required, urine can be collected from a baby by:

- placing a cotton ball by the urethra and after micturition, squeezing the urine into a container for dipstick
- applying a special 'urine collection bag' – usually a small plastic bag with adhesive edges which can be applied around the urethral area
- supra-pubic puncture – undertaken by a neonatologist and not usually done in a ward environment

Key point

As with all actions undertaken by the midwife, the effectiveness of urinalysis is directly related to the skill of the practitioner, underpinned by knowledge and record keeping.

Midwifery Skills at a Glance, First Edition. Edited by Patricia Lindsay, Carmel Bagness and Ian Peate.
© 2018 John Wiley & Sons, Ltd. Published 2018 by John Wiley & Sons, Ltd.

Urinalysis, testing of urine, is an assessment of wellbeing. When abnormalities are detected, the midwife may need to refer these to medical personnel, as well as undertake vital signs monitoring and/or blood tests to aid diagnosis.

Urine can be screened for many reasons, either routinely or selectively, during pregnancy, labour and the puerperium. Although it is a common test, it is still important to ensure the woman's permission for this procedure.

A specimen of urine should be free of contamination and consequently a midstream specimen is recommended (Box 50.1). When assessing urine, sight and smell is important. Visually it may be cloudy due to pyuria and bacteria, and it may contain visually apparent blood. The colour may be influenced by foods or medications ingested, or dark urine may indicate dehydration. The urine is also frequently malodourous when infection is present.

Dipsticks are the most usual way urinalysis is carried out. The dipstick should be dipped in the urine. After waiting the appropriate amount of time for each component, the dipstick is cross-referenced against the manufacturer's chart (usually on the container) for each individual colour change, which will then give a result. Familiarity with specific manufacturer's instructions should be ensured before undertaking the test. Because visual dipsticks are associated with a high level of false-positive results, automated readers are increasingly being introduced. Care of dipsticks will optimise their effectiveness – for example dating bottles when opened, replacing the cap and storing within temperatures advised by the manufacturers.

All testing should be done on fresh urine in a clean container – urine constituents change as it ages, and contamination can alter results. Also, bacteria can multiply at room temperature, which will compromise results. All specimens for laboratory analysis should be collected in a sterile container and sent immediately (and ideally examined within 2 hours) or placed in a medical specimen fridge.

If testing a specimen from an indwelling urinary catheter, urine should be obtained via the sampling port. These will differ between manufacturers (Figure 50.1). The sampling port should be cleaned with an alcohol pad for 10–30 seconds and allowed to dry. Using a sterile syringe and avoiding contamination, the tip of the syringe (or sterile needle attached to a syringe) is inserted into the sampling port at a 90 degree angle, aspirated and the contents transferred to a prelabelled sterile container. The port needs to then be cleaned again. If the woman is on strict fluid balance monitoring, it should be ensured that the amount of urine removed is charted appropriately.

Documentation should include the time, date, appearance, odour, colour, results and the legible signature of the midwife. All relevant information should be included on accompanying requests, including any current antibiotic treatment, when sending samples to laboratories, whilst ensuring that the laboratory request is accurately labelled as a 'CSU' (catheter specimen of urine) rather than the more normal 'MSU' (midstream specimen of urine).

Routine testing is undertaken regularly during the antenatal period for various infections (Boxes 50.2 and 50.3) and pre-eclampsia (PET) (Box 50.4); urine is also frequently tested during labour and the postnatal period for these reasons. Tests on the urine can also be carried out for individual concerns, as a result of a medical condition or to screen for drugs.

A dipstick examination will demonstrate varying levels of protein, and perhaps blood, as well as possibly neutrophils and leucocytes in the presence of infection. The gold standard test for both symptomatic and asymptomatic bacteriuria is laboratory urine microscopy, culture and sensitivity (M, C & S).

Proteinuria is often found when there is a urinary tract infection or renal system disease. In pregnancy it can be a sign of pre-eclampsia (often preceding other signs).

Physiological changes to how glucose is utilised in pregnancy means that **glycosuria** can be normal, particularly in late pregnancy. NICE (2008) diabetes guidelines recommend that 2+ or above on one occasion or 1+ on two occasions is an indication for further investigation to assess for gestational diabetes.

Ketones result from the breakdown of stored fat and can occur physiologically in small, transient amounts in normal pregnancy and labour. When detected in the urine the midwife should assess the woman's hydration and nutrition. However, **ketonuria** in diabetic women can be an indication of ketoacidosis. The smell of ketones is typically described as 'pear drop', 'nail polish remover' or sweet, and this smell on a woman's breath should alert the midwife to the possibility of ketoacidosis, which is a serious complication.

Neonatal urine screening can be undertaken for many reasons, the most common being as part of a sepsis screen or as an indication of underlying renal conditions. See Box 50.5 for collection methods.

51 Specimen collection – stool specimen

Figure 51.1 Faeces pot and integral spatula.

Figure 51.2 Collection of faeces specimen from bedpan.

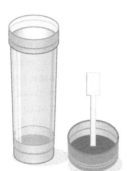

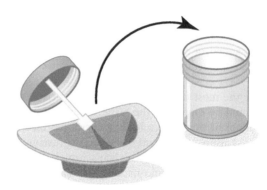

Figure 51.3 Example of a stool chart, based on the Bristol Stool chart Types 6 and 7 suggest diarrhoea with type 5 indicative of 'loose stool'.

Bristol stool chart		
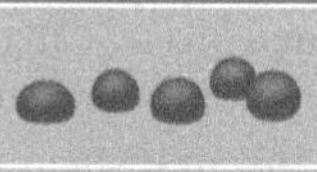	**Type 1**	Separate hard lumps, like nuts (hard to pass)
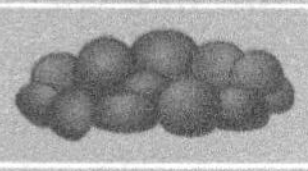	**Type 2**	Sausage-shaped, but lumpy
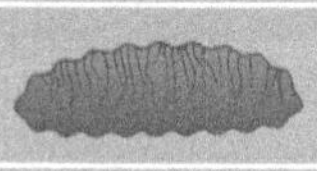	**Type 3**	Sausage-shaped, but with cracks on surface
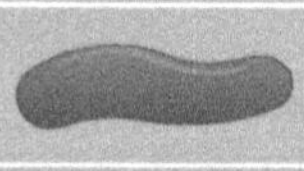	**Type 4**	Sausage or snake like, smooth and soft
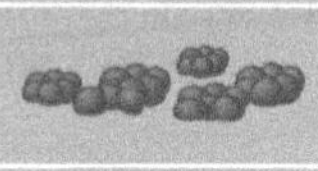	**Type 5**	soft blobs with clear-cut edges (easy to pass)
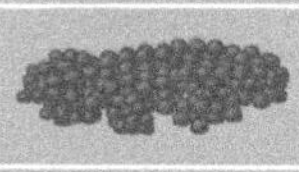	**Type 6**	Fluffy pieces with ragged edges, mushy
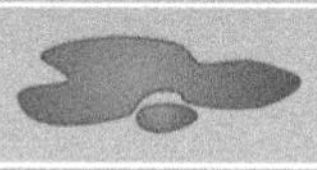	**Type 7**	Watery, no solid pieces (entirely liquid)

Box 51.1 Equipment required for specimen collection.

The following are required for collection of all specimens
- Accurate completion of laboratory request forms including all current treatment such as antibiotic therapy
- Positive identification of the woman/baby
- Use of Personal Protection Equipment (PPE) such as gloves and aprons (masks may be required for sputum inducing procedures in high risk women) for the collection or handling of specimens if contact with blood/body fluids is anticipated
- Hand hygiene before contact with the woman/baby
- Hand hygiene following removal of gloves on completion of specimen collection
- Hand hygiene after contact with the woman/baby
- Disposal of waste or sharps in line with waste risk assessment

Key point

The importance of engaging and supporting the woman to understand the importance of collecting specimens in the correct manner cannot be underestimated as specimen quality directly affects the results and subsequent decisions and actions taken.

Midwifery Skills at a Glance, First Edition. Edited by Patricia Lindsay, Carmel Bagness and Ian Peate.
© 2018 John Wiley & Sons, Ltd. Published 2018 by John Wiley & Sons, Ltd.

specimens are taken to support decision making with regard to treatment; in maternity care common specimens include blood, urine, faeces, sputum and wound, umbilical or 'screening' swabs.

The quality of the specimen collected has a direct impact on the accuracy of laboratory results. This can impact on treatment decisions; therefore it is important that the midwife:

- Is assured that there is a definite clinical need for the specimen.
- Gains consent to take the specimen and explains why the specimen is being taken, and the possible consequences/ treatment.
- Collects the specimen at the appropriate time (some specimens are time dependent).
- Advises the woman on how to collect the specimen.
- Collects the specimen in a way that avoids contamination – see Chapter 5 (aseptic technique).
- Arranges transportation to the laboratory in a timely way or stores appropriately if necessary.
- Checks and acts on all results once they are available.
- Documents results of all specimens.

Collecting a faeces specimen from an adult

Specimens are usually requested due to the presence of diarrhoea or suspicion of a gastrointestinal infection such as *Clostridium difficile*, *Salmonella*, *Campylobacter* or the presence of parasites. The specimen may be collected by a midwife or the woman if appropriate (Figures 51.1 and 51.2). See Box 51.1 for the equipment required for specimen collection.

If a specimen is requested due to the reporting or confirmation of diarrhoea then a stool chart should be instigated to capture the frequency and type of stool being passed. Each organisation has its own documentation; however, most stool charts are based on the Bristol Stool Chart (Figure 51.3).

Some women may find the procedure embarrassing. Use language that is appropriate to suit the woman's understanding.

Collection in a healthcare setting

- Be familiar with and adhere to local policy and procedure.
- Positively identify the woman.
- Explain the procedure.
- Ensure privacy and promote dignity.
- Provide the woman with either a commode and bedpan, or a foil tray to collect the faeces if a toilet is used.
- Encourage the woman to urinate first; however, a small amount of urine in the pan should not affect processing of the sample.
- Ask the woman to inform you once they have opened their bowels.
- Record on a stool chart if used.
- Put on gloves and undo the screw top on the faeces specimen container (Figures 51.1 and 51.2).
- Taking care not to contaminate the outside of the container, using the spatula provided in the pot place a small amount of faeces into the pot and tighten the lid. Do not attempt to fill the pot – a small amount only is required, for example a quarter of the pot.
- Discard gloves and perform hand hygiene.
- Ensure the woman is comfortable.

- Complete the identification details on the pot and laboratory form.
- Place the specimen in the dedicated collection point – inform the laboratory if notice is required.
- Document in the notes.

Collection in the home setting

- Positively identify the woman.
- Explain the procedure and provide any information available.
- Provide the faeces sample pot (the woman may require the laboratory request form and bag).
- The following may be used to collect the sample:
  - a commode or bedpan (if used)
  - a disposable plastic or foil container, e.g. take away container placed in a toilet (this does not have to be sterile just clean).
- Demonstrate to the woman how to transfer a small amount of the stool into the container (as above) and to perform hand hygiene afterwards.
- Place any remaining stool in the toilet and flush.
- Place the container used to collect the sample in a plastic bag, seal and place in household waste.
- Inform the woman about where to take the specimen and timescales required for this (some samples require rapid transfer to the laboratory to prevent degradation of pathogens, e.g. amoebic dysentery).

Storing a stool sample

After the faeces sample is collected it needs to be transported to the microbiology laboratory for processing. In the hospital environment each clinical area usually has a sample collection point where specimens can be left for collection. In community settings such as the home the woman will need to take the specimen to either the laboratory reception (usually at the local hospital) or GP reception. Where to take the specimen should be explained at the time of requesting the specimen in line with local procedures.

Collecting a faeces specimen from a neonate

Stool specimens can be requested from neonates. Indications for the need to collect a specimen include investigating for the presence of blood or infection.

The same principles apply as with adults; however, neonatal stool specimens are frequently collected from nappies. Always check local policies as, for example, some organisations advise the use of a non-absorbent liner to avoid liquid stools soaking into the nappy. Semiformed stools can be transferred from the nappy to the specimen pot using the integral spatula.

Service user's view

'But I didn't know what to do. I thought "how do you, how do you catch it here," I thought, "without it ending up in the water?"'

Lecky *et al.* 2014

52 Taking a wound swab

Figure 52.1 Example of a wound swab and tube containing transport medium.

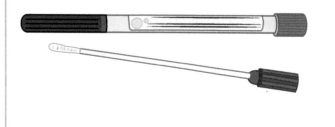

Figure 52.2 Wound being swabbed using a zig-zag motion.

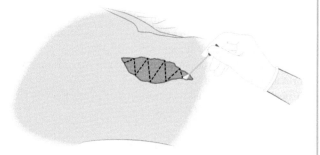

Figure 52.3 Insert swab back into container without touching edges.

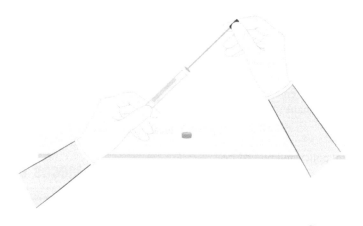

Key points

Wound swabs should only be taken when there is clinical evidence of infection. The swab must be taken correctly to produce a meaningful result.

Midwifery Skills at a Glance, First Edition. Edited by Patricia Lindsay, Carmel Bagness and Ian Peate.
© 2018 John Wiley & Sons, Ltd. Published 2018 by John Wiley & Sons, Ltd.

The principles of specimen collection are set out in Chapter 51. A wound swab is required if there is a clinical suspicion that infection is present. 'Just in case' wound swabs are not helpful and the midwife should be confident that clinical signs of infection are present – this includes redness, heat, pain and the presence of pus. If a discharge is present from the wound the following should be recorded:

- Colour
- Smell
- Consistency
- Presence of pus.

Wound swabs should be collected and sent to the laboratory in a timely way for culture and sensitivity testing.

Indications include infected surgical wounds, for example perineum, umbilicus, and invasive device insertion site (e.g. central line insertion site, drain site, suprapubic catheter site). Infected chicken pox pustules would also meet the definition of a wound.

The midwife should:
- Correctly complete the laboratory request form.
- Gain patient consent to take the specimen and inform the patient of the rationale for it.
- Ensure the patient is comfortable, and their privacy and dignity is maintained.
- Collect the specimen in a way that avoids contamination – see Chapter 5 (Asepsis and sepsis).
- Use the correct transport medium.
- Arrange transportation to the laboratory in a timely way or store appropriately if necessary.
- Check and act on results once they are available.
- Document collection of the specimen and the results together with any resulting actions.

Storing specimens

Once the swab has been obtained it should be placed in a plastic specimen bag together with the laboratory form in line with local policies and procedures. Specimens should be sent to the laboratory as soon as possible and should not be left for long periods at ambient temperatures as this may result in overgrowth of commensal bacteria, which can impact on the accuracy of the laboratory result.

If transport to the laboratory will be delayed the specimen should be refrigerated (not in a food fridge) until the next available laboratory collection.

The swabbing procedure

Note: this procedure requires an aseptic technique to avoid contamination of the swab or wound, which could lead to incorrect laboratory analysis due to contamination of equipment or the specimen.
- Positively identify the patient.
- Ensure all necessary equipment is available (including correct swab and laboratory form).
- Explain the procedure to the patient.
- Obtain patient consent.
- Obtain the swab before antibiotics are commenced wherever possible.
- Perform hand hygiene before patient contact.
- Remove old wound dressing if present – use personal protective equipment (PPE – gloves and apron) if required.

- Dip swab in transport media included in swab container or moisten with sterile saline (do *not* use tap water) (Figures 52.1).
- Rotate the swab over the area to be swabbed using a zig zag motion, ensuring you make contact with the area of the wound showing signs of infection (Figure 52.2).
- If a wound sinus is suspected or present do not probe the tract as exploration of the sinus should only be undertaken with a dedicated sinus probe. Cotton tips/ swabs or applicators should not be used for exploration. Swabbing of the sinus, if requested, should be undertaken by or with the support of tissue viability or surgical specialists.
- If pus is present swab pus.
- Replace swab in the container (Figure 52.3).
- Redress wound if necessary.
- Remove PPE and perform hand hygiene.
- Make the woman comfortable.
- Complete patient identification labels and send to laboratory. Document in patient records.

Pus

Pus usually presents as a white/yellowish discharge. It comprises dead leucocytes, which are produced by the body in response to the presence of infection.

Swabbing large wounds

Large wounds may include chronic wounds. In the maternity setting chronic wounds may include pressure ulcers or diabetic foot wounds. Large wounds may include areas of debridement (for example following breakdown of a caesarean section wound) or burns. It is not possible or necessary to swab the whole wound – attention should be paid to areas where inflammation or exudate/ pus are present.

Swabbing chronic wounds

Chronic wounds, as described above, are often heavily colonised with bacteria and do not require regular or 'just in case' swabbing. Swabs should only be taken if the presence of infection is suspected. In chronic wounds infection is characterised by increasing pain, inflammation/cellulitis and a pyrexia. If a sample of the wound is required, a tissue biopsy rather a wound swab is the preferred microbiological sample.

If a swab is required:
- Cleanse the wound by irrigating with sterile/tap water or saline to remove surface bacterial contaminants in line with local policies.
- Remove any slough and necrotic tissue if easily dislodged.
- Swab viable wound tissue only (do not take swabs from necrotic areas) on the edge of the wound or from areas showing signs of infection.

For complex wounds the expertise of tissue viability specialists should be sought.

Service user's view

'I was really nervous about having my wound swabbed as it was so painful but the midwife made sure I had pain killers beforehand and explained everything she was going to do. This really helped me and I never felt a thing. The results showed I did have an infection and once I started my antibiotics I felt much better.'

Mary, verbal communication, service user, Yorkshire

53 Use of a vaginal speculum and taking a vaginal swab

Figure 53.1 Cusco vaginal speculum blades open.

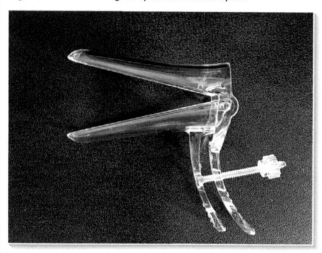

Figure 53.2 Cusco vaginal speculum blades close.

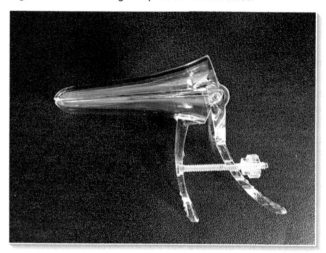

Figure 53.3 Part labia, insert speculum.

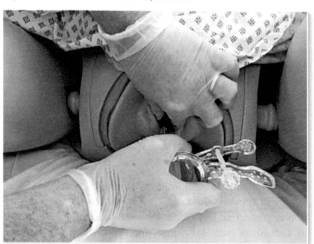

Figure 53.4 Rotate speculum 90 degrees.

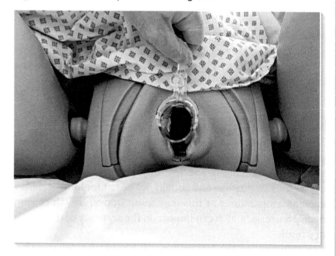

Box 53.1 The indications for speculum.

Examination during the antenatal period are:
- To assess the cervix in suspected preterm labour
- To assess the presence of liquor when prelabour spontaneous rupture of membranes (PROM) is suspected
- To assess the cause of antepartum vaginal bleeding
- When a high vaginal swab (HVS) is required to screen for infection in the presence of vaginal discharge

Box 53.2 Equipment required for speculum examination.

- Gloves (sterile if membranes have ruptured) apron
- Vaginal examination or aseptic examination pack which should contain swabs/cotton balls and a bowl
- Antiseptic solution or warm water (depending on local Trust policy)
- Speculum and lubricating gel.
- Swab
- A good light source

Key point

When spontaneous rupture of membranes (SROM) is suspected aseptic technique and sterile gloves must be used.

Midwifery Skills at a Glance, First Edition. Edited by Patricia Lindsay, Carmel Bagness and Ian Peate.
© 2018 John Wiley & Sons, Ltd. Published 2018 by John Wiley & Sons, Ltd.

The vaginal speculum has been in use for over 2000 years. It is used for both obstetric and gynaecological examinations. Midwives will carry out examinations using a speculum in certain circumstances during pregnancy and need to be competent in this skill.

The insertion of the speculum can be uncomfortable and may cause anxiety or embarrassment for some women. The level of anxiety may also be related to the reason for the examination so this should be taken into consideration. It is essential the midwife gives a full explanation of the indications for the speculum examination and procedure so as to obtain informed consent. Any queries or anxieties the woman has must be addressed at this time. It is probable that the woman has at some point had a cervical smear, which is obtained using a speculum, so it can be useful to use this as part of the explanation of the procedure so the woman knows what to expect.

A Cusco vaginal speculum is used for examination in pregnancy. Figure 53.1 shows the speculum with blades open; Figure 53.2 shows the blades closed. In pregnancy the midwife should use an aseptic technique if the membranes have ruptured; sterile gloves should be used. The speculum blades will require lubrication prior to use and the woman needs to be positioned correctly as described below.

The indications for speculum examination during the antenatal period are given in Box 53.1. Equipment required is listed in Box 53.2.

Examination procedure

• Wash hands.
• Prepare the woman; the midwife must ensure the indications for examination and procedure have been explained and informed consent gained.
• Position the woman; heels/ankles together, draw up towards the buttocks then relax the knees outwards so legs are open. Ensure privacy and dignity whilst woman is in the appropriate position with a cover over her. She can move this up when you are ready to begin.
• Open pack and gloves. Open all necessary equipment onto pack (gel, speculum, swab, cleaning fluid). Put on your apron, wash hands and put on gloves.
• Lubricate the outer aspect of the blades; ensure blades are closed to avoid gel going inside the speculum.
• Identify your clean/ dirty hand and clean perineum and vulva using aseptic technique, swabbing downwards with the 'dirty' hand.
• Part labia with 'dirty' hand and insert speculum (blades closed) in the AP diameter in a slightly downward direction (Figure 53.3).
• During insertion rotate the speculum until the handle is upwards towards the clitoris (Figure 53.4).
• Open the blades using the mechanism present (often a screw but may vary between models) and hold the speculum in place.
• Using the light source you should be able to inspect the vagina and cervix. You may need to insert the speculum further or

ask the woman to tilt her pelvis upward (put her fist under her bottom) if the cervix cannot be visualised. Take high vaginal swab (HVS) if indicated.
• If spontaneous rupture of membranes is suspected and no liquor is seen, ask the woman to cough. This raises the intra-abdominal pressure and can push liquor out. It can also help to ask the woman to lie on the bed for up to 30 minutes before examination to allow time for the liquor to pool in the vagina.
• When the examination is complete close blades slightly and remove. Ensure blades are gradually closed as speculum is rotated back to AP diameter as you remove it. It can be very painful if the vaginal wall is trapped whilst doing this.
• Assist the woman in removing the disposable sheet and replacing her sanitary towel and underwear.
• Ensure all equipment is disposed of in the correct clinical waste bin.
• Wash hands.
• Ensure you communicate all findings to the woman and her partner, including plan of care, then document all accurately. If any deviations from the norm, then escalate to the senior midwife and senior obstetrician.

Vaginal swab

A vaginal swab can either be a high vaginal swab (HVS) or low vaginal/vaginal swab (LVS). A speculum must be used to enable an HVS to be taken (Evans and Morgan, 2012). This is then sent to the laboratory for microscopy and then culture and sensitivity if indicated by microscopy examination. It can be used for diagnosis of vaginal infections such as bacteria vaginosis, Group B streptococcus and candidiasis. Some texts do not specify HVS, only vaginal swab and also advocate the woman being able to take the swab herself. Care must be taken to ensure the swab is not contaminated before placing it into the vagina to ensure that organisms detected are vaginal rather than from the perineum or anus.

The swab should be taken and then placed in the transport medium within the receiver provided, adhering to local policy and procedure. The transport medium is normally Amies transport medium with charcoal. The purpose of the charcoal is to protect the bacteria from the light and the transport medium provides a moist environment to keep the bacteria alive during transport to the laboratory. It is the responsibility of the midwife to ensure that the swab is clearly labelled and documented in the notes so that the result can be followed up and appropriate treatment given if required.

Service user's view

'It really helped that the midwife knew I was anxious and put me at ease before starting. Telling me it was like having a smear examination was really helpful.'

Verbal communication, service user, Berkshire

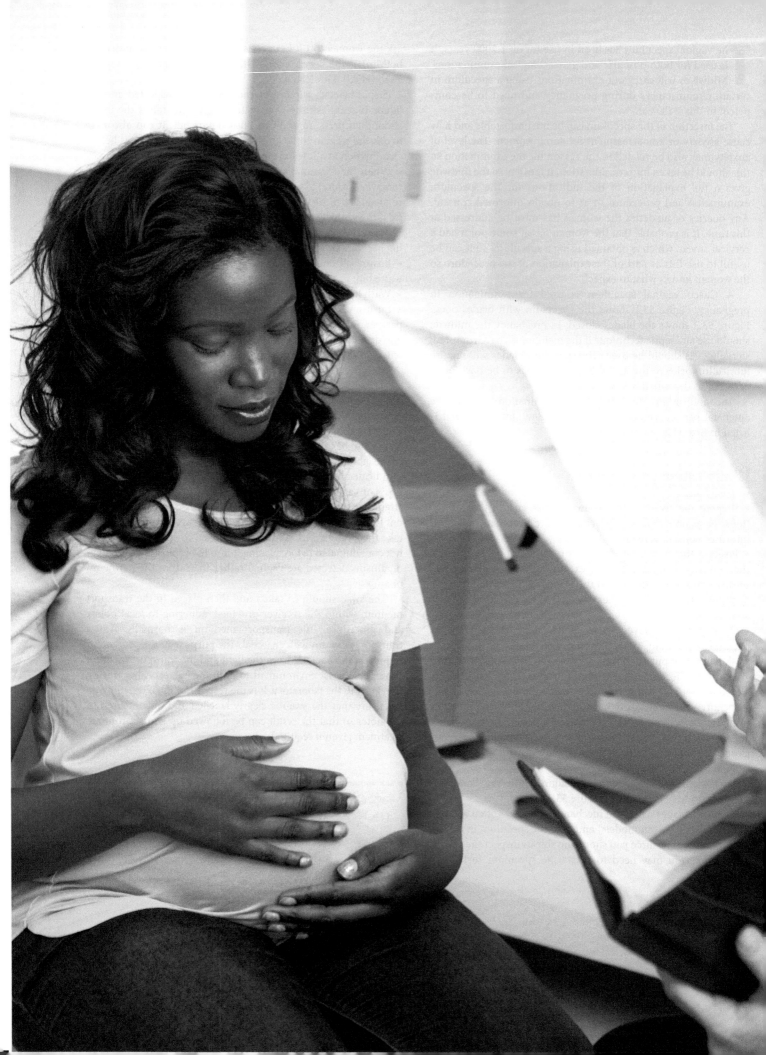

The woman or neonate with different needs

Part 3

54 Membrane sweep

Figure 54.1 Equipment for membrane sweep.

- Sterile gloves
- Water-based lubricant
- Pinnards stethoscope/hand held sonicaid/CTG

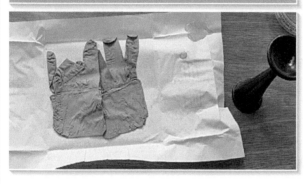

Table 54.1 Modified Bishop's score.

Cervix	0	1	2	3
Position	Posterior	Mid	Anterior	–
Consistency	Firm	Firm	Medium	Soft
Effacement	>2cm	1–2cm	<1cm	–
Dilatation	Os closed	1–2cm	3–4cm	<4cm
Station of PP	Spines –3	Spines –2	Spines –1, 0	Spines +1

Figure 54.2 Position the mother semirecumbent.

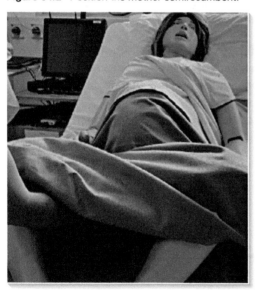

Ensure privacy and dignity maintained throughout procedure

Figure 54.3 Position of fingers.

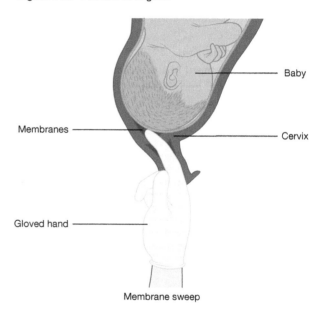

Baby

Membranes

Cervix

Gloved hand

Membrane sweep

Box 54.1 Indications for membrane sweep.

- Post dates 40 and 41 weeks for primparous women; 41 weeks for multiparous women
- As part of the induction of labour process
- In early labour at vaginal examination
- Maternal request when there are no contraindications

Box 54.2 Contraindications/cautions for membrane sweep.

- No fully informed maternal consent
- Placenta praevia
- Low lying placenta
- Less than 40 weeks – unless discussion with obstetrician

Key points

- Informed consent must be obtained before the procedure.
- The woman's discomfort and other side effects must be balanced against the expected benefits before subjecting the woman to membrane sweeping.

Midwifery Skills at a Glance, First Edition. Edited by Patricia Lindsay, Carmel Bagness and Ian Peate.
© 2018 John Wiley & Sons, Ltd. Published 2018 by John Wiley & Sons, Ltd.

Membrane sweeping or stripping is thought to increase the probability of physiological onset of labour by encouraging the local release of prostaglandin. Evidence suggests that the process of undertaking this procedure, during which the examining fingers are introduced into the cervical os and detach the membranes from the decidua using a circular movement of the fingers, releases prostaglandins. This, in turn, increases the likelihood of spontaneous labour within 48 hours. However, it is an uncomfortable procedure that is associated with vaginal bleeding and irregular contractions.

Membrane sweeping is commonly offered to primparous women at 40 and 41 weeks gestation and multiparous women at 41 weeks.

Evidence in regard to membrane sweeping is inconclusive and women and midwives must take this into account in order to make a fully informed choice. There has been debate as to the frequency at which membrane sweeping should be repeated. Undertaking the procedure three times a week at 48-hour intervals has been found to be effective in encouraging spontaneous labour. For indications and contraindications for membrane sweep see Boxes 54.1 and 54.2.

When undertaking a membrane sweep it is important that the Bishop's score is calculated (Table 54.1). The Bishop's score considers five factors. These are: the position, consistency, effacement and dilatation of the cervix, along with the station of the presenting part. Although it is accepted that a score of 5 or more deems the cervix to be favourable or 'ripe', and thus the greater likelihood of the sweep being successful. It is possible to undertake a membrane sweep with lower Bishop's scores as this may aid in the ripening of the cervix. If the cervix is closed or unfavourable and therefore the midwife is unable to undertake the membrane sweep, it is suggested that cervical massage is considered. This can be achieved by using the forefinger and middle finger to make gentle massaging circular movements on the cervix for about 15 seconds.

Procedure for undertaking a membrane sweep

- Ensure that the mother has given fully informed consent.
- Gather equipment (Figure 54.1).
- Ensure that you have privacy and maintain her comfort and dignity throughout.
- Encourage the mother to have emptied her bladder prior to the procedure.
- Wash hands.
- Undertake a full antenatal examination including abdominal examination and auscultation of fetal heart with a pinnards stethoscope or hand-held sonicaid.
- Encourage the mother to adopt a semirecumbent position with her knees bent, ankles together and knees apart (Figure 54.2).
- Wash hands. Maintaining asepsis put on sterile gloves and undertake a vaginal examination to locate the cervix and determine the Bishop's score.
- If cervix is closed then gently massage for 15 seconds.
- Do not proceed if you detect any abnormalities, i.e. vaginal infection, presence of the cord or the placenta in the cervical canal or close to the os, fetal malpresentation.
- Insert one or two fingers into the cervix and aim to gently dilate the os.
- Place examining fingers between the lower uterine segment and the membranes (Figure 54.3).
- Sweep your finger(s) in a 360-degree circular motion firmly but swiftly as this is uncomfortable for the woman. You must stop if the woman requests this.
- Remove examining fingers.
- Ensure the mother is clean, comfortable and not exposed following the procedure.
- Dispose of gloves correctly – wash hands.
- Auscultate fetal heart with Pinard stethoscope or hand-held sonicaid.
- Discuss findings with the mother and what to expect and when to contact the midwife/hospital, i.e. possible blood stained 'show', irregular contractions.
- Document all discussions, procedures, findings and advice given.
- Ensure documented plan of management is in place that mother is in agreement with.

Service user's view

'Even among the 239 women who described sweeping as painful, 210 (88%) reported that they would choose membrane sweeping again in the next pregnancy.'

De Miranda et al. 2006

55 Insertion of vaginal prostaglandin E2

Figure 55.1 Equipment for insertion of prostaglandin E2 (Prostin)®.

- Sterile gloves
- Prostin® – prescribed dose of gel, vaginal tablet or Propess®
- Pinard stethoscope/hand held sonicaid/CTG

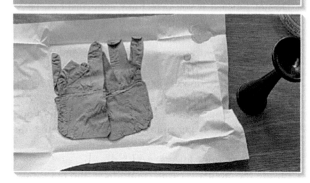

Figure 55.2 Prostin® gel/tablet.

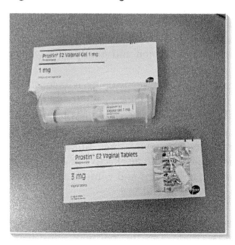

Figure 55.3 Propess® 24-hour delivery retrievable system.

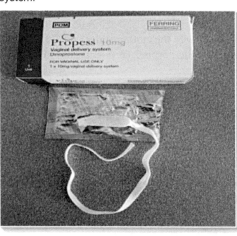

Figure 55.4 Insertion of Propess®.

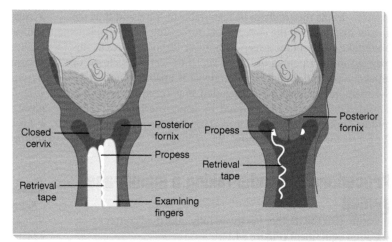

Closed cervix
Posterior fornix
Propess
Retrieval tape
Examining fingers

Propess
Posterior fornix
Retrieval tape

Box 55.1 Indications for induction of labour (IOL).

- Post maturity
- Concerns about fetal wellbeing
- IUG
- Existing maternal conditions e.g. diabetes
- Prelabour ruptured membranes
- Pre-eclampsia/eclampsia
- Multiple pregnancy
- Macrosomia
- Fetal death
- Fetal anomaly not compatible with life
- Maternal request -- psychological /social reasons – the mother must be fully informed of implications where there are no clinical indications for IOL

Box 55.2 Contraindications/cautions for induction of labour (IOL).

- No informed consent of mother
- Transverse lie
- Cord presentation
- Malposition/compound presentation
- Previous lower segment caesarean section (LSCS)/uterine surgery
- HIV-positive women not receiving antiretroviral therapy or whose viral load is 400 copies/mL or more
- Known cephalo-pelvic disproportion
- Active genital herpes
- Placenta praevia

Key points

- Must be prescribed by doctor – these drugs are not part of the midwives exemptions.
- Both mother and fetus must be appropriately monitored throughout the process.
- Accurate documentation must be made of all actions, discussions and observations.

Midwifery Skills at a Glance, First Edition. Edited by Patricia Lindsay, Carmel Bagness and Ian Peate.
© 2018 John Wiley & Sons, Ltd. Published 2018 by John Wiley & Sons, Ltd.

pproximately 1 in 5 labours are induced in the UK. Induction of labour can be a very frightening time for women and partner. The midwife is well placed to ensure that women receive evidence-based information to help them reach an informed choice about their care.

Currently, in the UK the most common method of induction utilises synthetic forms of prostaglandin, Prostin®. These come in the form of gels, tablets or 24-hour release formulations. For greatest efficacy these should be administered at regular intervals to maintain a therapeutic range of the drug within the system. Gels and tablets are commonly prescribed for administration at 6-hourly intervals with a maximum of three doses in 24 hours. There are many factors that can impact on the midwife's ability to adhere to this regimen. Capacity and staffing often delay or impede on the induction process. The single-dose Propess® delivers 0.3 mg per hour over the 24-hour period.

As with all medications it is vital that the midwife is aware of common side effects, indications and contraindications for administration of prostaglandin preparations (Boxes 55.1 and 55.2). The midwife must also ensure that the drug has been prescribed, checked and dispensed correctly.

Procedure for insertion of prostaglandin gels, tablets, Propess

- Ensure that the mother is fully aware of the process and gives informed consent.
- Encourage mother to empty bladder.
- Ensure privacy and comfort is maintained throughout the procedure.
- Wash hands.
- Undertake full antenatal examination, including abdominal palpation and auscultation of fetal heart with Pinnards stethoscope/hand-held sonicaid.
- Monitor fetal wellbeing via cardiotocograph (CTG) for 30 minutes.
- Do not undertake the procedure if any abnormalities identified with CTG or antenatal examination/ palpation.
- Gather all equipment (Figure 55.1) and the prescribed prostaglandin (Figures 55.2 and 55.3).
- Wash hands and put on apron.

- Maintaining asepsis, put on sterile gloves and undertake a vaginal examination.
- Ascertain Bishop's score (see Chapter 54). If 0–6 administer the prescribed prostaglandin.
- For Prostin tablet –secure tablet between index and middle fingers of examining hand. Insert lubricated fingers gently into the vagina in a downwards and backwards direction along posterior vaginal wall.
- Deposit the tablet high into the posterior vaginal fornix.
- For Prostin Gel – this comes in a syringe applicator. Locate posterior fornix as above, guide syringe applicator along examining fingers, squirt the gel into the posterior vaginal fornix.
- For Propess this needs to be placed crosswise, high in the posterior vaginal fornix (Figure 55.4). In order to achieve this, place the Propess between index and middle finger, enter vagina, once posterior fornix located manoeuvre the Propess into a transverse position, remove fingers, being careful not to pull retrieval tape and thus inadvertently removing Propess.
- Ensure woman is left clean and comfortable post procedure.
- Monitor fetal heart via CTG for 30 minutes postinsertion of prostglandin.
- Document fully all actions and observations.
- Ensure documented management plan in place that the woman is in agreement with.
- Monitor maternal and fetal condition in line with national/ local guidelines.
- Inform the woman of signs and symptoms to report to midwife, e.g. regular contractions, vaginal bleeding, ruptured membranes or Propess fallen out.
- Ensure that she has call bell in easy reach and anything else she may need.
- Remove Propess if indicated, i.e. ruptured membranes, regular painful contractions, vaginal bleeding.
- Ensure accurate, contemporaneous documentation is maintained.

Service user's view

'My advice is not to expect it to happen straight away. I thought that full labour would start immediately but this is often not the case.'

Mumsnet.com

56 Artificial rupture of membranes

Figure 56.1 Equipment for artificial rupture of the membranes.

- Sterile vaginal examination pack
- Sterile gloves
- Sterile amnihook
- Pinard's stethoscope/hand held sonicaid/CTG

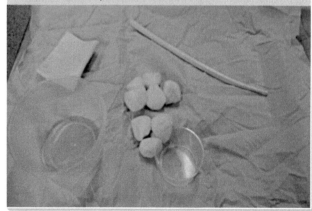

Table 56.1 Modified Bishop's score.

Cervix	0	1	2	3
Position	Posterior	Mid	Anterior	–
Consistency	Firm	Firm	Medium	Soft
Effacement	>2cm	1–2cm	<1cm	–
Dilatation	Os closed	1–2cm	3–4cm	>4cm
Station of presenting part	Spines – 3	Spines – 2	Spines – 1, 0	Spines + 1

Figure 56.2 Insertion of amnihook.

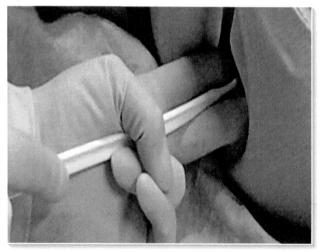

Figure 56.3 Twisting amnihook to tear membranes.

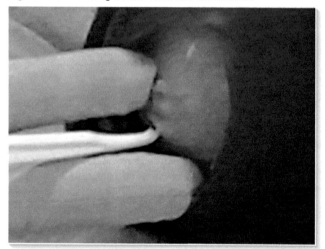

Box 56.1 Indications for ARM.

- As part of the Induction of labour process
- Augmentation of labour
- Assessment of liquor colour
- Application of fetal scalp electrode
- Maternal request
- Often prior to birth of second twin

Box 56.2 Contraindications/cautions for ARM.

- No fully informed maternal consent
- Premature labour
- Known vaginal infection such as Group B streptococcus
- High presenting part as risk of cord prolapse
- Placenta praevia
- Vasa praevia
- Malposition/malpresentation
- Polyhydramnios – risk of cord prolapse
- Maternal HIV infection/positive status

Key points

- Intact membranes provide protection from infection for the fetus and mother as well as cushioning for the presenting part.
- Artificial rupture of membranes should only be undertaken following fully informed consent.

Midwifery Skills at a Glance, First Edition. Edited by Patricia Lindsay, Carmel Bagness and Ian Peate.
© 2018 John Wiley & Sons, Ltd. Published 2018 by John Wiley & Sons, Ltd.

Artificial rupture of membranes (ARM) is one of the most commonly performed midwifery procedures. The argument often given in favour of ARM is that of 'speeding up labour'. The suggestion is that labour may be shortened by 1 hour. However, this procedure is often associated with an increase in intervention due to fetal heart rate abnormalities and changes in the mother's ability to cope. In line with Nursing Midwifery Council (NMC) guidance this procedure should only be undertaken following the fully informed consent of the mother.

Indications and contraindications for ARM are outlined in Boxes 56.1 and 56.2.

Obstetricians may choose to undertake a controlled ARM in the presence of polyhydramnios (increased amniotic fluid) or a high presenting part. This is when the presenting part (most commonly the fetal head) is above the ischial spines (a landmark on the maternal pelvis). The risk of cord prolapse is increased in these situations.

As an advocate for the woman, the midwife should ensure that this is undertaken in the safest environment, that is access to an obstetric theatre or in an obstetric theatre in the event of cord prolapse and the procedure carried out by the most experienced clinician. In the event that a more junior obstetrician is undertaking the procedure the midwife should ensure they are supported/ overseen by senior colleagues.

The amnihook is an instrument that resembles a long crochet hook. However, the end has a sharp hook and as such can cause tissue damage so care must be taken to protect the mother from injury during the procedure (Figure 56.1).

Procedure for undertaking ARM

• Discuss with the mother the indication for wishing to undertake the procedure allowing enough time for her to ask questions.
• Gain her informed consent.
• Wash hands.
• Undertake an abdominal examination and auscultation of the fetal heart.
• If any deviations from normal are detected the midwife must not carry out the ARM but refer to the obstetrician.
• Gather all necessary equipment (Figure 56.1).
• Ensure the mother has had opportunity to empty her bladder prior to procedure.
• As the mother will need to adopt a semirecumbent position with legs apart and ankles together you must ensure dignity, comfort and privacy is maintained throughout.
• Wash hands and maintaining an aseptic non-touch technique (ANTT) open pack and set out equipment and put on sterile gloves.

• Ensure mother is ready for you to commence procedure.
• Undertake vaginal examination and locate cervix to ensure conditions are suitable for ARM, i.e. no high presenting part, no suspected cord presentation, favourable Bishop's score (5 or more) (Table 56.1).
• Maintaining sterility of the amnihook – hold with the non-examining hand and slide between index and middle finger of examining hand and the anterior vaginal wall 'hook down' – the aim is to protect the woman from injury.
• Guide the hook into position against the membranes with the non-examining hand (Figure 56.2).
• Press the hook against the membranes and rotate it with the non-examining hand so that the point then tears the membranes (Figure 56.3).
• Success is marked by obvious drainage of amniotic fluid.
• Leaving the examining hand in situ, remove the amnihook, again taking care not to injure the mother.
• The examining hand may then locate the tear and if needed digitally enlarge the hole.
• It is vital that the midwife ensures that she reassess the cervix, position and station of presenting part before removing her fingers and excludes cord presentation and cord prolapse.
• Remove hand.
• Auscultate fetal heart with Pinard's stethoscope or hand-held sonicaid.
• Ensure that the mother is clean and dry, offer fresh sanitary towel.
• Discuss findings with the mother. Ensure she knows what is normal and what she needs to alert you to, i.e. blood/meconium-stained amniotic fluid.
• Correctly dispose of all equipment.
• Wash your hands.
• Document discussions, indications, procedure and findings in line with NMC 2015 and Trust guidelines.
• Inform midwife in charge and obstetrician if appropriate, and ensure plan of care in place.
• Monitor the maternal and fetal wellbeing in line with your national/local guidelines.

57 Recognising the deteriorating woman

Figure 57.1 Stages of shock.

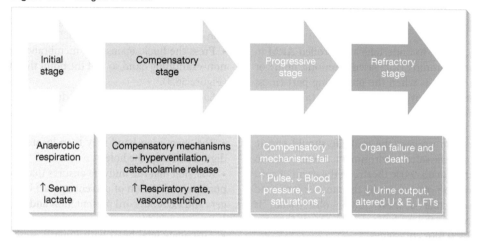

Initial stage → Compensatory stage → Progressive stage → Refractory stage

Anaerobic respiration

↑ Serum lactate

Compensatory mechanisms – hyperventilation, catecholamine release

↑ Respiratory rate, vasoconstriction

Compensatory mechanisms fail

↑ Pulse, ↓ Blood pressure, ↓ O₂ saturations

Organ failure and death

↓ Urine output, altered U & E, LFTs

Figure 57.2 Care of the deteriorating woman.

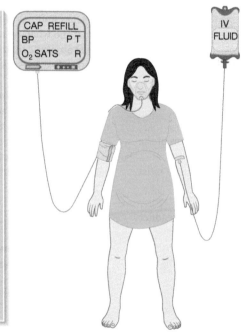

Call for help
Assessment every 3–5 minutes until stable:

Airway
- Assess airway – 'chin lift, head tilt' if airway compromised
- Give high-flow oxygen (15 litres per min)
- Oxygen saturations (keep > 94%; < 91% requires immediate action)

Breathing
- Count respiratory rate (12–20 breaths/min normal range, >20 breaths/min indicates shock, >25 breaths/min requires immediate action)
- Look for respiratory distress

Circulation
- Check for sources of haemorrhage
- Measure capillary refill (>2 seconds requires immediate action)
- Measure pulse rate (>100bpm indicates shock, >130bpm requires immediate action)
- Measure BP (systolic <90 mmHg or 40 mmHg drop from baseline requires immediate action)

CAP REFILL
BP   P T
O₂ SATS   R

IV FLUID

- Insert 2 × wide bore cannula
- Take bloods – FBC, G & S, U & E, LFT, serum lactate (≥2.0 mmols indicates anaerobic respiration, ≥ 4.0 mmols/L usually indicates septic shock – immediate action needed)
- Measure hourly urine output via indwelling catheter
- Fluid replacement in discussion with multiprofessional team

Disability
- Assess mental state – AVPU score
- Check drug chart
- Blood glucose measurement (hyperglycaemia may indicate sepsis)

Exposure
- Temperature (>38.3°C, or <36°C indicates sepsis)
- Check for rashes
- Take blood cultures
- Swab potential infection sites
- Administer broad-spectrum intravenous antibiotics

Document on HDU/ MEOWS chart

Key points
- Pregnant women compensate for being severely unwell for a long time. When they start to show signs of shock they are *dying*.
- Although hypovolaemic shock is common in maternity, the midwife must consider other types of shock such as septic shock.
- When a woman's observations start to change she is no longer compensating for a lack of oxygen and is *dying* rather than deteriorating if not treated appropriately.

Midwifery Skills at a Glance, First Edition. Edited by Patricia Lindsay, Carmel Bagness and Ian Peate.
© 2018 John Wiley & Sons, Ltd. Published 2018 by John Wiley & Sons, Ltd.

The most recent confidential enquiries into maternal death in the UK have identified that practitioners fail to recognise the deteriorating woman. This has far reaching consequences for the woman and her family because this failure can result in severe morbidity or mortality. In order to recognise the deteriorating woman, it is essential to understand and recognise the different stages of shock (Figure 57.1). Childbearing women generally compensate for shock very well, because they are (usually) young and fit their bodies physiologically adapt to cope well with shock, but will show subtle signs that they are becoming unwell. In order to recognise the deteriorating woman, the different stages of shock must be understood. Effective history taking antenatally will help to identify women who may have known risk factors that predispose them to shock and so allow decisions to be made through discussion with the multiprofessional team about appropriate place of birth.

Physiological shock occurs when there is a deficit in the oxygen available compared to the oxygen that is required by the cells to allow normal cell function. In childbearing women, the most common type of shock is **hypovolaemic** shock following an antepartum or postpartum haemorrhage, where the cells do not receive enough oxygen because there is not enough blood volume to get the oxygen to all cells. In **septic** shock, bacterial infection causes an acute inflammatory response that results in vasodilation and hypotension; again there is inadequate blood pressure to circulate oxygen to where it is needed. In midwifery care, we see **neurogenic** shock during a uterine inversion as the stretching of broad ligaments that support the uterus normally disrupts the sympathetic nervous system, which means that compensatory mechanisms cannot take place and the pulse and blood pressure will drop rapidly. **Anaphylactic** shock and **cardiogenic** shock are rare in maternity but the midwife should consider them if a woman has had a new drug administered (particularly an antibiotic or anti-D) or if she has a known cardiac disorder.

The **initial stage of shock** occurs in the absence of a sufficient oxygen supply, when cells begin to respire anaerobically. A by-product of this anaerobic respiration is lactic acid (measured as serum lactate in blood tests). At this early stage it is unlikely that the practitioner will be able observe changes.

In the **compensatory stage of shock**, the body's compensatory mechanisms begin to function. Hyperventilation reduces carbon dioxide levels and neutralises the acidic conditions that have begun to occur. Hyperventilation also serves to increase the oxygen levels that are available for cell function. Catecholamine release is triggered by hypotension and serves to increase the heart rate and blood pressure to maintain it at normal levels. Vasopressin is released and triggers fluid retention and vasoconstriction. This means that the first observations that the midwife will make indicating change are an increased respiration rate and a degree of vasoconstriction that may manifest as an increased peripheral capillary refill time. Anecdotally, these observations are often routinely omitted in practice so the opportunity to recognise the compensatory stage of shock is missed.

The **progressive stage of shock** occurs when shock is not corrected and compensatory mechanisms begin to fail. At this stage, the practitioner will observe an increasing pulse rate, a drop in blood pressure and a drop in oxygen saturation levels. It is essential that the severity of these observations are noted, reported and action taken if it has not been initiated already. A rising pulse rate, dropping blood pressure and oxygen saturation levels indicate a critically unwell woman and immediate action should be taken.

The **refractory stage of shock** occurs when organ failure begins due to the inability of cells to function effectively. Kidney function is the most sensitive to hypoxia, so although some women will have a reduced urine output if they are dehydrated, the midwife must consider reduced urine output may indicate a degree of renal failure. If the shock is not managed effectively, and more than one organ fails, then the woman will die because she cannot survive with multiple organ failure.

Regular observations are essential in recognising the deteriorating woman. In addition to changes in these observations, the midwife needs to consider the woman holistically, and extended assessment (ABCDE) is helpful (Figure 57.2). Her general appearance and cognitive function need to be considered. Once the deterioration has been recognised, prompt referral to senior midwifery and medical colleagues needs to be prioritised; failure to do this increases maternal mortality and morbidity. Immediate treatment of the deterioration will require input from the multiprofessional team. Early referral to a high-dependency or intensive care unit will also improve the outcome for the critically unwell woman.

High-flow facial oxygen needs to be applied and combined with intravenous access for blood tests and fluid replacement until the cause of the deterioration is identified and managed appropriately. An indwelling urinary catheter will allow accurate assessment of urine output and recording of fluid balance. A complete set of observations, including respiration rate, pulse rate, blood pressure, oxygen saturations and peripheral capillary refill should be repeated every 3 to 5 minutes to monitor deterioration until her condition stabilises.

Top tips

- Record a full set of observations, including respirations and capillary refill regularly.
- Document your findings on a Modified Early Obstetric Warning Score (MEOWS) or High Dependency Unit (HDU) chart.
- Look for trends in observations.
- Early referral to senior colleagues is essential.

Service user's view

'Because [of] the haemorrhage I was still seeping a lot of liquids and they were having to be changed, and almost feeling like I was a baby myself having my nappy changed. You know, it was quite humbling in a way. You felt very out of control. I've never felt like that before. That was quite hard.'

Hinton et al. 2015

58 CVP, S_pO_2 and ECGs

Figure 58.1 Triple lumen CVC.

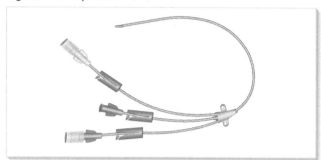

Figure 58.2 Right internal jugular central venous catheter.

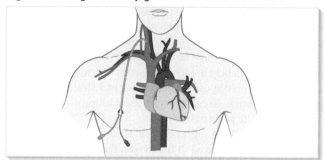

Figure 58.3 Pulse oximetry.

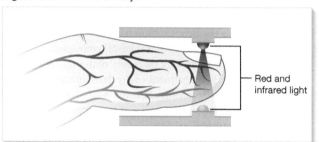

Red and infrared light

Figure 58.4 Top, probe; bottom, display.

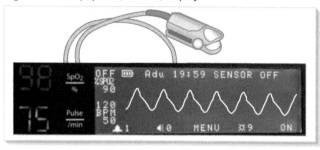

Figure 58.5 Position of ECG leads.

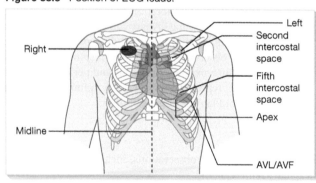

Right
Left
Second intercostal space
Fifth intercostal space
Apex
Midline
AVL/AVF

Figure 58.6 P, Q, R, S and T waves.

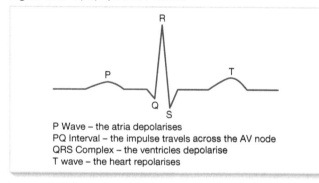

P Wave – the atria depolarises
PQ Interval – the impulse travels across the AV node
QRS Complex – the ventricles depolarise
T wave – the heart repolarises

Figure 58.7 Einthoven's Triangle.

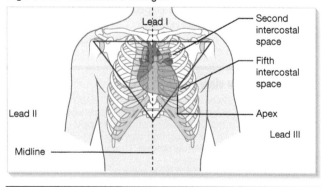

Lead I
Lead II
Lead III
Second intercostal space
Fifth intercostal space
Apex
Midline

Figure 58.8 Left axis deviation.

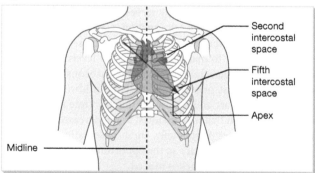

Second intercostal space
Fifth intercostal space
Apex
Midline

Key points

- CVP: transducer sets and monitors differ between manufacturers, and so it is vital you follow your local policy, ensure that you have achieved the relevant competencies before undertaking the procedure of priming a transducer, connecting it to a patient and beginning monitoring.
- Pulse oximetry: a pulse oximeter is simply an adjunct to care and focus remains on the person, not the machine.
- ECGs: The most important thing for a new midwife to learn about three-lead ECG monitoring is what normal looks like and to report and document anything which looks different.

Midwifery Skills at a Glance, First Edition. Edited by Patricia Lindsay, Carmel Bagness and Ian Peate.
© 2018 John Wiley & Sons, Ltd. Published 2018 by John Wiley & Sons, Ltd.

Central venous pressure

A central line or central venous catheter (CVC; Figures 58.1 and 58.2), is a catheter placed into a large vein, usually in the neck (internal jugular vein), chest (subclavian vein) or groin (femoral vein). It is used to measure central venous pressure, administer drugs or fluids that need to be administered rapidly or would damage peripheral veins, or to take blood samples.

Triple-lumen CVCs have proximal, medial and distal ports. The distal end lies in the superior vena cava (unless placed femorally) and should always be monitored using a transducer. The monitor produces a numerical value and a waveform. An accurate central venous pressure (CVP) measurement needs to be taken with the patient lying supine and the transducer aligned with the phlebostatic axis. The number (normal CVP is 2–6 mmHg) indicates right ventricular function and systemic fluid status.

Reasons why CVP may be elevated are:
- Over hydration increases venous return
- Heart failure or pulmonary artery stenosis limiting venous outflow
- Positive pressure breathing due to straining.
  A reason why CVP may be decreased is:
- Hypovolaemic shock.
  CVCs have potentially serious complications:
- Pneumothorax
- Bloodstream infections
- Thrombosis
- Misplacement – placing the catheter usually requires the patient adopting a Trendelenburg or at least supine position. This may be difficult in pregnancy as it may cause aortocaval compression.
- Air embolus – lines attached to a CVC must be kept air free
- Haemorrhage and formation of a haematoma.
  The use of CVCs is becoming increasingly rare in maternity care.

Pulse oximetry

Pulse oximetry provides continuous and non-invasive monitoring of the oxygen saturation of haemoglobin in arterial blood. It works by emitting light and then measuring the light after it has passed through capillaries, usually in the fingertip (Figure 58.3). Arterial oxygenated blood is red due to the quality of oxyhaemoglobin contained, and it absorbs light of certain wavelengths. Pulsatile arterial blood causes a flood of oxyhaemoglobin to tissues, absorbing more infrared light and allowing less light to reach the photodetector. Oxygen saturation of the blood determines the degree of light absorption.

The pulse oximeter displays two values (Figure 58.4):
1 The oxygen saturation of haemoglobin in arterial blood. The value of the oxygen saturation is given together with an audible signal varying in pitch depending on the oxygen saturation. A falling pitch indicates falling oxygen saturation. The figure shown is peripheral capillary oxygen saturation (S$_p$O$_2$) expressed as a percentage.
2 The pulse rate in beats per minute, averaged over 5 to 20 seconds.

Use of the pulse oximeter

- Turn the machine on, wait for it to go through its internal calibration and checks.
- Select the correct size of probe. Ensure the area is clean with any nail varnish or enamel nails removed, as this may interfere with the reading. The probe may be a hinged finger probe, a rubber finger probe or an ear sensor.
- Connect the probe to the pulse oximeter.
- Ensure the probe fits well without being too loose or too tight (either can produce a poor reading).
- Avoid using the arm being used for blood pressure monitoring (intermittent cuff inflation will interrupt the pulse oximeter signal).
- Once the unit has detected a good pulse, the oxygen saturation and pulse rate is displayed.
- Ensure the alarms are on and set; normal saturation is between 94 and 100% and the alarm should be set to occur if the S$_p$O$_2$ falls below 94%.

Trouble-shooting

If you cannot get a signal, or the signal is poor/intermittent, after the probe has been placed on a finger, check:
- Size and position of probe
- Peripheral perfusion
- Patient's temperature as cold peripheries are a common issue
- High levels of ambient light
- Excessive movement, possibly due to pain, anxiety or shivering
- Nail varnish, artificial nails, dirty nails.

Points to consider

While pulse oximeters function normally in anaemic patients, in severe anaemia oxygen saturation will still be normal (94–100%) but there may not be enough haemoglobin to transport sufficient oxygen to the tissues.

Continuous use of the probe may cause pressure damage to the skin or nail bed, and so the probe must be repositioned every 2–4 hours.

Three-lead ECG monitoring

For continuous monitoring, a three or five-lead electrocardiography (ECG) is often used. The leads are colour-coded red, yellow and green and placed as in Figure 58.5. Cardiac depolarisation and repolarisation can be seen, using an ECG, as an electrical force which has a direction and magnitude. This is shown below with each point labelled P, Q, R, S and T waves (Figure 58.6), depicting normal sinus rhythm. The lead placement creates what is known as Einthoven's triangle (Figure 58.7), enabling a view of the heart's electrical activity from the perspective of a particular lead.

The ECG for a pregnant woman may show some differences from that of their non-pregnant state; however, it is not necessarily abnormal and includes:
1 Left axis deviation (Figure 58.8). The heart depolarises from upper right to lower left in normal physiology. In pregnancy, this can be shifted upward and to the left; the image on the screen may look a little flatter or pointing away from you.
2 Small Q waves and inverted T wave in lead III. T wave inversion is usually a sign of ischaemia; however, strenuous exercise tests in pregnancy have shown this to be normal unless associated with other symptoms.
3 ST depression and inversion or flattening of the T wave in inferior and lateral leads are also signs of ischaemia. This is normal unless associated with other symptoms.
4 Atrial and ventricular ectopics. These are extra beats or missed beats, which are usually harmless. However, the woman may feel them as palpitations and require reassurance. If she has other symptoms such as breathlessness and reduced blood pressure, this may indicate that further treatment is required.

59 Fluid balance monitoring

Figure 59.1 Example of a fluid balance chart.

SURNAME ....

FIRST NAME ....

HOSPITAL NUMBER ....

DATE OF BIRTH ....

DATE ....

WEIGHT ....

INDICATION/INSTRUCTIONS FOR RECORDING
FLUID BALANCE

TIME	ORAL	FLUID INPUT			HOUR TOTAL IN	TOTAL IN	URINE	FLUID OUTPUT			HOUR TOTAL OUT	TOTAL OUT	FLUID BALANCE
		ENTERAL	IV	OTHER				GASTRIC	BOWEL	DRAINS			
01:00													
02:00													
03:00													
04:00													
05:00													
06:00													
07:00													
08:00													
09:00													
10:00													
11:00													
12:00													
01:00													
02:00													
03:00													
04:00													
05:00													
06:00													
07:00													
08:00													
09:00													
10:00													
11:00													
12:00													
01:00													
02:00													
03:00													
04:00													
TOTAL INTAKE							TOTAL OUTPUT						

FLUID BALANCE

Key point

Best practice maternity care includes the recognition of factors that contribute to optimal homeostatic fluid balance. Healthcare professionals should be competent in assessment, management, escalation and documentation skills in fluid balance monitoring in order to detect complications and ensure access to timely and appropriate care and expertise.

Midwifery Skills at a Glance, First Edition. Edited by Patricia Lindsay, Carmel Bagness and Ian Peate.
© 2018 John Wiley & Sons, Ltd. Published 2018 by John Wiley & Sons, Ltd.

Fluid balance is described as the balance of the input and output of fluids in the body to allow metabolic processes to function correctly. The Mothers and Babies Reducing Risk through Audit and Confidential Enquiries in the United Kingdom report (MBRRACE 2014) recognises the significant impact that midwives have in the prevention of maternal and neonatal mortality and morbidity, especially where there are known pre-existing pathologies such as metabolic, cardiac or renal disease. Early clinical assessment and treatment can be crucial for women requiring fluid balance monitoring as part of diagnostic assessments or as part of higher dependency care interventions.

Assessments should include client reports and observations of signs and symptoms associated with abnormal fluid balance, which may relate to pre-existing or acute conditions. For example, late-stage dehydration may be suspected if a client reports feeling dry, thirsty, passing infrequent dark urine, constipation, headaches or dizziness. Similarly, late-stage dehydration in babies may be suspected through observations of increased pulse and respiration rate, drowsiness, infrequent urination and bowel movements and sunken fontanelles. Over hydration may be detected through systemic generalised puffiness, pulmonary changes such as rales or wheezing and excessive urinary excretion. Fluid balance monitoring awareness is a fundamental skill in effective maternity care and is relevant to all care settings whether it be a home or level 1–3 care environments.

Recommendations from triennial confidential enquires outline the clinical importance of accurate fluid balance in the management of pathological conditions of childbirth and the prevention of associated morbidities. In addition, basic clinical skills such as fluid balance monitoring underpin best management in Practical Obstetric Multi-Professional Training (PROMPT) and in situations such as basic life support, anaesthetic emergencies, pre-eclampsia/eclampsia, sepsis and major obstetric haemorrhage.

Fluid balance monitoring can be an important step in detecting deviations from normality at any stage in the childbirth continuum. The promotion of professional, holistic woman and baby-centred clinical decision making are essential features of effective care and fluid monitoring may be required as part of antenatal, intrapartum and postnatal care planning, assessment, management and evaluation. For example, in antenatal care, fluid monitoring may be required in the management of: pre-existing medical conditions; hyperemesis gravidarum; pre-eclampsia/eclampsia; hemolysis, elevated liver enzymes, low platelet count (HELLP) syndrome; gestational diabetes; or antepartum haemorrhage. Intrapartum fluid balance may be required during epidural analgesia, augmentation of labour and instrumental or surgical births. In addition, fluid management may be required in postnatal care in acute situations such as postpartum haemorrhage, neonatal and maternal collapse, sepsis, urinary retention or where there has been maternal trauma to the bladder or genital tract.

The national guidance recommends that a documented individualised care plan is developed with the woman and that healthcare professionals demonstrate competencies in recognising abnormalities. In assessing the need for managed fluid balance care, the client's clinical history and observations such as temperature, pulse, blood pressure and skin condition may be considered. NICE guidance specifically addresses the prevention of urinary retention, recommending that if urination has not occurred within 6 hours after birth that bladder volume should be assessed with catheterisation considered. In addition, urinary output may be measured to evaluate morbidities and interventions to treat urinary incontinence.

Various tests are undertaken in maternal and neonatal fluid balance management and aim to assess information on systemic acid base balance and kidney function. Urinalysis may be done to determine pH, protein, blood, glucose content and osmolality. Assessments of blood chemistry is often done to evaluate full blood count and haemocrit profiles, creatinine, glucose, urea and electrolytes levels of sodium, potassium, chloride and bicarbonate. Accurate record keeping, charting and handover reviews are imperative responsibilities of care.

How to undertake accurate fluid balance

- Note the ambient care temperature – hot environments exacerbate sweating and moisture loss through respiration.
- Explain the rationale and indication with the client or parent.
- Encourage questions and participation in monitoring processes.
- Establish the time parameters for recording and review, e.g. hourly, 4 hourly, daily.
- Maintain infection control through before and after hand washing.
- Measure all oral intake.
- Urinary output is measured either by collecting urine in a calibrated jug or via temporary or self-retaining closed drainage catheter.
- Oliguria less than 30 mL output per hour is an indication of poor renal perfusion.
- Note intravenous intake and output.
- Drain output.
- Record findings on fluid balance chart (Figure 59.1) and/or in contemporaneous notes as per local policy and procedure.
- Maintain observations such as temperature, pulse, respirations and blood pressure as specified.
- Review clinical situation with relevant healthcare professionals in the multiprofessional team.
- Assess for complications and response to clinical care, e.g. hypo- or hypervolemia, pulmonary oedema, altered blood pathology.
- Review any associated medication requirements, e.g. women with hypertensive conditions may need adjustments in the dose and timing of drugs such as methyldopa, labetalol, hydralazine and calcium antagonists.
- In critical care, central venous pressure assessments may be used to avoid over perfusion.
- Report and document all findings.

60 Peak flow measurement in the woman

Figure 60.1 Peak flow meter.

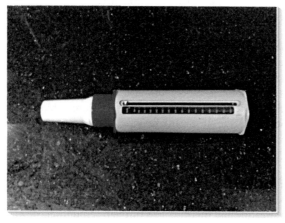

Figure 60.2 Taking a peak flow measurement.

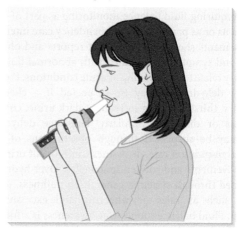

Figure 60.3 Example of a peak flow chart.

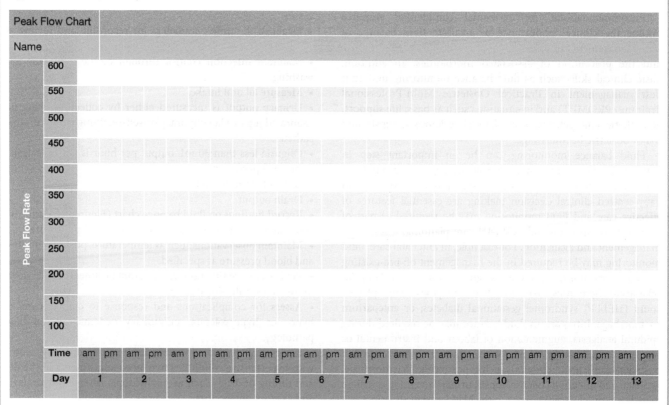

Peak Flow Chart		
Name		

Peak Flow Rate	Time	am	pm	am	pm	am	pm	am	pm	am	pm	am	pm	am	pm	am	pm	am	pm	am	pm	am	pm	am	pm	am	pm
600																												
550																												
500																												
450																												
400																												
350																												
300																												
250																												
200																												
150																												
100																												
	Day	1		2		3		4		5		6		7		8		9		10		11		12		13	

Key point

Midwives play an important role in supporting women in taking their peak flow readings and discussing with the woman the implications of the results for her pregnancy and ongoing care.

Midwifery Skills at a Glance, First Edition. Edited by Patricia Lindsay, Carmel Bagness and Ian Peate.
© 2018 John Wiley & Sons, Ltd. Published 2018 by John Wiley & Sons, Ltd.

This chapter overviews care in relation to taking a peak flow reading. The chapter explores principles of professional practice when supporting a woman to take a peak flow reading; it also provides a step by step approach to peak flow measurement.

Healthcare practitioners have an important role in promoting evidence-based practice and understanding the physiological basis of care is an essential professional accountability. As the result of hormonal, biochemical and skeletal adaptations in childbirth, the maternal respiratory system undergoes significant adaptations during pregnancy and childbirth. Progesterone is known to affect the biochemical function of the respiratory centre by regulating metabolic processes through detection of carbon dioxide and increasing arterial oxygen uptake. In addition, the effect of progesterone and relaxin on intercostal muscle elasticity enhances mechanical skeletal changes such as the displacement of the diaphragm and ribcage by the gravid uterus.

Usually, physiological changes to the respiratory system during childbirth do not cause any serious complications. However, in some cases midwives are supporting women who may experience an exacerbation or acute onset of respiratory pathology. National clinical guidance identifies the importance supporting those with asthma, a chronic long-term disease of the respiratory tract. Furthermore, the Confidential Enquiries into Maternal Mortality reports have noted the importance of detecting and treating asthma in childbirth as it is an attributable cause of maternal deaths (De Swiet 2011).

Clinical assessments to measure respiratory function include the following:

• Minute volume – the amount of air per minute taken into and out of the lungs
• Tidal volume – the amount of inspired and expired air in a breath
• Vital capacity – the maximum amount of air that can be forcibly exhaled with maximum inspiration
• Functional residual capacity – the amount of air at resting expiration
• Blood gases – serum arterial oxygen, carbon dioxide, bicarbonate and pH.

Woman-centred approaches to care enable midwives to assess, plan, diagnose, implement and evaluate appropriate interventions. The support of a woman to take their peak flow may be a useful parameter to assess any deterioration or stabilisation in condition. It is important to assess her knowledge of the reason and process of taking a peak flow and to allow sufficient time for instruction, demonstration and clarification of any questions. Women are often anxious to discuss any implications for their unborn baby and informing them of informational resources, including websites, is an important consideration.

Commonly, a peak flow reading is taken to assess the woman's vital capacity – the measurement of how well air is blown out of the lungs. Lower readings can indicate a blockage or narrowing of airways and further discussion may be required to explore treatment options, which may range from a conservative 'watch and wait' approach to more active treatment interventions.

How to assist a woman in doing a peak flow reading

See Figures 60.1 and 60.2.
• The midwife washes hands.
• Take a clean mouthpiece and attach to the peak flow meter.
• Make sure the dial marker is set at zero.
• Ensure the woman is in a comfortable standing or sitting position.
• Ask the woman to breathe in as much air as possible and hold the inspiration.
• Ask her to form a tight lip seal around the mouthpiece.
• Ask her to breathe out as much air as possible.
• Note the position of the dial.
• Record and if appropriate report the measurement.
• Repeat the steps above and take the 'best of three' recording, if the woman's condition permits.
• Compare the reading with previous measurements.
• Document findings (Figure 60.3).
• Raise any questions with an expert healthcare professional.
• The midwife washes hands.
• Clean and store equipment for next use.

Ongoing care may involve the implementation of a personalised care plan and/or referral for further tests and diagnostics such as spirometry, X rays and lung function tests. Peak flow measurements may be an important factor in deciding options, which may include initiation of treatment with bronchodilators, steroids or beta2 antagonist medication. Midwives have an important role in promoting holistic health strategies that potentiate maternal, fetal and neonatal health.

MEOWS, AVPU, GCS and SBAR

Figure 61.1 An example MEOWS chart.

A HOSPITAL MEOWS CHART

Name									
Hospital No.		Date of birth							
		Ward							

Date									
Time									

Temp	39								
	38								
	37								
	36								
	35								

Systolic BP	200								
	180								
	160								
	140								
	120								
	100								
	80								
	60								

Diastolic BP	140								
	120								
	100								
	80								
	60								
	40								

Heart rate	160								
	140								
	120								
	100								
	80								
	60								
	40								

Resp rate	> 30								
	21–29								
	11–20								
	0–10								

O₂ sats	> 95%								
	< 95%								

Urine urinalysis									

Pain score									

NEURO	Alert								
	Voice								
	Pain								
	Unresponsive								

Table 61.1 AVPU.

Alert	Are they awake and alert?
Voice	Do they only respond when you speak?
Pain	Do they only respond to a painful stimulus?
Unresponsive	Are they unresponsive to all stimuli?

Table 61.2 Glasgow Coma Scale.

EYES	VOICE	MOVEMENT	
		Obey commands	6
	Orientated	Localising	5
Spontaneous	Confused	Normal flexion	4
Move to sound	Words	Abnormal flexion	3
Move to pressure	Sounds	Extension	2
None	None	None	1

Key points

- All charts, scores and handovers are only as good as the person undertaking them.
- Be meticulous in completing all aspects.
- Make sure to document findings and refer appropriately.

Table 61.3 SBAR Handover.

SBAR	Example
Situation	Hi, is that the obstetric reg? It's Louise, midwife on LW. I'm phoning about Jane Smith who was admitted feeling unwell. I am concerned that she may have sepsis.
Background	She is a 27 years old, para 2, and previously fit and well. She is 5 days postnatal, following a forceps delivery. She reports flu-like symptoms for a couple of days, but felt very unwell this morning. She has been referred by her GP and arrived on LW 10 minutes ago.
Assessment	Airway – Can speak Breathing – Resps 27, 90% sats on 15 litres O₂ Circulation – Pulse 100, BP 100/60 Disability – she is a bit argumentative, BM 7.7mmols Exposure – Temp 35.8°C and says she is feeling cold.
Recommendation	I have started 15 litres of O₂, please come and review her immediately.

Midwifery Skills at a Glance, First Edition. Edited by Patricia Lindsay, Carmel Bagness and Ian Peate.
© 2018 John Wiley & Sons, Ltd. Published 2018 by John Wiley & Sons, Ltd.

Modified Early Obstetric Warning System (MEOWS) charts (Figure 61.1) were recommended by the UK Confidential Enquiry into Maternal Death in 2007 as a visual aid to detect trends in observations for women in the childbirth continuum. Many NHS Hospital Trusts in the UK have adapted these charts for their own use and this means that there is no standardisation of MEOWS charts; however, we will look at some of their common elements. The principle of a MEOWS chart is that a score is allocated to the findings of the observations to inform what action needs to be taken by the midwife. This can either be a numerical score or a traffic light system.

Most MEOWS charts contain an area to note the time and dates of the observations and chart respirations, temperature, pulse, diastolic and systolic blood pressure and oxygen saturations. As discussed in Chapter 57, timely completion and documentation of observations is essential in recognising trends that may indicate a woman whose condition is deteriorating. In addition to the observations, urine output and urinalysis, pain score and neurological response using AVPU or GCS are often documented.

Alert, Voice, Pain, Unresponsive (AVPU, Table 61.1) is a simple scale that allows a rapid assessment of the consciousness level of a patient, which is recommended by the UK Resuscitation Council. It is easily used by midwives who are unfamiliar with more comprehensive neurological assessment tools such as the Glasgow Coma Scale. It assesses whether a patient is *alert*; this means that they are conscious, coherent and able to maintain their own airway and are physiologically compensating for any illness. If a patient is only responding to *voice* stimuli they are likely to be feeling very unwell and need referral to a senior member of the multiprofessional team. If they only respond to *pain* (or pressure) stimuli such as a trapezium (the muscle that runs between the neck and the shoulder on either side) squeeze they are becoming unconscious and, again, urgent referral is needed. If the patient is *unresponsive* to all stimuli then it is likely that basic life support measures such as airway, breathing and circulation should be implemented until the multiprofessional team arrives.

The **Glasgow Coma Scale** (GCS) (Table 61.2) was developed in 1974 to provide a structured method of assessing patients with brain injuries, but has been adopted by the World Health Organisation as the standard for neurological assessment. Although the overall score is important, the individual categories must be considered and changes referred to the appropriate senior staff for action even if the overall score remains the same. Its use allows trends to be identified and communicated within the multiprofessional team and it is widely used worldwide.

The GCS assesses three aspects of neurological function and allocates a number to each function and responsiveness. The numbers from each aspect are combined to give an overall score. The first element are the eyes. The practitioner needs to assess whether they open spontaneously, or open to sound, to pressure or not at all. Next, the patient's verbal response is assessed. Are they well orientated? Can they have a confused conversation? Do they respond to speech with some words, some sounds or not at all? Finally, the patient's motor control is assessed. Can they obey commands to move? Are they moving towards localised stimulus of pain or pressure? Do they have normal flexion to be able to withdraw from stimulus? Are limbs abnormally flexed? Are limbs abnormally extended? Do they have no motor control?

A GCS of 15 usually indicates someone who is healthy with no brain injury, while a score of 8 or lower indicates someone who is comatose and early referral to senior staff is essential. At this level the patient would need to be cared for in a high-dependency or intensive care setting. A score 3 is a patient that is totally unresponsive.

Situation, Background, Assessment, Recommendation (SBAR) (Table 61.3) is the handover tool recommended by the UK Resuscitation Council on their courses. It provides a systematic approach to handover between different members of the multiprofessional team and ensures that the important information is communicated. Some organisations have developed their own handover tools using different acronyms, but it is likely that they contain similar information.

When a handover begins the midwife should explain the *situation* and ensure who they are speaking to, introduce themselves and identify which patient they are handing over with an indication of why they are concerned about them. *Background* gives an overview of the reason for their admission and an overview of their medical history. The use of an extended *assessment* tool such as ABCDE (airway, breathing, circulation, disability, exposure) will give a clear picture of the current observations. The last element of the handover tool is a *recommendation*. This will ensure that the midwife makes it clear what they have done already, and what action they want to be taken by the person they are handing over to, and gives a time frame for this action.

62 Care of the deceased

Figure 62.1 Flow chart.

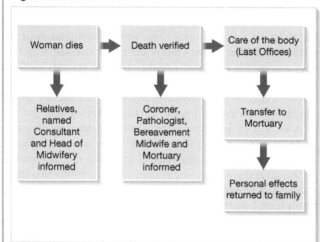

Woman dies → Death verified → Care of the body (Last Offices)

↓ ↓ ↓

Relatives, named Consultant and Head of Midwifery informed

Coroner, Pathologist, Bereavement Midwife and Mortuary informed

Transfer to Mortuary

↓

Personal effects returned to family

Box 62.1 Equipment.

Personal protective equipment (PPE)

Disposable washing bowl

Toiletries: soap, flannel, towel, mouth-care equipment, brush or comb

Clean bed linen including a sheet to wrap the body

2 Identification labels

Dressings, surgical tape and waterproof tape

Shroud or woman's own clothing

Plastic bags, sharps bins and linen skips

Record book and bag for woman's personal property

Documentation required e.g. notification of death forms

Figure 62.2 Hospital shroud.

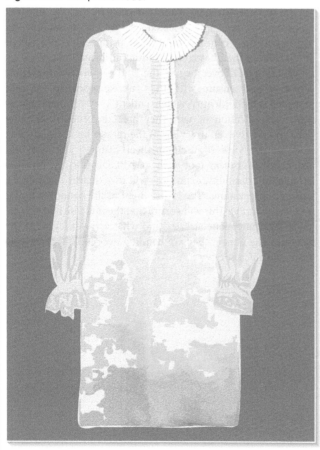

Box 62.2 Personal care of the deceased.

1. Ensure privacy and dignity of the woman at all times. Any religious requirements must be ascertained.
2. Collect all equipment required and don PPE.
3. Roll the woman onto her back, straighten the limbs and close the eyes. Ensure compliance with local manual handling policy at all times.
4. Remove all pillows except one and support the jaw.
5. Remove all jewellery unless otherwise requested. If rings are left in place they must be fixed with tape.
6. Cover wounds or open drainage sites with an absorbent dressing. These should then be covered with an occlusive dressing or waterproof tape.
7. Leave intravenous access lines or drainage tubing, including urinary catheters, in place, sealed with a cap or spigot to prevent leakage. Complete a body map to mark the sites.
8. Wash the body, clean the mouth and brush / comb the hair.
9. Dress the woman in either her own clothes or a white hospital shroud (Figure 62.2).
10. One identification label is attached to a wrist and another to an ankle. Toe tags are not used.
11. A notice of death / body identification form (or other similar document) is taped to the outside of the clothing.
12. Wrap the woman in a sheet, ensuring that the face is covered and the limbs are straight. Tape the sheet closed, but not too tightly.
13. If the body is leaking fluids it must be placed in a cadaver bag.
14. A second notice of death / body identification label is taped to the sheet or cadaver bag.
15. A label indicating that cannulae and/or lines are in situ is also fixed to the outer covering.

Key point

Last Offices is the final care maternity staff give to a deceased woman. It is a privilege to undertake and must be carried out respectfully, competently and in compliance with legal and policy requirements. The management of care of the deceased has a lasting impact on the family and the process of mourning.

Midwifery Skills at a Glance, First Edition. Edited by Patricia Lindsay, Carmel Bagness and Ian Peate.
© 2018 John Wiley & Sons, Ltd. Published 2018 by John Wiley & Sons, Ltd.

Care of a deceased woman

The death of a woman in childbirth is a tragedy, which requires sensitive and careful management. While this is a rare event it is essential that staff caring for the deceased know how to do so (Figure 62.1). The term 'last offices' refers to care of a deceased patient prior to transfer to the mortuary. All legal and cultural requirements must be complied with and all care recorded in the notes.

The Coroner's Office is informed of the death and any Coroner's Office instructions must be observed. Staff should refer to local policy for managing a maternal death and handling of the deceased. The procedure of last offices is not carried out until death is verified.

As the body may present an infection risk, careful hand hygiene must be observed and cuts covered. Personal protective equipment must be used when carrying out last offices (Box 62.1). Care must be taken to avoid cross-infection of other patients and not to contaminate the environment. Last offices are carried out before rigor mortis starts (Box 62.2) (2–4 hours after death) and by two members of staff. Avoid actions that may leave long-lasting marks such as binding the jaw. Body orifices are not packed and in the case of a maternal death all venous access and drainage tubes must be left in situ. The site of each device should be marked on a body map, which should accompany the deceased to the mortuary. A label indicating that access or drainage lines are still *in situ* should also be attached to the outer sheet or cadaver bag.

The personal belongings are checked and recorded by two members of staff. These are returned to the relatives. When recording jewellery or other potentially high-value items it is usual practice to avoid naming gems or precious metals. For example a gold ring would be described as 'yellow metal'.

The identity of the patient is checked again before transfer. The body is transported to the mortuary in a concealment trolley. Staff should ensure that other patients and visitors are guided away from corridors and other public spaces while the body is removed.

Care of a deceased infant

Staff may be involved in care of a deceased baby if there has been an intrauterine death, stillbirth or early neonatal death. The wishes of the parents must be ascertained. Many parents wish to see and hold their baby but they should not be persuaded to do so if they appear reluctant. Staff should remember that in cases of intrauterine death maceration begins within hours. (Maceration means softening by soaking and refers to the degenerative changes that begin after death *in utero*. The fetal skin may peel and become discoloured. Over time other tissues are affected.) This may affect the appearance at birth. Memory building is important and photographs and other mementoes such as hand and foot prints may be taken. If the parents do not want to keep these at the time they should be stored in the notes. The baby is cared for, washed and dressed in accordance with the parents' wishes, and must be treated with gentleness and respect at all times. The infant's name (if given) must be used when speaking of the baby. The baby is usually kept on the ward with the parents and some hospitals have a cold cot, that is, a refrigerated cot, for infants who die around birth. If the baby is transferred to the mortuary a Moses basket or suitably sized transport coffin should be used. Before transfer the baby must be clearly labelled and a label attached to the Moses basket or coffin. Unless this is a Coroner's case, the parents may take the baby home if they wish. The parents will want an explanation as to why the baby died and they will be asked for consent to a post-mortem examination. They may refuse and their wishes should be respected.

The correct registration procedures must be followed after the death and options for funeral arrangements explained. The woman should be informed that she will start to lactate and simple care/comfort remedies discussed. She should be offered a lactation suppressant.

If there was any sign of life at birth the case is referred to the Coroner, regardless of gestation.

In all cases, whether a mother or baby has died, all conversations and decisions must be recorded in the notes. The Bereavement Officer must be informed. Parents must be offered support and given contact details for groups such as SANDS.

Service user's view

'Bereavement isn't an illness and it never goes away, you just have to learn to live with it.'
  Ben Palmer, whose wife died of septicaemia. Jessica's Trust 2008

63 Recognising deterioration in the neonate

Table 63.1 Neonatal observations.

Parameter	Normal Values	Deviations	Comments
Heart Rate	120–160 beats/min	<100 bradycardia >180 tachycardia	Measure apical beat by using a stethoscope (bell side) between the nipples and to the left of the sternum
Respiratory Rate	40–60 breaths/min	Apnoea (cessation of breathing >20 seconds) >60 tachypnoea	Infants have periodic breathing, therefore always count for 1 full minute
Temperature	36.5–37.2°C	36–36.4°C cold stress 32–36°C moderate hypothermia <32°C severe hypothermia	Axilla temperature Use digital thermometer
Capillary Refill Time	<2 seconds	Prolonged if > 3 seconds	Press or blanch skin for 5 seconds and then count how many seconds it takes for perfusion or colour to return
Urine Output	≥ 1 mL per hour	< 1 mL per hour oliguria	A neonate should have at least 4 wet nappies a day

Figure 63.1 Signs of the deteriorating or unwell neonate.

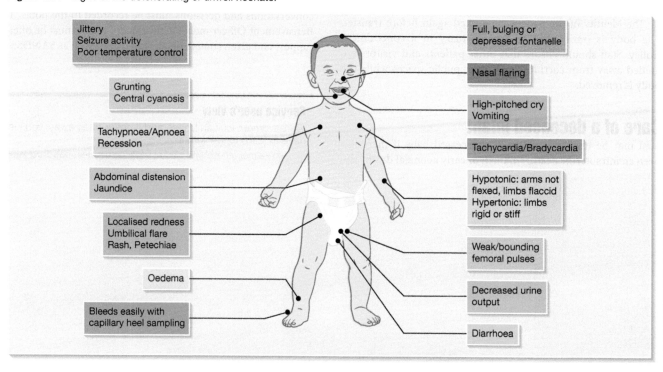

Jittery
Seizure activity
Poor temperature control

Grunting
Central cyanosis

Tachypnoea/Apnoea
Recession

Abdominal distension
Jaundice

Localised redness
Umbilical flare
Rash, Petechiae

Oedema

Bleeds easily with
capillary heel sampling

Full, bulging or
depressed fontanelle

Nasal flaring

High-pitched cry
Vomiting

Tachycardia/Bradycardia

Hypotonic: arms not
flexed, limbs flaccid
Hypertonic: limbs
rigid or stiff

Weak/bounding
femoral pulses

Decreased urine
output

Diarrhoea

Key point

Parental observations and concerns about their baby's behaviour, temperature, feeding and bodily functions should *not* be ignored.

Midwifery Skills at a Glance, First Edition. Edited by Patricia Lindsay, Carmel Bagness and Ian Peate.
© 2018 John Wiley & Sons, Ltd. Published 2018 by John Wiley & Sons, Ltd.

Early recognition of the unwell and/or deteriorating neonate is essential to ensure a timely referral, diagnosis, treatment and management to prevent problems that can lead to increased morbidity and even death.

Signs of deterioration

Deterioration can be very obvious or initially non-specific. Neonates can deteriorate very quickly, so early recognition is essential. The midwife must have the knowledge and skills to recognise normal and to be able to identify deviation from the normal or what is normal for a particular baby (Table 63.1).

In adults and children early warning scoring systems are well developed to assist the practitioner to identify deterioration. The Neonatal Early Warning (NEW) tool is an example of tools being developed to assist midwives in recognising deterioration in neonates following delivery, on the postnatal wards and during community visits.

The signs of deterioration will be discussed using a systems approach. Parental observations of changes in their infant's behaviour, temperature, feeding and bodily functions should not be ignored (Figure 63.1).

Neurological presenting signs could include:

- Irritability
- Sucks poorly
- Unresponsive
- High-pitched cry
- Jitteriness
- Full, bulging or depressed fontanelle
- Listlessness/lethargy
- Vomiting
- Hypo/hypertonic
- Seizure activity
- Temperature change.

Parents may observe and report an increase in their baby's sleepiness, decrease in activity, the baby lies not flexed but with arms at their side, baby feels hot or cold and the temperature cannot be explained by the baby's environment. Their baby may cry a lot and appears inconsolable.

Cardiovascular presenting signs could include:

- Tachycardia
- Pale
- Mottled
- Decreased urine output
- Oedema
- Poor cutaneous circulation resulting in a delayed capillary refill time
- Weak/bounding femoral pulses.

Parents may observe and report a decrease in the number of wet nappies their baby produces (less than four wet nappies in 24 hours should cause concern and should be reported).

Respiratory presenting signs could include:

- Tachypnoea
- Apnoea
- Nasal flaring
- Recession
- Grunting
- Cyanosis.

Parents may observe and report that their baby is breathing faster than usual and that they have noted blueness around the mouth. They may note that the baby makes an unusual noise when breathing.

Gastrointestinal presenting signs could include:

- Not interested in feeding
- Vomiting
- Diarrhoea
- Poor weight gain/weight loss greater than 10%
- Abdominal distension.

Parents may observe and report a decreased interest to feed and if bottle feeding the baby taking less than 50% of the usual volume in 24 hours, stools become watery and have passed at least six in the past 24 hours, an episode of vomiting or frequent vomiting, which could be digested, undigested, bile-stained and contain fresh or dark blood. They may have also noted that the baby's mouth and gums have become dry.

Hepatic presenting signs could include:

- Jaundice
- Altered coagulation (heel stabs for glucose sampling, bilirubin levels and blood spot screening do not readily stop bleeding).

Parents may observe and report that their baby looks yellow, especially the nose and white of the eyes.

Skin presenting signs could include:

- Petechiae
- Rash
- Localised heat and redness.

Parents may comment that the base of the cord is red or the cord is 'mucky'.

Additional signs

Midwifery is guided by evidence that includes knowledge gained from experience/continuity in care, resulting in the midwife suspecting a problem or all is not well, even though there are no overt or even non-specific signs yet to be observed. These are described as tacit or intuitive signs and can also be expressed by parents. Common expressions of concern include:

- 'She's just not right'
- 'He handled better yesterday'
- 'She doesn't seem to want to feed'
- 'Very sleepy, yesterday he was full of beans'.

Referral

Any concerns should be brought to the attention of appropriate personal such as a mentor/senior midwife, a paediatrician, neonatologist or advanced neonatal nurse practitioner. The referral, depending upon the condition and degree of concern, should be made in a timely manner. Effective interprofessional working and communication can be achieved by using the SBAR framework (situation, background, assessment, recommendation).

Causes of deterioration

Deterioration of an infant can be as a result of a variety of problems or conditions. These include infection, hypoglycaemia, respiratory conditions and congenital abnormality (e.g. bowel obstruction, congenital heart disease).

Neonatal infection is a leading cause of deterioration during the neonatal period. Midwives need to be knowledgeable of the risk factors and red flags that can result in early-onset infection (neonate is <72 hours old) associated with group β streptococcus (NICE 2012).

Service user's view

'All was well at birth, we cuddled, we had a good breastfeed. While feeding on the postnatal ward, he suddenly turned blue and stopped breathing. My midwife took him and he started breathing. He had to go to the neonatal unit. I was very scared.'

Verbal communication, service user, London

64 Neonatal jaundice

Table 64.1 Bilirubin metabolism.

Stage	Where	What happens
Production	Liver & spleen	Bilirubin is a by-product of the breakdown of haem mostly from old, immature or malformed red blood cells removed from circulation. This bilirubin is unconjugated and fat soluble.
Transport	Circulation	Unconjugated bilirubin which is free or unbound in the blood will readily deposit in fatty tissues (skin and brain). Unconjugated bilirubin binds to albumin molecules, where together it is unable to move out of circulation into fatty tissue. Albumin safely transports unconjugated bilirubin to the liver for conjugation. If billirubin production increases, all the sites on the albumin for binding get used up. This can result in free unconjugated bilirubin in the blood that can move into fatty tissues.
Conjugation	Liver	Unconjugated bilirubin is transported into the liver by intercellular proteins via carrier-mediated diffusion to the smooth endoplasmic reticulum for conjugation. Unconjugated bilirubin, glucose, oxygen, glucoronic acid and enzyme results in the formation of bilirubin glucoronide or water-soluble bilirubin which can now be excreted.
Excretion	Bowel	95% of bilirubin glucuronide is excreted into bile and eventually into the gut where it is catabolised by intestinal bacteria into urobilinogen. Most urobilinogen (99%) is excreted in the stools as stercobilinogen and 1% is reabsorbed from the colon and excreted via the kidneys as urine. In the small bowel, conjugated bilirubin can be cleaved by the enzyme β-glucuronidase converting it back to unconjugated bilirubin. A small portion of this unconjugated bilirubin is then reabsorbed from the small bowel into the bloodstream, where it rebinds to albumin, travels to the liver and undergoes the process of conjugation again. This process is called enterohepatic shunting (EHS).

Red Blood Cell
Haem — Globin & Iron (stored)
Biliverdin
Unconjugated Bilirubin
Binds with albumin — Skin / Brain — EHS
Liver – for conjugation / – excreted in bile
Bowel — Kidney
Stercobilinogen (stool in nappy)   Urine in nappy

Table 64.2 Causes of physiological and pathological jaundice for each stage of metabolism.

Stage	Physiological Jaundice	Pathological Jaundice
Production	Shortened RBC lifespan. Neonates have more RBCs per kg than adults. RBC production is inefficient therefore more immature, malformed cells. Enterohepatic shunting	Conditions that lead to haemolysis e.g. infection; congenital abnormalities like spherocytosis, ABO, Rh disease; enzyme deficiencies like G6PD and galactosemia; enclosed haemorrhage like bruising, cephalohaematoma and polycythaemia
Transport	Neonates have less albumin, especially those born premature	Albumin levels are even lower in malnourished infants. Drugs that compete for albumin binding sites. Hypothermia and acidosis interfere with albumin binding. Total parenteral nutrition
Conjugation	Neonates are initially low in intracellular carrier proteins. Conjugation enzyme activity is low for the first 24 hours after birth. The activity level is even lower in the preterm baby	Hypoxemia (oxygen is required for liver function/conjugation). Hypoglycaemia (glucose is needed for conjugation). Decreased liver perfusion (hypoxic and ischaemic episodes). Sepsis can alter the liver's ability to function/conjugate. Endocrine disorders can affect conjugation enzyme activity
Excretion	Enterohepatic shunting is increased due to decreased gut flora, resulting in less conjugated bilirubin converting to urobilinogen and available to be cleaved to unconjugated bilirubin by β-glucuronidase	Any cause of gut obstruction e.g. atresia, meconium ileus. Hepatic obstruction e.g. biliary atresia, cystic fibrosis. Biliary stasis caused by hepatitis or other obstruction. Saturation of protein carriers that carry conjugated bilirubin into the biliary tree (backlog)

Key point

To help ease parental anxiety, ensure parent's questions are answered and that they are kept up to date of their infant's progress, using language and literature that is parent friendly.

Midwifery Skills at a Glance, First Edition. Edited by Patricia Lindsay, Carmel Bagness and Ian Peate.
© 2018 John Wiley & Sons, Ltd. Published 2018 by John Wiley & Sons, Ltd.

Jaundice occurs when bilirubin accumulates in the extravascular fatty tissues (skin and brain). Jaundice in the newborn is common, occurring in over two-thirds of term infants and even more frequently in the preterm infant. In order to provide informed care for a jaundiced baby and parents it is important to have an understanding of bilirubin metabolism. There are four stages involved in bilirubin metabolism. Alterations at any of these stages can result in jaundice (Table 64.1).

Physiological versus pathological jaundice

Jaundice is classified as physiological or pathological. Physiological jaundice is normal. It does not present on day 1. Serum bilirubin (SBR) levels will peak by day 4 and reduces by day 14. Pathological jaundice, on the other hand, should raise concern and always requires further investigation. Pathological jaundice can present on day 1 or it can be prolonged, persistent after day 14 in the term infant or day 21 in the preterm infant. Causes of physiological and pathological jaundice can be linked to each stages of metabolism (Table 64.2).

Breast milk jaundice

There is controversy in the literature as to how to classify breast milk jaundice. It is important not to imply that breast milk jaundice is harmful, thereby influencing a mother's choice not to breastfeed. The use of early versus late onset is preferred by many over using the terms physiological or pathological jaundice.

Early onset

The impact of feeding frequency can be a contributing cause of jaundice in the breastfed baby. Feeding stimulates the gastrocolonic reflex and increases intestinal motility, clearance of meconium and conjugated bilirubin from the gut. Mothers do not initially produce sufficient quantities of milk for the demand-fed infant unlike bottle-fed infants who are given calculated amounts at regular intervals. Small-volume feeds result in less frequent and smaller stools, increasing enterohepatic shunting, and a caloric deficiency, increasing circulating free fatty acids which can displace unconjugated bilirubin from albumin.

Late onset

Breast milk inhibits the development of bacterial gut flora and the making of urobilinogen. Breast milk contains high levels of β-glucuronidase, increasing the cleaving of conjugated bilirubin/urobilinogen back to unconjugated bilirubin. As the breastfed baby is more efficient at absorption, the overall result is an increase in enterohepatic shunting.

Toxicity

High levels of unconjugated bilirubin can result in damage to the basal ganglia in the brain causing kernicterus and damage to the 8th cranial nerve, resulting in sensorineural hearing loss. Assessment and management is essential to prevent these complications. National guidelines are available and include treatment thresholds/graphs and algorithms on investigations, management of jaundice, including phototherapy and exchange transfusions.

Assessing for jaundice

Jaundice can be assessed by examining the skin and eyes. The sclera or 'white' of the eye and skin when pressed will be yellow.

Jaundice develops in a 'head to tail' direction – first the head, then body and finally the limbs. Jaundice should be quantified and this can be done by transcutaneous devices and blood sampling.

Management of neonatal jaundice

If the underlying cause of jaundice is treatable then this should be treated. It is also important to ensure that the infant's stages of metabolism are supported by ensuring the baby is given adequate food (glucose is needed for conjugation) and drink (to ensure excretion and minimise enterohepatic shunting). Careful plotting of SBR levels on treatment threshold graphs for the infant's gestation will indicate the when the baby requires phototherapy or an exchange transfusion. Babies with rapidly increasing SBRs or potentially in need of an exchange transfusion should be cared for on the neonatal unit.

Phototherapy is the usual treatment for neonatal jaundice and it is used to curtail the rise of unconjugated bilirubin therefore preventing kernicterus. Phototherapy simply converts unconjugated bilirubin into photoisomers of bilirubin, which are water soluble and excretable via the liver into the small bowel. The effects of phototherapy are reversible, so when the light is turned off, the bilirubin transforms back to a fat-soluble molecule.

Two types of phototherapy devices are available. They are conventional or fibre optic. The type of light used is determined by the type and levels of jaundice. Multiple lights or devices can be used to manage high SBR levels. Phototherapy must be delivered effectively and safely. Therapeutic phototherapy is dependent upon the colour or wavelength/spectrum used. Blue-green light is most effective. The irradiance or measurement of the light beams used is determined by the quality of lights used and the distance of the light from the baby. Irradiance decreases as the distance[2] increases, therefore follow manufacturer's advice. Maximum skin exposure to the light is important. The baby ideally should just wear eye pads and a 'bikini' nappy. Unless a baby is at risk of an exchange transfusion, phototherapy can be interrupted for care and feeding.

Babies under phototherapy are at risk of a number of potential problems. Eye pads worn to prevent retinal damage can slip and obstruct the baby's airway causing apnoea. Eyes should be closed prior to applying the eye pads to prevent corneal abrasions and changed daily and if soiled to prevent conjunctivitis. Depending on whether the baby is nursed in an incubator or cot, the baby can develop hypo- or hyperthermia. Conventional phototherapy increases gut transit time and with the increase in radiant heat generated by the light, can increase transepidermal water loss resulting in dehydration, decreased nutrition and weight loss. Phototherapy also causes local histamine release from skin mast cells resulting in a skin rash. Babies under phototherapy tend to be less interested in feeding, providing challenges for the breastfeeding mother. Unlike fibre optic phototherapy, conventional phototherapy creates a barrier and can temporarily increase parent–baby separation.

Service user's view

'A mother stated on seeing her baby for the first time: "She looks more like a neonate than a baby." She later added, "I wanted to hold her but she needed the light. The midwife made sure I had opportunities to hold and feed her."'

Verbal communication, service user, Surrey

65 Hypoglycaemia

Table 65.1 Infants at risk of hypoglycaemia.
Source for pictures: *Neonatology at a Glance*, Third Edition. Edited by Tom Lissauer, Avroy A. Fanaroff, Lawrence Miall and Jonathan Fanaroff. © 2016 John Wiley & Sons, Ltd. Reproduced with permission of John Wiley & Sons.

What babies?		Why at risk?
Preterm (<37 weeks)		<Glycogen stores, therefore unable to counter-regulate Elevated insulin: glucose ratio Glucogenic pathway less mature
Small for gestational age (term twin on left)		<Glycogen stores High brain: body mass ratio ↓ Fat stores Hyperinsulinism leading to failure to counter-regulate
Stress hypoglycaemia due to: Infection Perinatal asphyxia Hypothermia		Despite an ↑ in catecholamines, there is a ↓ ketogenic response Peripheral vasoconstriction can result in availability of substrate needed for gluconeogenesis ↑ In glucose requirements
Transient hyperinsulinism For example infants of diabetic mothers (IDM) For example altered maternal metabolism due to: Intrapartum administration of glucose Maternal drug treatment such as terbutaline, ritodrine or propranolol		Maternal hypoglycaemia leads to fetal hyperglycaemia and ↑ levels of insulin, resulting in hypoglycaemia when separated from placenta Deficient in catecholamines, ↓ of free fatty acids and ketone bodies Can result in an increase in fetal insulin
Fetal hydrops due to: ABO incompatibility Rhesus disease		Red blood cell breakdown leads to release of glutathione which causes increase levels of insulin
Large for gestational age (LGA)		Without evidence of maternal/gestational diabetes, these infants do not require routine blood glucose monitoring

Box 65.1 The signs of hypoglycaemia.

Apathy and hypotonia
Abnormal cry
Feeding difficulties
Tremor, 'jitteriness'
Cyanosis
Tachypnoea
Irritability
Temperature instability
Convulsions

Figure 65.1 Shaded areas show sites for capillary sampling.
Source: *Neonatology at a Glance*, Third Edition. Edited by Tom Lissauer, Avroy A. Fanaroff, Lawrence Miall and Jonathan Fanaroff. © 2016 John Wiley & Sons, Ltd. Reproduced with permission of John Wiley & Sons.

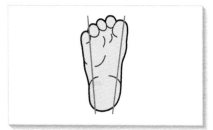

Key points

- If a full term infant is 'not feeding' a blood glucose measurement alone will not be helpful. The infant requires a full clinical assessment.
- Guidance is available to enable midwifery units to develop evidence-based guidelines and review existing guidelines to ensure that they are coherently written.
- It is important that those infants at risk are recognised quickly and managed appropriately as prolonged, severe hypoglycaemia is associated with neurological dysfunction and long-term neurodevelopmental sequelae.

Hypoglycaemia in the newborn occurs when normal metabolic adaptation does not occur in the first few hours after birth. Immediately after birth, newborns experience a transient drop in blood glucose, but this is normal and self-limiting. In utero the fetus consumes glucose in order to grow and concentrate glycogen in the liver. Once born the neonate must produce its own glucose or alternative fuels to supply and meet organ needs (such as the brain) and at the same time adjust to intermittent milk feeding. In order for the infant to maintain metabolic function in the 'fasting state', the infant must counter-regulate. The initial counter-regulatory process is glycogenolysis, or the breakdown of glycogen. When the glycogen stores are exhausted the neonate will form glucose from non-carbohydrate substances such as lactate, pyruvate, glycerol and alanine by releasing hormones such as glucagon, catecholamines, growth hormone and cortisol. This process known as gluconeogenesis takes place in the liver and produces ketone bodies. Ketone bodies are an alternative fuel that can be used by the body. As glucose levels in the well term neonate decrease, ketone bodies have been observed to increase. The brain has an enhanced capacity in the term neonate to utilise ketone bodies for metabolic energy. Therefore, monitoring glucose alone in a well neonate, provides an incomplete picture and any action in response to a low glucose alone can lead to inappropriate action.

Midwifery units should have guidelines available to inform practice on the assessment, investigation and management of infants at risk of hypoglycaemia (Table 65.1).

Normal healthy term infants commonly feed infrequently in the first 24–48 hours of life and cope with low glucose levels because they are able to counter-regulate. Therefore infants who do not have risk factors do not require glucose monitoring providing they are assessed as well. These infants at birth should be offered skin-to-skin contact with mother at delivery and should be put to the breast within an hour of birth to promote metabolic adaptation.

However, the infant who does want to feed should be assessed for wellbeing. This assessment should consider the following:

- Infant's muscle tone
- Temperature
- Colour/perfusion
- Respiration rate
- Level of consciousness.

If any concerns are raised by the assessment or the infant is symptomatic of hypoglycaemia, the infant should be urgently referred to the paediatric team. A blood sugar alone is not helpful, but should be a part of the full assessment undertaken by the paediatric team. Active treatment will be required with a blood glucose of less than 2.6 mmol/L. Please note there is no agreement in the literature as to what is a normal blood glucose. WHO defines hypoglycaemia as a blood glucose less than 2.6 mmol/L, while NICE uses 2.0 mmol/L for infants of diabetic mothers. Whatever value is used, WHO/NICE/locally agreed value, it should be communicated and used by all healthcare team members.

The signs of hypoglycaemia, like infection can be subtle and non-specific or absent (Box 65.1). Signs of hypoglycaemia are often neurological as this is a reflection of the brain's needs for glucose. If any of these signs are observed or reported by parents, the infant should be referred immediately for assessment to the paediatric team.

Managing infants at risk

Managing infants at risk commences at birth and continues until discharge. The infant who is able to enterally feed should be fed ideally within the first hour and observations to assess wellbeing should commence. The paediatric team should be informed of the infant's birth and care to date.

The infant should then be fed again within 3 hours from the initial feed and then continue to feed 3 hourly until blood glucose levels stabilise and are maintained. Prior to the second feed, the midwife must commence blood glucose measurements. These measurements should continue for 48 hours and can be stopped once the infant demonstrates at least two blood glucose levels within the normal range, remains well and continues to feed. The infant's wellbeing should also be assessed and documentation of results and time of feed recorded in the infant's notes. It is important to ensure the parents are kept informed throughout.

Infants with persistently low results (less than what has been locally agreed, for example less than 2.6 mmol/L) will require an urgent consultation from the paediatric team and subsequent transfer to the neonatal unit.

Parents should be provided with ongoing feeding support regardless of feeding methods chosen. Breastfeeding mothers may need support with actual feeding or with expressing breastmilk to ensure colostrum is available for the baby. Whether breast or bottle feeding, parents should be taught to recognise behavioural feeding cues or signs of hunger to enable an early response. These include:

- Waking up
- Restlessness
- Smacking of lips
- Sucking on a fist
- Rooting
- While feeding, opening mouth.
- Short pitched cry, with clear rises and falls

Infants who are unable to maintain their blood glucose may require admission to a neonatal unit. There they may receive additional feeding support, that is, tube feeding or require an IV bolus of glucose followed by a maintenance infusion of dextrose.

Monitoring of glucose should be done by capillary heel sampling and by means of a quality-assured bedside monitoring device. Low values should be confirmed by the laboratory as plasma glucose results may be higher than blood glucose readings.

Care must be taken when performing capillary heel sampling. A precision device appropriate for the size of the baby can avoid complications such as infection, osteomyelitis and bruising. Ensure only the areas shaded on Figure 65.1 are used to prevent these complications. In order to manage pain from heel sampling, consider procedural pain measures such as sucrose, use of a pacifier and skin-to-skin contact with parent.

Service user's view

'He was not keen to feed, he was very sleepy, so the midwife taught me to express my first milk and this was given to him by a tube down his nose to his stomach. It did the trick, his blood sugars stayed normal.'

Verbal communication, service user, London

66 Hypothermia

Figure 66.1 (a, b, c and d) How newborn infants lose heat.
Source: *Neonatology at a Glance*, Third Edition. Edited by Tom Lissauer, Avroy A. Fanaroff, Lawrence Miall and Jonathan Fanaroff. © 2016 John Wiley & Sons, Ltd. Reproduced with permission of John Wiley & Sons.

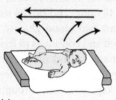

(a)
Convection
Heat is lost to currents of air

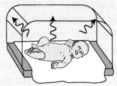

(b)
Radiation
Heat loss via electromagnetic waves from skin to surrounding surfaces

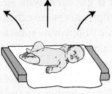

(c)
Evaporation
Heat loss when water evaporates from skin or breath

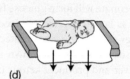

(d)
Conduction
Direct heat loss to solid surfaces with which they are in contact

---

Box 66.1 Recognising hypothermia in the newborn.

		Signs of respiratory distress:		
• Feet and trunk feels cold to touch • Axilla temperature less than 36.5°C	• Poor feeding • Weight loss or poor weight gain • Hypoglycaemia	• Tachypnoea • Nasal flaring • Grunting	• Recession • Cyanosis	• Apnoea • Bradycardia • Lethargy

Figure 66.2 Consequences of cold stress.
Source: Adapted from Thomas K (1994) Thermoregulation in Neonates. *Neonatal Network* 13(2): 15–22.

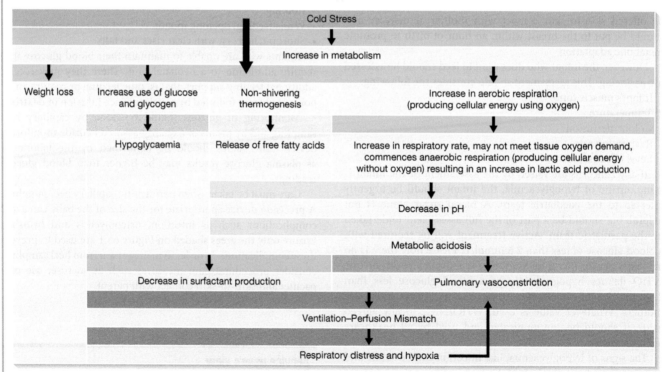

Cold Stress

Increase in metabolism

Weight loss — Increase use of glucose and glycogen — Non-shivering thermogenesis — Increase in aerobic respiration (producing cellular energy using oxygen)

Hypoglycaemia — Release of free fatty acids — Increase in respiratory rate, may not meet tissue oxygen demand, commences anaerobic respiration (producing cellular energy without oxygen) resulting in an increase in lactic acid production

Decrease in pH

Metabolic acidosis

Decrease in surfactant production — Pulmonary vasoconstriction

Ventilation–Perfusion Mismatch

Respiratory distress and hypoxia

Key points
Skin-to-skin contact between mother and baby creates a thermal synergy and is an excellent way of maintaining a baby's temperature or warming a cold preterm/term baby.

Midwifery Skills at a Glance, First Edition. Edited by Patricia Lindsay, Carmel Bagness and Ian Peate.
© 2018 John Wiley & Sons, Ltd. Published 2018 by John Wiley & Sons, Ltd.

Thermoregulation is a critical physiologic function that is closely related to the transition and survival of the infant. An understanding of transitional events and the physiological adaptations that neonates must make is essential to helping the nurse provide an appropriate environment and help infants maintain thermal stability.

Thomas 1994, p.15.

The above quote, a message originally meant for neonatal nurses, is equally apt to midwives working in labour ward or in postnatal care.

Adaptation

Circulating catecholamines are increased in both mother and fetus in response to the stress of labour. This increase in catecholamines helps prepare the fetus for transition to life outside of the uterus by promoting the absorption of fetal lung fluid into the pulmonary interstitium, stimulating the release of pulmonary surfactant, triggering essential metabolic changes and non-shivering thermogenesis. The placenta has a high capacity for inactivation of maternal catecholamines, limiting transfer to the fetus. At delivery once separated from the placenta, a catecholamine surge occurs to initiate non-shivering thermogenesis, enabling the infant to immediately produce heat in response to the lower environmental temperature. Despite this fetal preparation, unless immediate thermal attention is given to maintain the infant's temperature, the infant will be at risk of hypothermia.

Temperature control

Thermoregulation is controlled by the hypothalamus. It receives thermal information from the body skin, deep thermal receptors and receptors found in the preoptic area of the hypothalamus. The hypothalamus compares this information with what is described as the 'set point' (temperature it wants to maintain the body at) and responds by stimulating the pituitary or the sympathetic nervous system (SNS) to allow the infant to conserve, produce or lose heat.

Heat is conserved by:
- Peripheral vasoconstriction
- Flexing extremities towards body.

Heat is produced by:
- Normal metabolic activity
- Muscular activity
- Shivering (at low environmental temperatures only)
- Non-shivering thermogenesis or the metabolism of brown fat/ brown adipose tissue (BAT) in the infant.

BAT starts to develop in the late second trimester and can be found down the vertebral column and around the scapulae, neck, sternum and the adrenal glands. It is well innervated by the SNS and has a rich blood supply resulting in its dark appearance.

Heat is lost by:
- Vasodilatation
- Stretched posture
- Sweating
- Lying very still
- Breathing faster.

Modes of heat loss/ transfer

In addition to physiology, the environment plays a role in how an infant loses or gains heat. Infants lose/ transfer heat by means of the following four modes of heat loss/ transfer:
- Conduction
- Convection
- Evaporation
- Radiation (Figure 66.1).

Understanding these four modes will enable you to prevent heat loss or use them to your advantage when you need to warm an infant. For example, an effective way to warm a term or preterm infant is to ask the mother to provide skin-to-skin or kangaroo care. Skin-to-skin contact uses the direct transfer of heat from the mother to her infant (conduction) to warm and then maintain the infant's temperature.

Why preterm losses are greater than that of term infants

- Immature hypothalamus
- Sweat glands initially do not work, and are functional by day 14
- Larger body surface area to weight ratio
- Produce less body heat per unit surface area
- No shivering
- Will metabolise what brown adipose tissue is available, depleting valuable energy stores
- Thinner skin with less subcutaneous fat
- Skin may only be two or three cells thick or less
- Skin has less keratin, therefore leaks water
- Evaporative heat loss exceeds ability for heat production
- Blood vessels just below skin surface
- Posture.

As a result of mainly the physical characteristics of the premature baby, heat loss/ transfer are different for the term and preterm infant. The full term baby will lose heat by radiation, convection and lastly evaporation. The preterm infant is most vulnerable to evaporation, convection and then radiation. As the surfaces babies are placed on are usually covered with, for example, a blanket or single-use cover, conductive heat losses are less of an issue today. Heat loss in very immature infants is mainly due to evaporation of water from the skin surface. Evaporative heat losses increase with decreasing gestational age, but then decrease as the skin matures and achieves near-term maturity by 2 weeks of age. Therefore, the midwife should remember the gestational differences between term and preterm when addressing thermal care needs at delivery and while delivering postnatal care.

Neutral thermal environment

There are two types of thermal stress. Infants can experience heat or cold stress, the latter being more common. A normal newborn's axillary temperature is 36.5–37.5°C. WHO (1997) defines cold stress as an axillary temperature between 36 and 36.4°C, moderate hypothermia as a temperature between 32 and 35.9°C and severe hypothermia as a temperature less than 32°C. See Box 66.1 for signs of cold stress/ hypothermia. To prevent thermal stress the midwife should nurse the infant in a neutral thermal environment (NTE) or the environment temperature that allows the infant to use the use the least amount of oxygen to maintain a normal temperature. The NTE will vary from baby to baby and is determined by gestational age, postnatal age and the infant's wellbeing. The consequences of thermal stress can increase a baby's morbidity and mortality (Figure 66.2).

67 Wound assessment

Table 67.1 The stages of wound healing.

The stages	Timing	What happens
Haemostasis	Occurs in minutes	Clotting cascade activated Bleeding stops as a result of vasoconstriction and platelet aggregation
Inflammatory response	1–5 days	Release of histamine, increasing capillary permeability and vasodilation Phagocytosis: process when macrophages engulf microbes and secrete growth factors that promote angiogenesis
Regenerative phase/ proliferation	2–21days	Cell recruitment, migration and proliferation Macrophages attract fibroblasts to produce a matrix of collagen, a strengthening protein of connective tissue Formation of granulation tissue
Tissue remodelling/ maturation	14 days to 2 years Timing may vary	Re-epithelialisation Wound contraction Scar tissue formation Avascular tissue, doesn't sweat, grow hair, or tan.

Table 67.2 Factors that may impair wound healing.

Local factors	Systemic factors
• Poor blood supply • Misalignment • Increased skin tension • Wound dehiscence • Poor venous drainage • Presence of foreign body • Infection	• Advancing age • Malnutrition • Obesity/emaciation • Shock of any cause • Immunosuppression • Smoking • Incontinence • Obesity • Vitamins deficiency • Medications (steroids) • Co-morbidities (diabetes) • Lack of adequate healthcare • Poor hygiene

Table 67.3 Promoting wound healing.

Warm compress	Cold compress
• Reduces pain and promotes healing through vasodilation • Increases oxygen and nutrients to aid in inflammatory response • Reduces oedema by promoting removal of excessive interstitial fluid • Promotes muscle relaxation	• Decreases pain by vasoconstriction • Decreased blood flow to the area decreased inflammation and oedema • Raises the threshold of pain receptors thereby decreasing pain • Decreases muscle

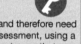

Key point

Midwives have a duty of care and therefore need to be competent in wound assessment, using a holistic approach to identify any issues that may be preventing the wound from healing well.

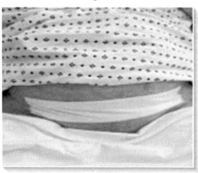

Figure 67.1 Day 1 caesarean section wound with dressing.

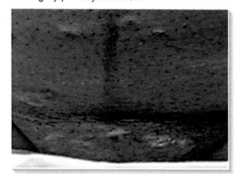

Figure 67.2 Day 8 post caesarean section, healing by primary intention.

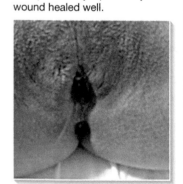

Figure 67.3 Four weeks after forceps delivery. Episiotomy wound healed well.

Figure 67.4 The shiny red area is the production of over granulation tissue, also known as granuloma. It is easily treated with silver nitrate.

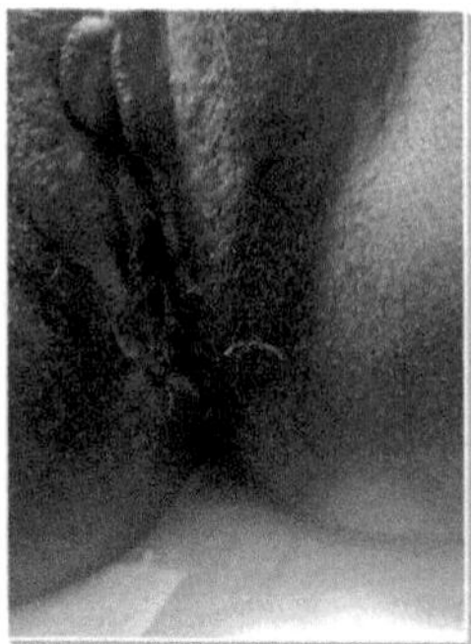

Figure 67.5 Episiotomy wound breakdown, day 4 after ventouse birth.

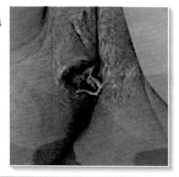

Midwifery Skills at a Glance, First Edition. Edited by Patricia Lindsay, Carmel Bagness and Ian Peate.
© 2018 John Wiley & Sons, Ltd. Published 2018 by John Wiley & Sons, Ltd.

Wound assessment is a vital and dynamic process that can ensure women receive appropriate care to optimise wound healing. It is part of the midwife's role to provide wound care for women who have had perineal trauma and caesarean section. Midwives need to be competent in wound assessment, using a holistic approach to identify any issues that may be preventing the wound from healing well. The use of a standardised assessment tool may be helpful. For example, the Southampton wound scoring system. Stages of wound healing are shown in Table 67.1.

Wound assessment

Assessment of the perineal wound is one area that is often neglected in practice leading, potentially, to ongoing health issues such as perineal wound infections and dehiscence. Similarly, the increase in caesarean births has also triggered a rise in wound care management issues for midwives, such as potential surgical site infections. The burden of wound infections includes maternal mortality, morbidity and lengthy hospital stay, all of which have cost implications. Like all wounds, the healing process is affected by physical, economic, social, psychological, emotional and environmental factors.

Perineal and caesarean section wounds should heal by primary intention as the edges are sutured soon after the trauma (Figures 67.1, 67.2 and 67.3). Factors impinging on wound healing are identified in Table 67.2. The time frame for wound healing is normally within 2–4 weeks (Figure 67.3). During the wound assessment, the following should be observed and recorded in the woman's notes. The list presented below is by no means exhaustive.

Skin: Redness of the surrounding skin, is usually normal. This is due to increased blood flow to the area. However, any redness around the wound lasting several days should be a cause for concern, particularly if the area is warmer and painful.

Exudate: Excessive amount of blood oozing from the wound is not normal and should be addressed. Pressure dressing should be applied over the initial dressing to stop the bleeding. If the bleeding does to stop, refer to the obstetrician for further management. Pus exudate is also a sign of infection.

Odour: Offensive smell is an indication of infection.

Hypergranulation tissue: Excessive growth of tissue beyond the amount required to replace the tissue deficit can delay healing. Hypergranulation is usually present in wounds healing by secondary intention. For example perineal wound dehiscence. It has a red shiny appearance above the level of the surrounding skin (Figure 67.4).

Slough: This is thought to be associated with bacterial activity (Figure 67.5).

Misalignments: The wound edges are not aligned correctly anatomically. This is commonly found with perineal wounds due to poor suturing technique. Misalignment can often cause pain and in some cases lead to wound dehiscence.

Dehiscence: This is when the wound burst open. It is usually treated with antibiotics and allowed to heal by secondary intention (Figure 67.4). In some cases, it may be debrided and resutured. Wound cultures may be taken to determine if there is an infection.

Pain: Pain occurs due to nerve ending damage or toxins from bacteria and pressure from oedema. Persistent pain that is not improving with analgesia is not normal.

Oedema: The occurrence of phagocytosis and increased blood flow to the wound area may cause oedema. This usually subsides within a few days.

Pyrexia. Maternal pyrexia may be an indication of wound infection.

Promoting wound healing

• The wound bed should be moist and the surrounding skin dry. Optimum wound healing occurs in a moist environment.
• Good nutrition is vital to wound healing. The woman should be encouraged to eat food rich in vitamin C and high in protein.
• Good personal hygiene should also be observed to reduce the risk of infection.
• Heat and cold therapy may be used (Table 67.3).
• During the assessment, midwives should be able to recognise their limitations and refer complicated wounds to the appropriate healthcare professional for further management.

68 Wound dressings and drains

Table 68.1 Wound dressings.

Dressing	Features
Low Adherent Dressings	These maintain a moist wound bed without adhering to the wound site, meaning additional trauma on removal is avoided. They are widely available, cost-effective and good for areas of sensitivity.
Semipermeable Films	Transparent sheets of flexible polyurethane which traps moisture, ensuring a moist wound area impermeable to bacteria. Transparency enables close monitoring of the wound which is a major benefit and they conform well to the body.
Hydrocolloid Dressings	These dressings contain ingredients with absorptive properties such as sodium carboxymethylcellulose, gelatine or elastomers. They form a gel on the wound surface ensuring a moist healing environment is achieved. Hydrocolloid dressings are occlusive (water and bacteria impermeable) meaning daily hygiene, including showering, can occur without the need for regular changing.
Hydrogel Dressings	Dressings made of insoluble polymers with high water content, meaning a moist environment is maintained. They can be transparent allowing close monitoring of wounds. These dressings are not suitable for wounds with a high volume of exudate.
Alginate Dressings	Highly absorbent dressings derived from phaeophyceae (brown seaweed). Due to the hydrophilic nature of these dressings they are unsuitable for dry wounds and can cause trauma on removal.
Foam Dressings	These normally consist of a hydrophilic layer, with a secondary hydrophobic layer. This results in excessive exudate being drawn away, whilst maintaining a moist environment. Some have an adhesive border facilitating fixation and conformity to the body.
Antimicrobial Dressings	The two most common antimicrobial dressings are those containing iodine or silver products with antimicrobial agents. Their purpose is to create the optimum healing environment for the wound.
Pressure Dressings	The purpose of these dressings is to minimise the risk of haematomas by eliminating dead spaces, with the use of pressure. They are often foam dressings applied with pressure and covered with a secondary dressing on top. They can be used in conjunction with wound drains and are also referred to as 'Topical Negative Pressure Dressings'.

Table 68.2 Types of wound drains.

Type	Features
Packs and Wicks	These drains comprise of gauze or sterile cloths being placed directly onto the wound surface to absorb exudate. They can be either dry, or soaked in an isotonic or antimicrobial agent to enable gentler removal, but need frequent changing.
Cigarette Drains	These are a variation of the packs and wicks. However the gauze is placed in a thin latex tube to prevent adherence to the wound surface.
Sheet Drains and Yeates Drains	These are formed of folded sheets of latex or rubber which form channels to allow any fluid or debris to escape and accumulate externally on gauze or an absorbent material. As these drains are positioned in a channel extruding from the wound, they need to be secured into position to ensure they do not fully penetrate the body cavity.
Tube Drains	These drains comprise of a piece of tubing with a hole at the end and often along the sides, which track down a separate pathway to the wound site. They are attached to a bottle or other suitable receptacle at the body surface, and therefore form a 'closed' drain system. These types of drain can either be passive, by working on the basis of gravity, or active whereby a vacuum is applied to actively draw fluid from the wound site. The tube drains with vacuums attached, e.g. Redivac® or Concertina drains, have more rigid tubing to counteract the pressure of the vacuum and avoid tube collapse and blockage.
Negative Pressure Wound Healing	These drains are non-invasive, as they do not penetrate the body cavity, but instead are inserted beneath a wound dressing on the wound surface. A vacuum is applied to remove any excessive exudate or wound debris. It has been suggested that this type of wound drain also encouraged blood flow to the wound site, which is conducive to healing.

Box 68.1 What constitutes an ideal dressing?

Features

Protective barrier, impermeable to bacteria

Ability to maintain humidity (moist environment)

Breathability for effective gaseous exchange

Removal of excessive exudate

Non-toxic

Non-allergenic

Non-adherent to the wound surface and easy to remove without causing further trauma

Comfortable

Cost and time effective by requiring infrequent changing

Key point

Wounds and drain sites should be carefully observed to monitor healing and identify signs of infection.

Midwifery Skills at a Glance, First Edition. Edited by Patricia Lindsay, Carmel Bagness and Ian Peate.
© 2018 John Wiley & Sons, Ltd. Published 2018 by John Wiley & Sons, Ltd.

The most common types of wounds encountered by midwives are perineal and caesarean section wounds. Perineal tearing is classified as a traumatic wound, whilst episiotomies and caesarean section wounds are classified as surgical wounds. Due to the positioning of perineal wounds, dressings are not applied but the perineum is observed throughout the postnatal period to ensure that healing is taking place and infection does not hamper the healing process.

In order to identify deviations from normal healing with regards to wound management and an understanding of the physiology of the healing process is essential. Healing involves a complex and systematic chain of events which, whilst divided into phases, often overlap. This process is outlined in Chapter 67. In midwifery care, most healing occurs by primary intention after successful suturing.

Wound dressings are used to mimic the properties of skin by providing a clean, protective barrier and removing exudate from the area. These properties are all conducive to the healing process. Work carried out by Winter in the 1960s has led to many criteria being suggested as to what constitutes an 'ideal' dressing (Box 68.1).

Dressings may be removed 24 hours postdelivery, with assessment of the wound for signs of infection, although, in practice, some will leave wounds covered for between 5 and 7 days and observe the external dressing surface for signs of excessive exudate. Due to the short-term nature of the dressing and lack of evidence surrounding choice of dressing, often the dressing used is dependent on the opinion and preference of the surgeon involved; therefore a variety of different dressings may be encountered.

Table 68.1 gives some of the common types of dressing. It is essential that decisions regarding dressing choice are made on an individual basis to ensure best care for the woman. Negative pressure wound therapy may be useful for managing some wounds.

Surgical site infections develop in at least 5% of all patients undergoing surgical procedures. Whilst extensive preventative measures for the pre- and intraoperative phases have been identified, the choice of wound dressing and the potential impact on infection rates have received limited attention other than by identifying an appropriate dressing postsurgery and consulting tissue viability experts for advice if healing is via secondary intention.

Whilst midwives need to be able to recognise signs of infection or abnormality and provide advice on intrinsic, extrinsic and social factors that may impact on the healing process, it falls outside their area of expertise to try to manage complex wounds. Appropriate referrals to tissue viability specialists, doctors and other relevant members of the multidisciplinary team should be made to ensure that the best evidence-based care is provided.

Wound drains

Common wounds encountered by midwives include caesarean section wounds and these should heal through primary intention, with little or no intervention. However, if complications arise during surgery and haemostasis is not achieved adequately, a drain may be inserted by the surgeon to avoid accumulation of fluid, haematomas or potential infection. Different drains are designed to either draw any additional fluid or debris passively away from the wound site or actively remove it via suction. Types of wound drains are described in Table 68.2.

Wound drains can themselves cause complications as they are foreign objects being inserted into the body cavity. Therefore, strict aseptic techniques need to be followed on insertion. The drain material used should be the least irritant possible and the drainage site needs to be observed closely for signs of infection. Often tube drains are inserted in through a separate 'stab' wound in order to avoid compromising the healing of the primary wound.

Wound drains can either be 'open' or 'closed' and work by 'active' or 'passive' drainage. Open drains are those whereby fluid is collected in gauze or other material placed into the cavity of the open wound; strict aseptic techniques need to be applied. Closed drains consist of tubing attached to an external bottle or bag to collect fluid and debris. Due to the closed nature of these drains, inward infection rates are thought to be lower than with open drains.

Care of wound drains

Wound drains need to be checked at regular intervals, dependant on the wound site and size, to monitor the amount and type of fluid that is being removed. Excessive drainage may indicate haemorrhage and should be escalated to a doctor immediately for review. It is essential that drains are secured in position, often done by a suture to avoid movement and dislodging, and the patient needs to be made aware of this. Bottles and tubes should be checked for patency, by ensuring the tubing is not kinked or trapped and should not be attached to beds or bed linen, because of the risk of dislodging. The drain site needs careful observation for signs of infection such as redness, swelling, offensive discharge and tracking, and patient comfort needs to be assessed with the use of pain scores. Drains should always be inserted and positioned below the wound site to allow gravitation effects and avoid 'back-flow' of drainage material.

Removal of wound drains

Wound drains should only be in situ whilst drainage is still occurring. Once drainage has stopped it should be removed to avoid increased risks of infection. Most wounds will drain for 24 hours and then the drainage material should decrease in volume over the next 24 hours. The risks associated with drain site infection and tissue damage increase after 3–4 days. Removal should be carried out using an aseptic technique. Ensure all sutures holding the drain in position have been removed and any suction has been disconnected. Ask the patient if they would like pain relief and give adequate time for this to work if administered. Once the drain is removed, cover the drain site wound with a sterile dressing and monitor closely for any excessive exudate.

The management of complex wounds should be referred to the specialist such as tissue viability nurses and doctors to ensure that the best evidence-based care is provided.

69 Wound closures

Table 69.1 Examples of suture materials.

Name	Type	Properties
Catgut	Absorbable	Withdrawn from UK use in 2002 Made from intestinal submucosa of sheep or cattle Natural Monofilament
Silk	Non-absorbable	Although non-absorbable can be acted upon by proteolysis Monofilament
Stainless steel	Non-absorbable	No tissue reaction – inert Difficult to handle Monofilament
Vicryl	Absorbable	Retains 70% of initial strength at 10 days Braided Complete absorption within 60–90 days
Coated Vicryl / Polyglactin	Absorbable	Vicryl coated with calcium stearate / polyglactin Retains 100% of initial strength at 45 days Braided Minimal tissue reaction
Vicryl rapide	Absorbable	Loses all strength within 14 days Rapidly absorbed Braided Recommended in the RCOG Green-top guideline No. 23 for use in perineal repair
PDS (Polydioxanone)	Absorbable	Retains 70% of initial strength for 14–21 days Monofilament Minimal tissue reaction Absorption complete within 180 days
Prolene (Polypropylene)	Non-absorbable	Used widely for abdominal wall closure Held in position with beads at either end More inert than nylon

Figure 69.1 Examples of interrupted and continuous sutures (a, b) and other wound closure techniques (c).

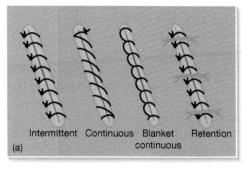

Intermittent Continuous Blanket continuous Retention

(a)

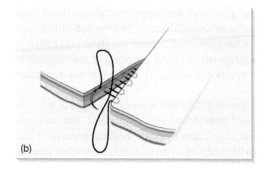

(b)

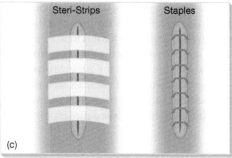

Steri-Strips Staples

(c)

Key point

Removal of wound closures should be carried out with informed consent and attention to patient comfort and dignity.

Midwifery Skills at a Glance, First Edition. Edited by Patricia Lindsay, Carmel Bagness and Ian Peate.
© 2018 John Wiley & Sons, Ltd. Published 2018 by John Wiley & Sons, Ltd.

Figure 69.2 Suture (a) and staple (b) removal.

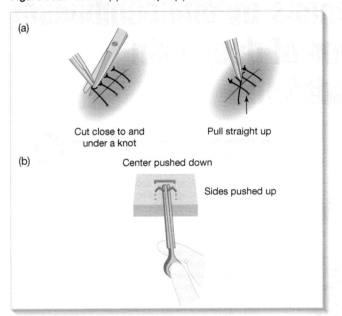

(a)

Cut close to and
under a knot

Pull straight up

(b)

Center pushed down

Sides pushed up

The mechanism of wound closure can either be through primary, secondary or tertiary intention. Primary intention involves the bringing together of skin edges into close apposition using sutures or other skin closure techniques, whilst ensuring there is no 'dead space' left in the tissue and muscle layers beneath. Secondary intention involves leaving the wound open to allow the healing processes of granulation, contraction and epithelialisation to occur, prior to closing the wound.

The most common types of wounds encountered by midwives are perineal trauma/tearing, episiotomies and caesarean section wounds. The type of wound closure depends on the wound and the preference of the obstetrician or midwife performing the repair. However, knowledge of other types of closure techniques is necessary as these may be encountered when dealing with prolonged or impaired healing, or wound drains.

The main purposes of using closure techniques are to:
• Produce a strong scar by bringing wound edges into close approximation
• Ensure the woman can continue with normal everyday functions with minimal disturbance
• Achieve a cosmetically acceptable result.

The types of suture material used fall into two categories; absorbable and non-absorbable (Table 69.1). They can be single stranded in nature (monofilament) or made of multiple filaments (braided) and the choice made is dependent on the wound, wound site and practitioner performing the repair. The major benefit of absorbable sutures is that they do not need to be removed. Absorbable sutures will hold a wound together for a definitive length of time, dependent on the material, before being digested by proteolytic enzymes or hydrolysis, whereas non-absorbable sutures require removal, otherwise they become embedded and may cause further trauma and pain.

Caesarean section wounds: These wounds are normally closed in layers starting with the uterus and finishing with the skin. The materials used for each layer are specific to the tissue being repaired and need to be documented. The skin can be closed with sutures, clips, staples or a continuous Prolene strand held in position with beads. Staples or clips are sometimes used to close caesarean section wounds. They are often used for their speed of application and painless removal and their use does not impact on the overall cosmetic results of the wound.

Suturing techniques: There are multiple suturing techniques and the technique used depends on factors including the site, size of the wound and the tissues involved. The two main categories of suturing techniques are continuous and interrupted (Figure 69.1).

Continuous sutures have the benefit of ensuring that the same tension is achieved along the wound site. However, should the suture break it can result in gaping and opening of the wound, which may require resuturing to achieve complete wound closure.

Interrupted sutures are individual sutures positioned and tied intermittently along the wound edge. These are thought to be more robust than continuous sutures and may be used for suturing areas of high mobility. Good suturing outcomes are dependent on use of the correct material and practitioner execution.

Adhesive skin tapes: These types of wound closures, often also called 'steri-strips' or 'butterfly closures' are used on superficial wounds, often when cosmetic appearance is of importance. They may be seen by midwives as additional support to sutures and staples on caesarean section wounds. Additionally, they may be used to close the wound site caused by wound drains. They only require changing if they become soiled by exudate from the wound site.

Tissue adhesives: This type of wound closure is not encountered in midwifery practice. It is excellent for treating minor lacerations and in children. Glue is applied to the wound surface whilst the wound edges are held in apposition.

Removal of sutures and staples

The timing of suture and staple removal is a balancing act. Consideration needs to be given to ensure sutures and staples do not become embedded, whilst ensuring adequate healing has occurred prior to removal. The main aim of removal is to ensure that that none of the external material is dragged through the wound site, potentially introducing micro-organisms and infection. Removal of any type of wound closures should be carried out under strict aseptic conditions with informed consent. Hands should be washed before and afterwards. Analgesia should be offered prior to removal of wound closures.

To remove interrupted and continuous sutures (Figure 69.2):
• Hold and lift the external part of the suture with a pair of forceps.
• Using either sterile scissors or a stitch cutter cut beneath the knot.
• Gently pull the suture through the skin to remove it, ensuring that none of the external material is pulled through the skin.
• Ensure all suture material is removed.
• With continuous sutures the lifting, cutting and pulling through steps are repeated until all the suture material is removed.

To remove staples and clips (Figure 69.2):
• The correct type of removal tool needs to be used for the closure material.
• Staple or clip removers need to be sterile and are single-use instruments.
• The lower blade is placed under the centre of the staple/ clip and uniform pressure is applied.
• This action pulls the ends of the staple or clip from the skin and allows safe removal.
• All staples or clips need to be accounted for and disposed of safely, along with the removing implement, in a sharps bin.

To remove skin tapes:
• Using forceps slowly peel back the skin tape from the outside edge.
• If the tape is difficult to peel away, sterile water can be used to make the removal easier and more comfortable for the woman.

To remove subcuticular sutures (Prolene beads):
• The bead at the end of the Prolene suture needs to be removed with a sterile stitch cutter or sterile scissors.
• The Prolene suture then needs to be pulled in a smooth continuous action from the opposite end.
• The pulling action should be in line with the wound not in an upwards motion and should not cause discomfort to the woman.

70 Assessment of venous thromboembolism risk and prevention of deep vein thrombosis in childbirth

Figure 70.1 Deep veins of the legs and development of embolus.

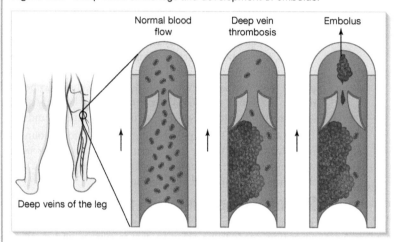

Key points

- Risk assessment and early recognition of VTE in all childbearing women with appropriate care interventions, are essential throughout pregnancy and the puerperium in order to significantly improve their health and birth outcomes.
- Clear documentation of the VTE risk assessment and subsequent management and care plans should be evident in the woman's records, reflecting decisions made by the multidisciplinary team.
- It is essential that women are given accurate and consistent information by all health professionals regarding the management of their VTE and the impact this may have on choice of infant feeding.
- It is recognised that some women have been misinformed that they could not breastfeed their baby because of the medication they were taking to treat the DVT. As a consequence, this can lead to further anxiety for the woman and disruption in developing the mother-infant relationship.

Table 70.1 Risk factors for venous thromboembolism (VTE).

Source: Royal College of Obstetricians and Gynaecologists (2015). *Thrombosis and embolism during pregnancy and the puerperium, reducing the risk*. Green-top Guideline No. 37a. London. Reproduced with permission of the Royal College of Obstetricians and Gynaecologists.

Pre-existing risk factors	Tick	Score
Previous VTE (except a single event related to major surgery)		4
Previous VTE provoked by major surgery		3
Known high-risk thrombophilia		3
Medical co-morbidities (e.g. cancer, heart failure, systemic lupus erythematosus (SLE), inflammatory polyarthropathy or inflammatory bowel disease, nephrotic syndrome, type 1 diabetes mellitus with nephropathy, sickle cell disease, current intravenous drug user).		3
Family history of unprovoked or oestrogen-related VTE in first-degree relative		1
Known low-risk thrombophilia (no VTE)		1[a]
Age > 35 years		1
Obesity		1 or 2[b]
Parity ≥ 3		1
Smoker		1
Gross varicose veins		1
Obstetric risk factors		
Pre-eclampsia in current pregnancy		1
Assisted reproductive therapy (ART) / in vitro fertilisation (IVF) [antenatal only]		1
Multiple pregnancy		1
Caesarean section in labour		2
Elective caesarean section		1
Mid-cavity or rotational operative birth		1
Prolonged labour > 24 hours		1
Postpartum haemorrhage (PPH) > 1 litre or transfusion		1
Preterm birth < 37 weeks in current pregnancy		1
Stillbirth in current pregnancy		1
Transient risk factors		
Any surgical procedure in pregnancy or the puerperium except immediate repair of the perineum (e.g. appendicectomy, postpartum sterilisation)		3
Hyperemesis gravidarum		3
Ovarian hyperstimulation syndrome (OHSS) [first trimester only]		4
Current systemic infection		1
Immobility, dehydration		1
TOTAL		

[a] If the known low-risk thrombophilia is in a woman with a family history of VTE in a first-degree relative, postpartum thromboprophylaxis should be continued for 6 weeks.

[b] BMI ≥ 30 = 1, BMI ≥ 40 = 2

In the Confidential Enquiry into maternal deaths from 2010-2012, thrombosis and thromboembolism were the leading cause, accounting for 30 deaths [1.26 / 100,000 maternities]. Although 62% of women with fatal VTEs die in the first trimester, the risk per day is actually greatest in the weeks following birth.

Midwifery Skills at a Glance, First Edition. Edited by Patricia Lindsay, Carmel Bagness and Ian Peate.
© 2018 John Wiley & Sons, Ltd. Published 2018 by John Wiley & Sons, Ltd.

All pregnant women have a risk of thrombosis from the first trimester until at least 6 weeks postpartum, the absolute risk being 1 : 1000 pregnancies.

The factors contributing to venous thromboembolism (VTE) include immobility, stasis of blood flow, alteration of the constituents of the blood (hypercoagulability) and abnormalities/damage to the vessel wall; all of these are affected by pregnancy. An increase in coagulation factors, with a decrease in natural inhibitors to anticoagulation, reduced venous tone and the pressure of the pregnant uterus all predispose to VTE. If left untreated, 25% of deep vein thrombosis (DVT) will be complicated by pulmonary embolism (PE), where a fragment of thrombus breaks away (Figure 70.1) and travels through the right side of the heart to lodge in the pulmonary circulation. The risk factors are listed in Table 70.1.

Antenatal assessment

NICE (2015), RCOG (2015) and SIGN (2010) recommend that all pregnant women should undergo a thrombotic risk assessment with numerical scoring at the first antenatal visit or prepregnancy wherever possible (Table 70.1). This assessment should consider personal and family history, the presence of any risk factors and any known thrombophilia, balancing with the risk of bleeding. If the woman's circumstances change, such as excessive weight gain, immobility or vomiting with dehydration, or admittance to hospital, then assessment should be repeated. Once the baby is born, a further risk assessment should be undertaken. All details should be documented in her records.

Preventing VTE

If assessment identifies a risk of developing VTE or bleeding, the midwife should refer the woman to a specialist haematologist. Based on the numerical scoring from the thrombotic risk assessment, NICE recommend pharmacological VTE thromboprophylaxis with low molecular weight heparin (LMWH) or unfractionated heparin (UFH) for those with renal failure, as follows:

- From the first trimester if the total score ≥4
- From 28 weeks, if the total score is 3 antenatally
- For at least 10 days, if the total score is ≥2 postnatally.
- If admitted to hospital antenatally
- If prolonged admission ≥3 days or readmission to hospital within the puerperium.

Anticoagulants are given to prevent formation of further blood clots in other locations, to allow existing clots to stabilise and to prevent fragmentation and embolisation of clots. Vessels partly occluded by blood clots become recanalised, with the clot being incorporated into the vessel wall. As this process occurs, the localised pain and swelling associated with thrombosis usually reduces. As warfarin and other vitamin K antagonists (VKA) freely cross the placenta and are known to be associated with increased risk of miscarriage, teratogenic effects in the first trimester and haemorrhagic complications in the fetus, they are not considered safe to use in pregnancy and thus LMWH is the anticoagulant of choice.

The midwife or specialist nurse should educate the woman into self-administering the subcutaneous heparin injections and advise her to carry a medical alert card with her at all times. The woman should be provided with a sharps bin at home for the safe disposal of the injection devices.

Advice regarding smoking cessation, eating a healthy diet and travelling long distances should also be provided. Maintaining hydration and mobility is essential, especially when the woman is in labour to minimise risk. For women who are hospitalised or have a contraindication to LMWH, the use of compression stockings/antiembolism stockings (AES)/thromboembolic deterrent stockings (TEDS) are recommended in pregnancy and the puerperium (Chapter 71). These include women who are postcaesarean section (combined with LMWH) and considered to be at high risk of VTE: (e.g. previous VTE, more than four risk factors antenatally or more than two risk factors postnatally, and women travelling long distances for more than 4 hours). As most DVTs in pregnancy are ileofemoral, thigh-length TEDS are recommended as a preventative measure.

Intrapartum care

If the woman has been prescribed LMWH in pregnancy, this should be omitted at the onset of labour and regional anaesthesia should be avoided within 12 hours of the last administered dose to reduce the risk of significant spinal bleeding and epidural haematoma. Furthermore, LMWH should not be given for 4 hours after spinal anaesthesia or after the epidural catheter has been removed and the catheter should not be removed within 12 hours of the most recent injection. It is important that labour is not prolonged so as not to further increase the woman's thrombotic risk. The third stage of labour should be actively managed with the oxytocin drug being administered intravenously (IV) to reduce the risk of haemorrhage. Should the woman require perineal suturing, the midwife should undertake this promptly to avoid the woman being in the lithotomy position for a prolonged time as this further increases the risk for DVT. If surgery is agreed upon, intermittent calf compression will be required in theatre.

Postpartum care

In the 6 weeks following birth, the woman is at highest risk (increasing by 20 fold) and should be encouraged to mobilise as early as possible following birth to reduce the risk of DVT and PE. The first thromboprophylactic dose of LMWH should be given as soon as possible after birth provided there is no postpartum haemorrhage and regional analgesia has not been used. Postnatal observations are vital, especially respiration rate, with particular vigilance given to the development of any swelling of the leg. Therapy includes hydration, mobility, use of TEDS and suitable form and length of postpartum anticoagulant therapy (usually for at least 6 weeks postpartum). If any deviation is noted, the woman must be referred urgently to a haematologist, or if at home, readmitted to hospital. Breastfeeding is not contraindicated with heparin or warfarin/ VKA therapy. Women who have experienced VTE should be offered prepregnancy counselling and a prospective management plan for thromboprohylaxis in a subsequent pregnancy (NICE 2015).

Women's experiences

One of the anxieties that childbearing women have following diagnosis of DVT relates to the self-administration of heparin and the resulting pain felt at the injection site (see www.healthtalk.org). The midwife has an educative role to discuss the importance of thromboprophylaxis/treatment with the woman and her family as well as supporting her in developing confidence in self-administration of the injection. In addition, the woman may need to take analgesia for a number of months after the diagnosis of a DVT as clots in the leg are known to be very painful.

71 Application and use of compression stockings

Figure 71.1 Blood flow velocity in the veins of the legs.

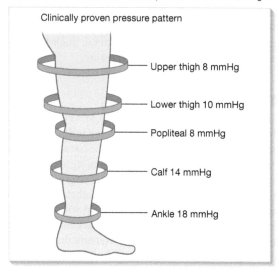

Clinically proven pressure pattern

- Upper thigh 8 mmHg
- Lower thigh 10 mmHg
- Popliteal 8 mmHg
- Calf 14 mmHg
- Ankle 18 mmHg

Key points
- Compression stockings are recommended to minimise the risk of VTE during the childbirth continuum.
- Correct measurement, fitting and application of the stockings are essential.
- The midwife is responsible for accurately recording specific details regarding the woman's risk of VTE and any subsequent treatment offered.

Figure 71.2 Application of compression stockings.

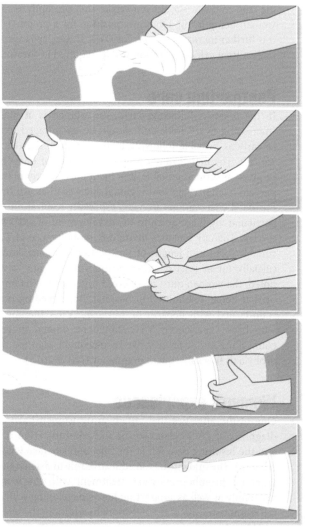

1 Insert hand into stocking as far as the heel pocket.

2 Grasp center of heel pocket and turn stocking inside out to heel area.

3 Carefully position stocking over foot and heel. Be sure heel is centered in the heel pocket.

4 Begin pulling body of stocking up around the ankle and calf. The stitch change (change in fabric sheerness) should fall between one and two inches below the bend of the knee.

5 As thigh portion of stocking is applied, start rotating stocking inward so the gusset is centered over the femoral vein. The gusset is placed slightly towards inside of leg and top band should rest in gluteal fold (line at bottom of buttocks). Smooth out any excess material. Pull toe section forward to smooth ankle and instep.

Midwifery Skills at a Glance, First Edition. Edited by Patricia Lindsay, Carmel Bagness and Ian Peate.
© 2018 John Wiley & Sons, Ltd. Published 2018 by John Wiley & Sons, Ltd.

The function of graduated compression stockings or thromboembolic deterrent (TED) stockings is to increase the main blood flow velocity in the leg veins and reduce venous stasis by applying graduated compression calf pressure of between 14 and 17 mmHg (Class I: light support). Such stockings are available in two lengths, below the knee and thigh length, and are designed to give a pressure gradient from the ankle to the knee or thigh that mimics the pumping action of the deep leg vein calf muscles, with the highest pressure being at the ankle. However, there is much debate about their use in the management of venous thromboembolism (VTE), albeit the National Institute for Health and Care Excellence (NICE) (2015) recommends their use in prophylaxis where there are no contraindications. Figure 71.1 shows the pressures.

In the American College of Chest Physicians (ACCP) guideline, Bates *et al.* (2008) recommend compression hosiery during pregnancy and in the puerperium for all women with a previous DVT and for women considered to be at high risk of VTE after caesarean section until mobility improves. As the woman becomes more ambulant after the baby's birth, the stockings may be of less benefit as hydrostatic pressures on standing appear to overcome venous compression from TEDS. In addition, studies comparing thigh-length with knee-length stockings are limited in determining whether or not there is equal effectiveness, albeit a meta-analysis suggested no major difference in efficacy in surgical patients (Sajid *et al.* 2006). Taking into consideration that in pregnant women most DVTs are iliofemoral, thigh-length TEDS should therefore be worn as a preventative measure.

If the woman is symptomatic, that is swelling, pain and tenderness, warm skin and redness particularly at the back of the leg below the knee, Class II (medium support) graduated compression stockings providing an ankle pressure gradient of 18–24 mmHg should be worn during the day for 2 years after giving birth to prevent post-thrombotic syndrome. For women with a greater risk of developing VTE, Class III compression stockings would be prescribed to provide a much firmer support of 24–35 mmHg.

Contraindications to the wearing of compression stockings:

- Massive leg oedema
- Major leg deformity
- Severe peripheral neuropathy
- Pulmonary oedema (e.g. heart failure)
- Severe peripheral arterial disease
- Dermatitis
- Latex allergy.

If the woman presents with, or develops, any of the above, there are alternative treatments available such as foot impulse devices, intermittent pneumatic compression devices (thigh or knee), as well as thromboprophylaxis (low molecular weight heparin [LMWH] or unfractionated heparin [UFH]) depending on the individual woman's VTE risk (RCOG 2015).

Application of compression hosiery

See Figure 71.2:

- Select correct size: measured around the ankle and calf or thigh (depending on type of stocking prescribed).
- Wash your hands and apply gloves.
- Greet the woman and explain what you will be doing.
- The woman should be in the supine position wherever possible.
- Legs should be horizontal.
- Ensure the woman's feet are dry before applying the stockings.
- Do *not* fold stocking down.
- Apply carefully, aligning toe hole *under* each toe.
- Remove gloves and wash hands after application.
- Remove stockings daily for no more than 30 minutes.
- Check fitting, signs of tissue damage and measure leg circumference daily for changes in size or appearance.

Remember

- The size of the stockings should be such that they properly fit the woman's legs.
- Stockings should be wrinkle free, otherwise they may cause discomfort to the woman.
- While applying stockings, ensure that the woman's peripheral blood circulation is good.
- The toes and feet of the woman should be checked daily for signs of decreased circulation, such as slow refill, discomfort or coldness.
- If the woman complains of loss of feeling in any part, numbness or tingling, report the same to the doctor immediately.
- Ideally the woman should be issued with two pairs of compression stockings, to allow for washing should they become soiled.

It is essential the midwife documents the following details in the woman's records:

- The VTE and bleeding risk assessment
- The absence of contraindications to using TED stockings
- The woman has consented to wearing TED stockings
- That the woman has been given written and verbal information about TED stockings
- The choice of stocking length – knee or thigh
- The leg measurements in cm (thigh circumference, length, i.e. buttock fold to heel or popliteal fold to heel, calf circumference)
- The size of stocking applied to the woman.

User compliance to wearing compression stocking can be influenced by the following:

- Their understanding of the actual need to wear the stockings
- The type and strength of stocking to be worn as may think they are the wrong size because they feel too tight
- The ease with which the stockings are applied – thigh length and those with firmer support are more difficult to put on
- Appearance, particularly if the woman prefers to wear skirts and dresses.

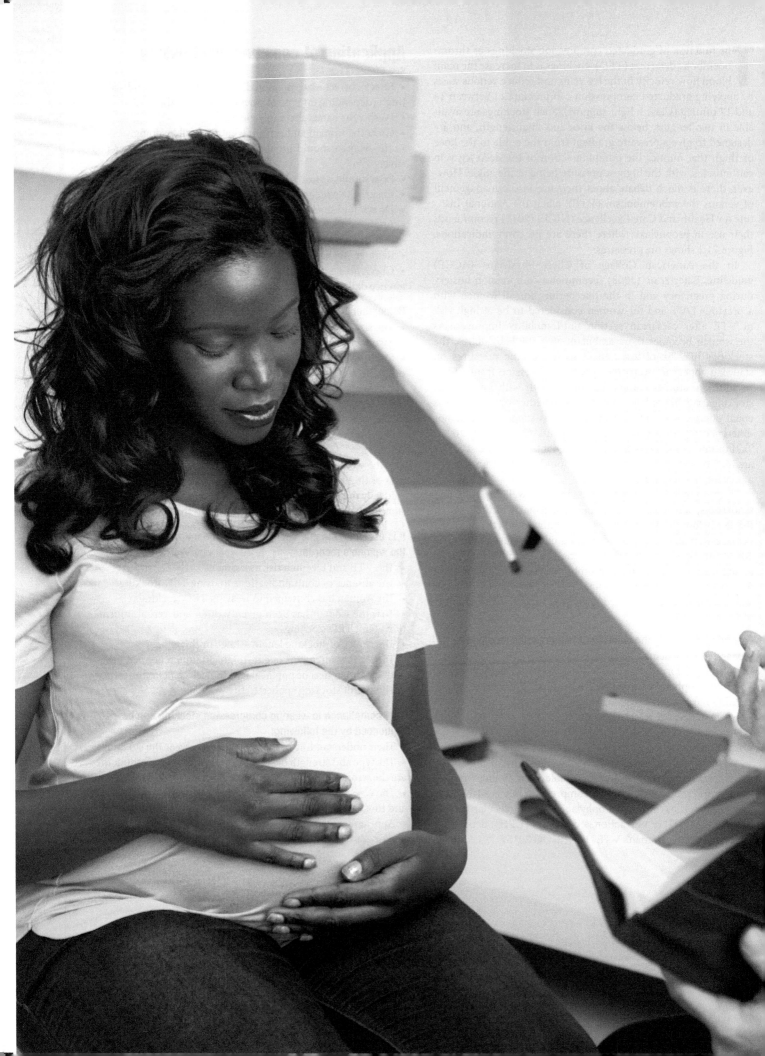

Drug administration in midwifery

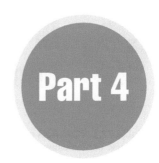
Chapters

Routes of administration

Pain relief

Drug administration, handling and storage

Table 72.1 Main Acts of Parliament that control the administration and use of medicines.

Legislation	Key Points
The Medicines Act 1968	Defines the three legal classes of medicines (see Table 72.2) and the supply of medicines.
The Misuse of Drugs Act 1971	The main purpose of the Act is to prevent the misuse of controlled drugs.
The Human Medicines Regulations 2012	Provides a complete regime for the authorisation of medicinal products for human use. These include the manufacture, import, distribution, sale and supply of medicinal products as well as their labelling and advertising and pharmacovigilance.

Table 72.2 Classes of medicinal products for humans.

Class	Description
General Sale List (GSL) medicines	These medicines do not require a prescription or pharmacy supervision. They can be obtained from retail outlets provided those premises are lockable and the medicines are prepacked.
Pharmacy medicine (P)	These medicines do not require a prescription but can only be sold from pharmacies, either by a pharmacist or by their staff under pharmacy supervision.
Prescription Only Medicines (POMs)	These medicines may only be sold or supplied via a prescription from an appropriate qualified practitioner.

Table 72.3 An overview of common methods of drug administration within midwifery.

Route and abbreviation	Action	Practice Notes
Intravenous (IV)	Medication placed directly into the vein	Reaches the blood supply very rapidly. Measures should be in place to ensure care of the cannula site. Be alert for signs of infection and extravasation and adverse reactions.
Intramuscular (IM)	An injection into the muscle	Be aware of optimal sites for injection, angle of injection and the need to avoid nerve injury.
Subcutaneous (SC)	Places the medication into the connective tissue and fat beneath the skin	Check instructions for angle of administration and consider individual needs. Generally an orange needle used to administer at an angle of 45 degrees and a pre-loaded syringe and needle at an angle of 90 degrees.
Oral (PO)	Medication taken via the mouth	The individual needs to be alert and able to swallow. May be taken before, with or after food in tablet, capsule, granules or liquid form – check manufacturer's instructions.
Per vaginum (PV)	Medication placed inside the vagina	Be alert for uterine hyperstimulation when vaginal PGE2 used for induction of labour. Can be administered as a gel, tablet or controlled-release pessary.
Per rectum (PR)	Medication placed into the rectum	Advise woman to adopt a left lateral position with flexed knees where possible. A useful route to administer analgesics if other routes unavailable.
Inhalational	Medication inhaled directly into the lungs	Rapid absorption due to the large surface area of the respiratory endothelium means that drugs can be delivered to provide fast relief of symptoms.

Box 72.1 Overview of the main principles of drug administration. Source: Standards for medicines management https://www.nmc.org.uk/globalassets sitedocuments/standards/nmc-standards-for-medicines-management.pdf (accessed February 2017). Reproduced with permission of the Nursing and Midwifery Council.

As a registrant, in exercising your professional accountability in the best interests of your patients:
- You must be certain of the identity of the patient to whom the medicine is to be administered
- You must check that the patient is not allergic to the medicine before administering it
- You must know the therapeutic uses of the medicine to be administered, its normal dosage, side effects, precautions and contraindications
- You must be aware of the patient's plan of care (care plan or pathway)
- You must check that the prescription or the label on medicine dispensed is clearly written and unambiguous
- You must check the expiry date (where it exists) of the medicine to be administered
- You must have considered the dosage, weight where appropriate, method of administration, route and timing
- You must administer or withhold in the context of the patient's condition, (for example, digoxin not usually to be given if pulse below 60) and co-existing therapies, for example, physiotherapy
- You must contact the prescriber or another authorised prescriber without delay where contraindications to the prescribed medicine are discovered, where the patient develops a reaction to the medicine, or where assessment of the patient indicates that the medicine is no longer suitable
- You must make a clear, accurate and immediate record of all medicine administered, intentionally withheld or refused by the patient, ensuring the signature is clear and legible. It is also your responsibility to ensure that a record is made when delegating the task of administering medicine.

Key point

The NMC provides guidance and sets out the professional standards expected for the administration of medicines. It is of paramount importance that midwives use their clinical judgement and professional accountability when storing, handling and administering medicines to ensure that they act safely at all times, putting the interests of the woman and her baby first.

Midwifery Skills at a Glance, First Edition. Edited by Patricia Lindsay, Carmel Bagness and Ian Peate.
© 2018 John Wiley & Sons, Ltd. Published 2018 by John Wiley & Sons, Ltd.

The aim here is to provide an opportunity to review and revisit the main principles of drug administration and consider the midwife's role in relation to medicine administration, handling and storage. Medicines should only be administered in pregnancy if the anticipated benefits for the mother are thought to outweigh the potential risks to the fetus, and all drugs should be avoided during the first trimester if possible.

Legal framework and professional standards

The control of medicines in the United Kingdom is primarily through the Medicines Act (1968) and The Misuse of Drugs Act (1971). Legislation regulating the authorisation, sale and supply of medicinal products for human use is laid out in the Human Medicines Regulations (2012) (Table 72.1). There are three main classes of medicinal products for humans (Table 72.2) although some medicines can be classified under more than one category depending on factors including their formulation, strength and quantity.

Within their professional role, registered midwives can supply and administer medicines without the need of a prescription or Patient Specific Direction (PSD) when there is a Patient Group Direction (PGD) or Midwives' Exemption (ME) for a particular drug. PGDs are written instructions for the sale, supply and administration of medicines to patients, usually in planned circumstances or an identified clinical situation. PGDs should be put together by a multidisciplinary group including a doctor, a pharmacist and a representative of any relevant professional group.

Midwives Exemptions refer to the medicinal products that midwives can supply and administer on their own initiative (without a prescription or PGD) provided it is appropriate and within the course of their professional midwifery practice. The list of medicines that midwives are able to supply and administer under the Midwives Exemptions legislation can be found on the Nursing Midwifery Council (NMC) website and was last amended in July 2011 to ensure that drugs commonly used within midwifery practice are included. It is important to note that if a medicine is not included in the ME list then a prescription, PSD or PGD will be required.

Ensuring safety and accountability

The NMC provides guidance and sets out the professional standards expected for the administration of medicines. These provide the benchmark by which practice should be conducted and measured. An overview of these main principles can be found within Box 72.1. It is of paramount importance that midwives use both their clinical judgement and professional accountability when administering medicines to ensure that they act safely at all times, involving the woman and putting the interests of the woman and her baby first. The process of drug administration can be fraught with potential errors. Healthcare organisations have a duty to ensure that clear protocols are in place for the administration of drugs and midwives must be proactive in following both organisational and professional guidance to ensure that the right patient receives the right drug, in the right dose, by the right route, at the right time. The NMC stipulate that where possible two registrants should check medication to be administered intravenously, one of whom should also be the registrant who then administers the IV medication. Student midwives should refer to the NMC guidance for details regarding drug administration and should only administer medicines under the direct supervision of their mentor.

Routes of administration

Ensuring that drugs are administered by the correct route is vital in ensuring that the drug works in an effective and timely way. Table 72.3 provides an overview of the commonly used routes of administration that may be used within midwifery practice. It is important that midwives are competent in the administration method required and the NMC (2010) points out the midwife has to ensure that they have undergone the correct training with regards to the administration of medicines, including those for which they are exempt. Following registration, midwives are required to undertake additional local training to be able to safely administer drugs via the intravenous and epidural routes.

Storage and handling

Medicines must be stored securely in an environment that will not affect their potency. All healthcare organisations should have Standard Operating Procedures and policies in place to ensure compliance with the manufacturer's storage recommendations and the relevant legislation, for example the storage of controlled drugs. Drugs must be stored in a locked cupboard or medical fridge according to the manufacturer's recommended temperature range. The appropriate temperature range should be monitored and both a room thermometer and fridge thermometer is required to enable this. Organisational policies should be available to ensure that medicines requiring storage within a medical fridge, for example Syntocinon, are stored appropriately when used within the community setting. Midwives must also follow organisational policy for the supply, storage, administration and disposal of controlled drugs that may be used in hospital and community settings.

Steps should be taken to prevent human error and potential harm. Drugs should be stored to minimise mix-ups between medications of a similar appearance, for example intravenous (IV) solutions bags and vials of sterile water, normal saline and lidocaine. Measures should also be in place to reduce distractions that may occur in a busy care environment during drug rounds and the making up of IV infusions. Midwives should never prepare substances for injection in advance of immediate use or administer medication drawn into a syringe or container by another practitioner when not in their presence.

Service user's view

'We were told it was really important for our baby to be given antibiotics at certain times each day – these times slipped by 5 hours and frequently we were having to find someone to remind them to come and give the drugs.'

www.patientopinion.org.uk/opinions/310023

73 Administration by injection to the woman

Figure 73.1 Intramuscular and subcutaneous injections.

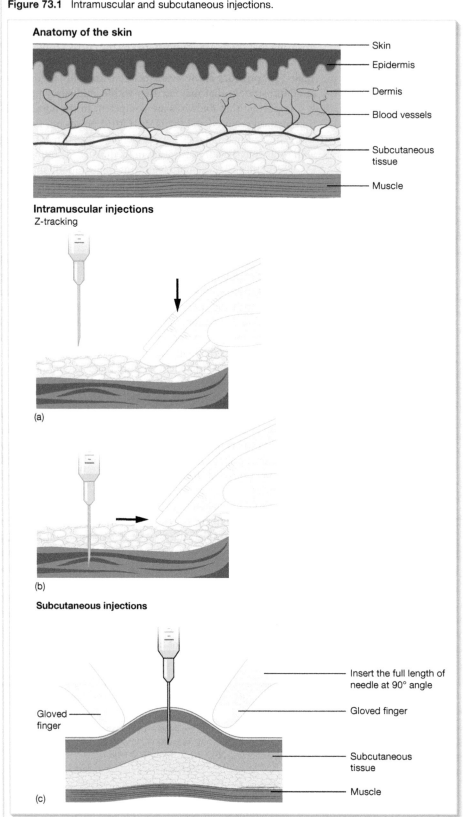

Anatomy of the skin

Skin
Epidermis
Dermis
Blood vessels
Subcutaneous tissue
Muscle

Intramuscular injections
Z-tracking

(a)

(b)

Subcutaneous injections

Insert the full length of needle at 90° angle
Gloved finger
Gloved finger
Subcutaneous tissue
Muscle

(c)

Key point

Midwives need to be proficient in giving injections and always remember to be compassionate as the woman may be frightened or at least concerned about pain and discomfort.

Midwifery Skills at a Glance, First Edition. Edited by Patricia Lindsay, Carmel Bagness and Ian Peate.
© 2018 John Wiley & Sons, Ltd. Published 2018 by John Wiley & Sons, Ltd.

All midwives must be proficient in the administration of medication by injection. An injection is the process by which medication is given using a needle and syringe and is most commonly given intramuscularly (IM) or subcutaneously (SC). Intradermal injections are given into the dermis and are not commonly given by midwives; however, some may administer the BCG vaccination to susceptible neonates using this method in accordance with local policy. The location of the injection depends on the amount of medication, the required speed of administration, accessibility to the site, how the drug has been manufactured and the manufacturers guidance. Consideration should also be given to the anatomical structures such as blood vessels, bones and nerves in the location.

Practitioners need to know how to prepare and administer the medication, and be aware of any side effects and contraindications to minimise the risk to the woman and themselves.

Nerve damage, pain and abscesses may be experienced by the woman if poor techniques are used. To reduce this risk it is important to consider the choice of equipment, choice of needle length and gauge (diameter).

The correct procedure should be followed to reduce the risk of a needlestick injury. Needles must never be resheathed and must be disposed of straight away in a sharps bin. Some needles and syringes now come with safety devices fitted to further reduce the risk of needlestick injuries and should be used as the first choice if they are available.

Best practice is to draw up the medication to be given with a filter needle that prevents any debris such as glass shards from entering into the syringe.

Intramuscular injections can be given in four different sites: the deltoid muscle, the quadriceps muscle (vastus lateralis), the dorsogluteal muscle and the ventrogluteal muscle. There is a rich blood supply to muscles and less pain receptors, which enables medications to be absorbed more quickly than with oral or subcutaneous administration but slower than intravenous administration. Most commonly, analgesics, antiemetics, antibiotics and vitamin K (for babies) are given via intramuscular injections. Skin cleansing is not routinely recommended; however, if alcohol swabs are used in accordance with local policy, the site must be completely dry before giving the injection.

Subcutaneous injections are made into the subcutaneous tissue beneath the skin. Medications are absorbed more slowly than intramuscular or intravenous injections due to the reduced blood supply of subcutaneous tissues. There are three sites for subcutaneous injections: the deltoid area of both arms, the umbilical area of the abdomen and the central region on thighs. Alcohol wipes are not recommended when carrying out this method of administration as they can harden the skin over time and interfere with the absorption of some medications. Common drugs such as insulin and low molecular weight heparin are given this way.

Procedure

Ensure the woman is comfortable and relaxed as this will help to reduce any discomfort during the injection. Gather together all the equipment required: prescription, medicine for injection, gauze swab, alcohol wipe (according to local protocols), appropriate sized syringe and needle, a blunt drawing up needle, sharps bin and a receiver to hold all the equipment in. It is vital that midwives adhere to the Nursing and Midwifery Council's Standards for Medicines Management (2010) and any local trust protocols.

Hands should be washed prior to the procedure. As there is a risk of exposure to blood, body fluids gloves should always be worn. The prescription should be checked and cross-checked against the medication to ensure the right drug, the right route of administration and the right dose are being given correctly at the right time to the right woman.

The midwife administering the drug must check with the woman that they have no allergies and obtain informed consent. The drawing up needle and syringe need to be assembled and the drug drawn up to the amount that is required on the prescription. Remove and dispose of the needle into the sharps bin and attach a new needle. A 21 G (green) needle is the usual choice for an intramuscular injection for an adult or 25 G (orange) or 23 G (blue) needle for a baby, and a 25 G (orange) for subcutaneous injections. Tap the side of the syringe to let any air bubbles rise to the top and expel any excess medication and air. This will leave the correct dosage in the syringe.

Sometimes more than one injection is given at the same time. If this occurs, the syringes must be clearly labelled. Take the medication in the receiver and prescription chart to the woman and confirm their identity verbally and by checking their wrist band. The injection site will determine where and how the woman is positioned. With intramuscular injections, the midwife should stretch the skin 2 or 3 cm and maintain this traction until the needle has been removed as this helps to reduce pain and leakage from the injection site. This is known as z-tracking (Figure 73.1). Insert the needle to its full length using a darting motion at 90° to the surface of the skin and depress the plunger slowly to inject the medication so the muscle fibres can gently stretch to accommodate the medication. There is no need to check for flashback of blood in the syringe unless injecting into the dorsogluteal muscle. If any blood appears when the plunger has been pulled back, then the procedure should be stopped as the injection is not in the correct site and is inadvertently being given directly into the blood stream.

After the injection it is best practice to wait 10 seconds before removing the needle and then the gentle traction on the skin can be released. Apply pressure to the site with dry gauze. Wash hands following the procedure and dispose of the needle and syringe into a sharps bin and clear away any other equipment. Any medication that is given must be documented on the prescription chart and the woman must be assessed for any adverse reactions.

The procedure for a subcutaneous injection is the same but the skin should be pinched between the thumb and forefinger of the non-dominant hand to raise the subcutaneous tissue away from the muscle layer and the needle can be removed quickly once the medication has been injected.

Service user's view

'I knew I was going to have to have an injection during my pregnancy and the midwife explained the procedure and made sure I understood why I was having the injection and what the medication was. She made me feel at ease with the whole thing which made it almost painless!'

Verbal communication, service user, Surrey

74 Intravenous administration of drugs

Box 74.1 Intravenous administration equipment.

Patient's prescription chart
Hand-wash solution (soap and water, alcohol)
Protective clothing: gloves, apron
Infusion stand
Aseptic tray
Sterile syringe and needles
Flush solution (usually 0.9% NaCl)
2% chlorhexidine swab
Intravenous administration set with a clamp
Extension sets
Drug label
Medication to be administered, with solute and solvent (if applicable)
If required: sterile cannula dressing, hypoallergenic tape, sharp bin
Intravenous pump (where indicated): volumetric, syringe or patient controlled analgesia pumps

Figure 74.1 Photograph of intravenous equipment.

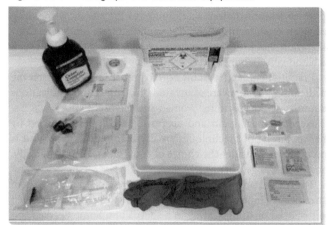

Key point

Administration of intravenous medication is relatively common in clinical practice. Midwives must ensure they are aware of any potential complications that can arise during the administration process. They need to ensure they use the appropriate equipment and follow the correct steps to avoid harm. They also need to work under their sphere of practice and be aware of their responsibilities when administering intravenous medication.

Midwifery Skills at a Glance, First Edition. Edited by Patricia Lindsay, Carmel Bagness and Ian Peate.
© 2018 John Wiley & Sons, Ltd. Published 2018 by John Wiley & Sons, Ltd.

Administration of intravenous medication can be defined as the process within which a solution or medication is introduced, using a vein, into the circulatory system. This route of administration began to emerge from the 1850s. Today, it is estimated that the number of patients receiving intravenous treatment is as high as 85% of the population using hospital services. These figures may differ in maternity services, where a significant number of women have an uneventful childbirth experience. In spite of this, there will be a proportion of women requiring intravenous medication. Therefore, it is important that midwives understand the safety implications and the principles behind optimum administration of intravenous medication.

Although essential at times, the use of intravenous drugs does not come without risks. National data highlights that there are more than 85 000 reported medication incidents in the NHS per year. The high proportion of incidents highlights safety concerns, with scope for potential errors in: prescribing, administering medication, patient monitoring, patient factors, human factors and environmental factors. Besides this, there are a number of complications that can also arise when administering drugs using the intravenous route. These include: phlebitis, speed shock and extravasation. Research shows that, although rare, the risk of death is increased when errors occurred using intravenous administration of medication. Studies have highlighted inconsistencies in clinical practice in reference to the preparation and/or administration of intravenous medication, which could partially be due to the lack of standardised guideline to use in practice. The National Institute for Health and Care Excellence (NICE) published general guidelines for hospital use of intravenous fluid therapy in adults, but there is not specific national guidance for using intravenous medication. Instead, different organisations may choose to design Trust-specific guidelines, instructing practitioners on preparation procedures, compatibilities/incompatibilities and safety precautions. It is important to take into account patient variables such as dose-response relationship and inter- and intraindividual variability to ensure safe practice.

Methods and equipment

Administration of intravenous medication can take place using a variety of methods, which include: intravenous bolus, intermittent infusion or continuous infusion. The choice for using one method over another will be determined by the drug to be administered, the manufacturer's advice, the medical prescription and the desired effect of the drug. The British National Formulary (BNF) has guidance on preparation of intravenous medication for all drugs licensed to be used in the UK. The equipment to use is as varied as there are manufacturers. Irrespective of this, the primary items required are included in Box 74.1 and Figure 74.1.

Procedure

The Royal Marsden Manual of Clinical Nursing Procedures provides extensive step-by-step guidance relating to administration of intravenous drugs (Dougherty and Lister 2015). Consent must be obtained and the records checked for drug allergy. The following process constitutes a summary:

- In the patient's prescription chart, check for patient's details, drug, dose, date and time of administration, route of administration, prescriber's signature and date, prescription advice and any potential interactions. Two qualified practitioners should undertake these checks.
- Wash your hands with soap and water or antibacterial alcohol gel.
- In an aseptic room, prepare the drug following the manufacturer's and/or BNFs advice.
- Prime the line.
- Prepare the flush solution.
- Place all equipment in a clean tray and dispose of all needles, unless it is strictly necessary to use these during the administration process.
- Wash your hands before approaching the patient.
- Ensure the five rights of medication administration: patient, medication, dose, route and time. Some experts expand these to 10 rights, adding right education, documentation, right to refuse, assessment and evaluation.
- Inspect the insertion site.
- Wash your hands and put on protective equipment (gloves, apron).
- Clean the cannula cap or extension with 2% chlorhexidine swab.
- Flush the line with 10 mL of 0.9% of NaCl for injection. Ensure patency and patient's response.
- Connect the primed intravenous line to the cannula whilst clamped. Insert the tubing into an infusion pump, if appropriate.
- Open the roller clamp and adjust the flow rate, as per prescription.
- Ensure the patient is comfortable.
- Remove gloves/apron; wash hands.
- Monitor the patient and the flow rate regularly.
- At the end of the infusion, disconnect equipment.
- Flush the line with 10 mL of 0.9% NaCl.
- Clean the injection site of the cap with 2% chlorhexidine swab.
- Safely discard the utilised equipment and document the intervention in the patient's notes.

Midwives are the lead healthcare professional with expertise to care for women during the childbirth period, when pregnancy is uneventful; they also work as part of the multidisciplinary team in delivering care for women in need of specialist care by a qualified doctor. Midwives must always apply the four principles as guided by the NMC Code. In regards to administration of intravenous fluids, midwives must work under their scope of practice, meeting practice standards as stated by their regulatory body. Medicines management is one of the essential skills clusters in the Standards for Competence for Registered Midwives and specific guidelines exist within the NMC to support midwives' practice. Midwives must ensure they adhere to the Trust's policy and undertake any training that is required prior to administering intravenous medication. They must adhere to documentation guidelines, which includes incident reporting.

Service user's view

'Before administering my antibiotic, the midwife explained what she would do and that put my mind at rest.'

A new mother, London

75 Medicine administration by oral, rectal, vaginal, topical and inhalation routes

Figure 75.1 Oral medicine syringe.

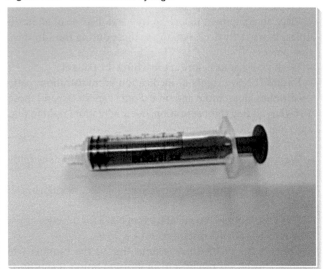

Figure 75.2 Position for rectal administration.

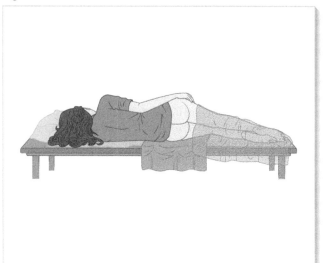

Figure 75.3 Position for vaginal administration.

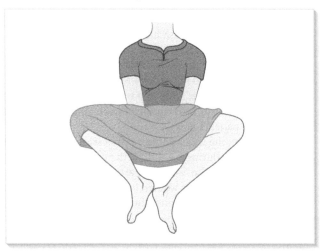

Figure 75.4 Oxygen administration. (a) Non-rebreather oxygen face mask with reservoir, (b) nasal oxygen prongs.

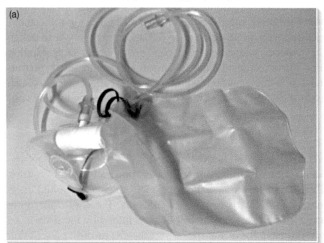

(a)

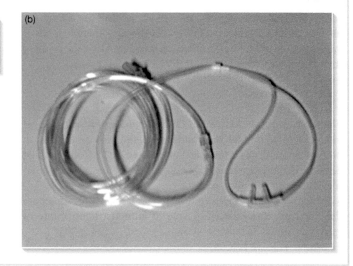

(b)

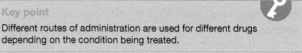

Key point

Different routes of administration are used for different drugs depending on the condition being treated.

Midwifery Skills at a Glance, First Edition. Edited by Patricia Lindsay, Carmel Bagness and Ian Peate.
© 2018 John Wiley & Sons, Ltd. Published 2018 by John Wiley & Sons, Ltd.

Medicines are administered by various routes depending on the condition being treated, the desired site of effect and anticipated speed of effect. The intramuscular and intravenous routes have a rapid, system-wide effect and, by bypassing the stomach, avoid the potential risk of enzyme breakdown of drugs within the gastrointestinal system. Those given by other routes are absorbed more slowly. The 'seven rights' of drug administration must always be observed (Chapter 76).

The woman's identity must be confirmed, drug allergies ascertained, and administration documented immediately. Self-administration of medicines is common in maternity care where the woman has been assessed as competent to do this and there are arrangements for safe storage of the drugs. Informed consent is essential and hands must be washed before and after giving any drug by any route.

Oral

Equipment includes drug chart, medicine to be administered, medicine pot or measure. An oral or medicine syringe is sometimes required for the administration of liquid medicines (Figure 75.1). Water to swallow should be provided.

This route is suitable where a rapid response to the drug is not required. It is not suitable for women who may have trouble swallowing or who are not fully conscious and alert.

The prescription must be checked to ascertain any specific instructions such as whether it should be given with food. Tablets must not be crushed or capsules broken. Sublingual preparations are placed under the tongue, buccal preparations in the buccal cavity.

Rectal

Rectal administration produces a faster effect than oral and reduces nausea. It also reduces 'first pass' metabolism and increases the bioavailability of the drug. Suitable when the woman cannot swallow or where direct local effect is required such as in the treatment of haemorrhoids, constipation or steroids for the treatment of inflammatory bowel disease. Postoperative analgesics may also be given in suppository form. The notes should be checked to exclude a history of anal or rectal damage, surgery or disease. If present, the preparation should be withheld and medical advice sought. Under normal circumstances a digital rectal examination prior to insertion is unlikely to be required in midwifery practice.

Equipment includes the drug in suppository or liquid (enema) form, drug chart, water-based lubricating gel, absorbent pad, gloves and apron, clinical waste bag, tissue to wipe. A bedpan or commode will be needed if the aim is bowel evacuation and the woman cannot get up to the toilet. An explanation must be given. Verbal consent must be obtained. Attention to privacy, dignity and comfort is essential, with exposure kept as brief as possible. The midwife must explain what she is doing at each step.

Explain the procedure to the woman, the woman lies on her left side, with knees flexed and right knee higher than left (Figure 75.2), the midwife may be required to assist with this. The buttocks only are exposed and safely positioned close to the edge of the bed. The absorbent pad is placed under the buttocks. Hands are washed and gloves and apron put on. The buttocks are gently separated to expose the anus. The anal area is examined for abnormalities such as anogenital warts. For suppositories, apply lubricant, ask the woman to relax and breathe deeply and insert into rectum to a depth of 2–4 cm. The suppository should be inserted according to the manufacturer's instructions. This is usually 'pointed' end first. There is limited evidence for insertion 'blunt' end first. Enemas should be warmed to body temperature and inserted with the tube well lubricated and air expelled from the pack. The container is slowly squeezed until empty. The woman should be gently cleaned and covered. She should be asked to retain the suppository or enema for as long as she can, if the purpose is to retain the medicine. The call bell should be given.

Topical

Topical medicines are applied directly to the affected area. Preparations of topical drugs include eye or ear drops, creams, lotions, gels and transdermal patches. When administering topical medications gloves must be worn. The skin is the largest organ in the body and readily absorbs drugs. Care must be taken to avoid over-dose of topical preparations such as steroids, which have significant side effects.

Vaginal

Common drugs given by the vaginal route in midwifery include preparations for treatment of vaginal infections and drugs for cervical ripening. They may be in gel or pessary form. Equipment includes sterile gloves, sterile vaginal examination pack, apron, absorbent pad, wipes, water-based lubricating gel, the drug and the prescription sheet. Informed consent must be obtained; attention to privacy, dignity and comfort are essential. The woman lies semirecumbent with legs flexed, ankles together and knees apart (Figure 75.3). The drug is inserted in accordance with the manufacturer's instructions and local policy. The fetal heart must be auscultated and documented before and after the procedure.

Inhalation

Entonox® is the commonest inhaled drug in midwifery practice. Midwives must be trained in its use, including the associated health and safety risks. Oxygen is the second most common inhaled drug and is often used in emergency situations, given by face mask or nasal prongs (Figure 75.4). Oxygen saturation levels must be monitored. It is a powerful drug, which should be prescribed. In emergencies it is often given unprescribed and its use must be clearly documented. Staff administering oxygen must be trained in its use and aware of the risks associated with this highly explosive gas. Inhaled drugs, used to treat chronic and acute respiratory disorders, are rapidly absorbed through the respiratory endothelium. The commonest means of drug administration for conditions such as asthma is through aerosol delivery in the form of dry powder inhalers (DPI), metered dose inhalers (MDI) or nebulisers. The effect is dependent on the woman's inhaler technique.

Inhalational administration of drugs is usually with the woman sitting upright or in a semirecumbent position.

Service user's view

'72.8 % women reported deliberately avoiding the use of certain medicines during pregnancy.'

Twigg et al. 2016

76 Neonatal drug administration

Source: Pape (2003).

Figure 76.1 The 'seven rights' of drug administration.

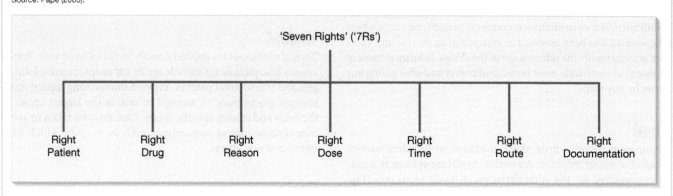

'Seven Rights' ('7Rs')

| Right Patient | Right Drug | Right Reason | Right Dose | Right Time | Right Route | Right Documentation |

Figure 76.2 Administration of oral medication.

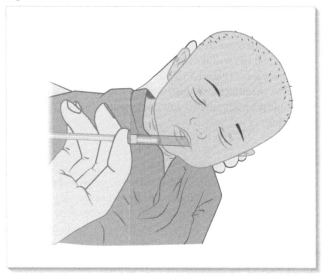

Figure 76.3 Intramuscular injection into vastus lateralis site.

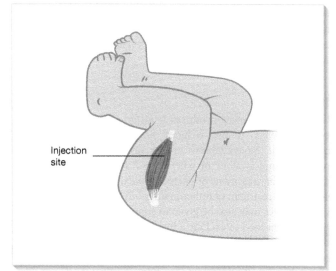

Injection site

Key point

Drug administration is complex; it involves essential phases and steps that midwives must follow to ensure good practice every time.

Drug administration is a complex system involving a number of essential phases and steps that midwives must follow to prevent mistakes (NMC 2010). A simple way to avoid error is to follow the 'seven rights' of medicine administration (Pape 2003) (Figure 76.1).

- **Right patient:** Check that the name, date of birth and hospital number of the baby match the prescription chart. Check for any known allergies.
- **Right drug:** Does the drug fit with the medical management plan for the baby? Is the drug correctly prescribed? Never administer a drug without an understanding of its usage and dosage, therapeutic action and potential side effects.
- **Right reason:** Question the reason for administration and assess if the drug is necessary. Midwives must perform an assessment of the baby's current condition and question if the baby is fit to have the required dose.
- **Right dose:** Does the dose take into account the baby's current weight? Underdosing can result in the medicine proving ineffective and overdosing can lead to adverse or fatal responses.
- **Right time:** Check the last dose (if relevant) and ensure that it is appropriate to administer the drug at the prescribed time.
- **Right route:** Check that the prescribed route of administration is appropriate for the baby. Routes of administration include oral, intramuscular, subcuticular, intradermal or topical. Although medicines are sometimes administered intravenously (IV) or via an umbilical venous catheter (UVC) these routes of administration are generally reserved for sick neonates. Additional training is required for midwives to gain this skill.
- **Right documentation:** Following drug administration the midwife needs to immediately document and sign on the appropriate drug administration chart.

Preparation for administration

The need to administer medications in neonates can generate significant anxiety for parents and carers. Time must be taken to explain the rationale and the potential adverse effects of treatment prior to administration. Effective communication skills are essential to not only prepare the parents but also to obtain consent for the drug to be given to the baby. Allow time for parents to ask questions. It is important to follow local infection control policies to minimise the risk of harm to the baby and others. This will require drugs to be checked and prepared in the designated drug preparation area where you are working. This should be a quiet and clean environment with no distractions; distractions can lead to significant errors.

Oral administration

Midwives will sometimes be required to administer oral medication to neonates and also, educate parents to give oral medication with safety and confidence.

Tips for oral liquid drug administration

- Equipment: prescription chart, neonatal oral drug administration syringe and prescribed medication. Oral drugs are administered using a 1 or 2-mL drug administration syringe dependent on total volume to be given.
- Follow the 'seven rights' of drug administration and obtain consent from parents. Wash your hands.
- Draw up the required volume of medication and take to bedside/cot side.
- Have the parent/colleague hold the baby wrapped in a blanket, in an upright position.
- Insert the hub of the syringe gently into the corner of the baby's mouth and direct towards the cheek (Figure 76.2). Up to 0.5 mL should be administered at a time to allow the baby time to swallow the medication slowly, and also prevent choking. If time is not allowed for swallowing the baby is likely to expel the drug out of his/her mouth. In this situation the doctor must be informed to advise appropriately.
- Following administration comfort and settle the baby. Dispose of equipment according to local policy and wash hands. Observe baby for effect/adverse reactions.

Intramuscular administration

The intramuscular (IM) route should only be used where no acceptable alternative exists for administration, due to the procedure causing pain for the baby. A maximum volume of 1 mL should be administered via this route. Reduction of pain is possible by using the vastus lateralis site (outer thigh; Figure 76.3). It may be useful to adopt distraction strategies such as breastfeeding, non-nutritive sucking and oral sucrose administration (Shah et al. 2009).

Tips for IM administration

- Equipment: prescription chart, IM medication ampoule, filter needle, 1-mL syringe, 25 gauge needle (term baby), cotton wool swab, gloves, sharps box.
- Follow the 'seven rights' of drug administration and obtain consent from parents.
- Wash hands. Draw up the required medication into the syringe using a filter needle. Discard filter needle appropriately and change the needle to a 25 gauge needle to reduce unnecessary trauma and pain.
- Take medication to the bed/cot side.
- With parental help position the baby appropriately and prepare baby with chosen distraction strategy. Expose and locate the vastus lateralis (Figure 76.3).
- Clean the injection site with cotton wool and tepid water. Allow to dry.
- Position the leg to relax the muscle and pierce the skin at a 90 degree angle into the vastus lateralis.
- Slowly inject the medication to minimise discomfort.
- Remove the needle and check the injection site for bleeding. Apply gentle pressure with cotton wool if necessary.
- Dispose of needle into sharps bin immediately.
- Comfort and settle the baby. Wash hands and observe baby for any reaction or adverse response to administration. Complete documentation.

Service user's view

'I knew that the injection would make her cry, but the midwife had explained why she needed it. I would never put my baby at risk, so I was happy to agree...'

Verbal communication, service user, Cambridge

77 Immunisation

Figure 77.1 Immunisation is very effective at reducing the incidence of infectious disease. This diagram from Public Health England (PHE) shows us how once common and potentially fatal infections are now very rarely seen in the UK following the introduction of vaccination. Source: Public Health England (2016). *The impact of vaccines: infographic* https://www.gov.uk/government/publications/the-impact-of-vaccines-infographic (accessed February 2017).

Timeline	Disease		Cases		% Reduction	
Vaccine introduced			Total number of cases per year before the vaccine was introduced	2014 total laboratory confirmed cases		Geography
1942	Diphtheria (Pre vaccine year 1941)		50,804*	3506	99.9%	England and Wales
1957	Pertussis (whooping cough) (Pre vaccine year 1956)		92,407*	3506	96%	England and Wales
1968	Measles (Pre vaccine year 1967)		460,407*	130	99.9%	England and Wales
1992	Haemophilus influenzae type b (Pre vaccine year 1991)		862**	28^	99%	England
1999	Group C invasive meningococcal disease (Pre vaccine year 1998/99)		883**	28^	97%	England
2006	Invasive Pneumococcal disease caused by 13 vaccine serotypes (Pre vaccine year 2005/06)		3552**	858^^	76%	England and Wales

1992: Haemophilus influenzae can cause serious invasive disease, especially in young children, Before the introduction of vaccination, type b (Hb) was the most common strain and frequently caused meningitis, ofen accompenied by blood poisoning

2006: Pneumococcal conjugate vaccine (PCV) was introduced to protect against 7 serotypes (PCV7) in 2006, these 7 serotypes have been reduced by 9596, A vaccine to protect against 6 additional serotypes (PCV13) was introduced in 2010. There are additional, less common serotypes that PCV13 does not protect against.

```
 * notified cases of disease        ^ 2014/15
** confirmed cases of disease      ^^ 2013/14
```

Box 77.1 Resources.

Country immunisation advice; access to the Green Book, Vaccine update, latest news, and publications and leaflets.
- Public Health England (PHE) http://immunisation.gov.uk
- Health Protection Scotland http://www.hps.scot.nhs.uk/
- HSC Public Health Agency Northern Ireland http://www.publichealth.hscni.net/directorate-public-health/health-protection
- Public Health Wales Health Protection http://www.wales.nhs.uk/sites3/home.cfm?orgid=457
- Current Immunisation schedule https://www.gov.uk/government/publications/the-complete-routine-immunisation-schedule
- NHS information for the public NHS choices and NHS leaflet *Pregnant? there are many ways to protect you and your baby* (Figure 77.2)

Box 77.2 Making every contact count.

Making Every Contact Count (MECC): making the most of all opportunities during pregnancy to check on vaccination status and to discuss immunisation.
- The maternal pertussis immunisation programme was introduced in October 2012 in response to a pertussis outbreak. Between January and October that year there were 14 recorded deaths in babies under the age of 3 months.
- Since the vaccine was implemented there have been 15 deaths from pertussis, in children under three months of age. In 13 of these the mother had no vaccine and in the other 2 the vaccine was given too late in the pregnancy.

Key point

Access to reliable and up to date information is key.

Figure 77.2 Helping to protect you and your baby.

Public Health England / NHS

Pregnant?

There are many ways to help protect you and your baby

Immunise against:
Flu (Influenza)
Whooping cough (Pertussis)
German measles (Rubella)

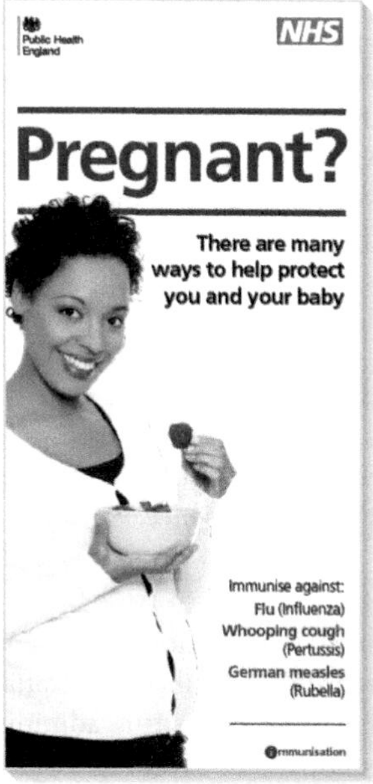

Source: https://www.gov.uk/government/uploads/system/uploads/attachment_data/file/510981/9738_PHE_Pregnancy_DL_16pp_leaflet_13_web.pdf (accessed February 2017).

The value of vaccination in preventing ill health globally is widely acknowledged (Figure 77.1). The vaccination schedule in the UK now includes vaccines to protect against over 20 infections (see links to resources in Box 77.1). The schedule changes as new vaccines are developed and understanding increases on how they can impact on the burden of disease to people at different stages in their lives.

Midwives are in an ideal position to discuss and promote immunisation with women and families at various stages during the antenatal period and postnatally. They need to make sure they know where to access the most recent schedule and how to get the most up to date advice on new vaccines (Box 77.2). The on-line version of the Green Book *Immunisation Against Infectious Diseases* (PHE 2016), contains all the up to date information with the rationale for each vaccine schedule.

There have been significant changes over the last few years in the way vaccines and immunisation advice in pregnancy is seen, and immunisation checks are part of the antenatal screening process (PHE/NHS 2016). Using the opportunities during pregnancy to make sure women get the best advice and to provide information for the future health of their baby has always been important (Figure 77.2). Box 77.2 emphasises making every contact count.

Midwives may have anxieties about actively immunising during pregnancy due to concerns about the potential teratogenic effects of vaccines to the fetus. The World Health Organization, Global Advisory Committee for Vaccine Safety (2014) have reviewed and evaluated the evidence on vaccines given in pregnancy, both intended and inadvertent use. The review showed no evidence of adverse pregnancy outcomes from vaccination with inactivated vaccines, therefore where it is appropriate vaccination should be available in pregnancy. They also concluded that although there is a theoretical risk to the fetus in using live vaccines there is a substantial body of literature describing their safety.

Some infections are known to cause complications to both the mother and fetus. Infants also benefit from the passive immunity acquired from giving the mother vaccines in pregnancy and boosting the antibodies. This provides protection in the first few months of life.

Influenza vaccination: Influenza is more likely to cause severe illness in pregnant women than those who are not pregnant. The reason for this is thought to be due to the normal physiological changes that occur during pregnancy, altered heat rate, oxygen consumption and immune response. The vaccine is offered during the flu season (October to February) to help protect the woman from infection. It can be given at any stage of pregnancy. The vaccine helps protect against influenza and its complications, including maternal pneumonia, premature birth, low birth weight and in rare cases maternal mortality. Influenza can also be serious for neonates and passive immunity from vaccinating women also protects the infant.

Pertussis vaccination: There has been an increase in pertussis infections in many countries. Waning immunity from the vaccine and natural infection mean that boosting of immunity is required for lasting protection. The disease can be fatal, particularly in babies too young to be protected by the primary immunisation schedule. Maternal vaccination boosts the maternal antibodies, which cross the placenta and provide protection to the baby for the first few months. The vaccine is offered in the second trimester from 16 weeks of pregnancy. In practice, the fetal anomaly scan, at 20 weeks provides an ideal opportunity although the vaccine can be given after this and midwives should always check the vaccine has been offered.

MMR status: The measles mumps and rubella vaccine was introduced into the UK in 1988. Rubella is normally a mild illness but can cause serious complications such as terminations and congenital rubella syndrome (CRS) if women contract the disease in the early stages of pregnancy. The vaccine is very effective with one dose providing protection in 95–100% of cases. Infections in the UK are now very rare since the introduction of universal vaccination. Those most at risk are women born overseas and particularly those from rubella endemic countries. Ideally, women should be asked about their vaccination history to check they have had the recommended two doses of vaccine preconception. MMR is a live vaccine and is not recommended during pregnancy; however, women should be reminded to go to their GP surgery postpartum and have missing doses to protect them in future pregnancies from rubella.

Hepatitis screening: Antenatal screening includes screening women for the presence of hepatitis B infection. The infants of infectious women are at risk of acquiring infection at the time of delivery and should be commenced on a course of hepatitis B vaccine at birth. Vaccinating susceptible infants can protect them from contracting chronic hepatitis B in 90% of cases. Midwives are in an ideal position to make sure that the importance of this vaccine is explained to the woman and her family and that this information is passed on the GP surgery and Health Visiting teams to make sure the course is completed.

The offer of vaccination in pregnancy will continue to evolve. New vaccines in development for group B streptococcus and respiratory syncytial virus (RSV) will help to prevent these neonatal infections in the future (Oxford Vaccine Group 2016).

'There is now a wealth of evidence on the efficacy and safety of vaccination in pregnancy and therefore, where recommended for whatever reason, midwives should recommend the appropriate vaccines and be able to confidently advise women and their families.'

WHO GAVS 2014

78 Regional analgesia

Figure 78.1 The midwife's role in supporting the woman who chooses regional analgesia to cope with her labour.

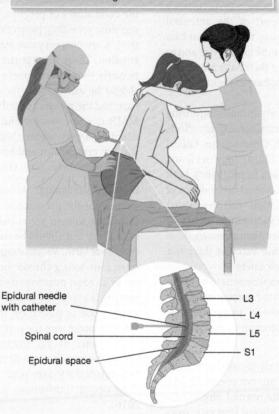

Before
- Discuss the benefits and risk with the woman prior to her being in established labour
- Assess and document the wellbeing of the woman including her blood pressure, pulse
- Assess and document the fetal heart rate
- Assess and document stage of labour

During
- Assist the anaesthetist to prepare the equipment for the sterile procedure
- Communicate with the woman and her partner to address any concerns and to ensure they remain informed
- Support the woman to maintain an appropriate position while assisting her to remain comfortable
- Monitor fetal wellbeing

After
- Record the blood pressure every 5 minutes for 15 minutes after first dose and every bolus dose
- Continuously monitor and document fetal heart rate
- Observe the woman's behavior for signs of discomfort
- Ask the woman how she feels
- Monitor her sensory and motor block hourly
- Monitor the epidural catheter site regularly to ensure it remains in place
- Monitor prone areas for developing pressure sores
- Maintain bladder care and document urine output
- Liaise with/call the anaesthetist if there are any concerns e.g. sudden hypotension after bolus dose
- Continue to monitor and document progress in labour
- Continue to provide individual support and care for the woman in labour

Epidural needle with catheter — L3
— L4
Spinal cord — L5
— S1
Epidural space

Box 78.1 Risks of regional anaesthesia include.

- increased use of oxytocin
- prolonged second stage resulting in instrumental delivery
- urinary retention
- raised temperature
- itching due the use of opioid
- respiratory depression
- reduced breastfeeding rates
- postpartum headaches resulting from unintentional dural punctures may also occur.

The woman should also be informed that there are indirect risks to the fetus as a result of the effect of the medication.

Key points
- Some women choose pharmacological forms of pain relief to cope with the challenges that often accompany this significant life experience.
- Complete analgesia in labour is possible with regional anaesthesia that involves a block in nerve sensation, achieved by the introduction of a local anaesthetising agent into the lumbar epidural space surrounding the spinal cord.
- The aim for all concerned, including the midwife, is provision of adequate comfort and analgesia for the woman who chooses to have regional anaesthesia in labour and provide the care that enables her to safely birth her baby.

Midwifery Skills at a Glance, First Edition. Edited by Patricia Lindsay, Carmel Bagness and Ian Peate.
© 2018 John Wiley & Sons, Ltd. Published 2018 by John Wiley & Sons, Ltd.

Childbirth is a natural phenomenon, but it is painful! Some women choose pharmacological pain relief to cope with the challenges that accompany this life experience. Complete analgesia in labour is possible with regional anaesthesia that involves a block in nerve sensation, achieved by introducing a local anaesthetising agent into the lumbar epidural space surrounding the spinal cord. Commonly known as an 'epidural', it is only available in obstetric-led units.

An anaesthetist is required to undertake this procedure, during which a catheter is inserted into the epidural space, usually between lumbar vertebrae 3 (L3) and lumbar vertebrae 4 (L4) (Figure 78.1). The anaesthetist must administer the first dose of anaesthetic agent, after which further bolus doses are given to maintain the analgesic effect. How these doses are given may vary as in some hospitals the woman is given the opportunity to control the administration of the maintenance dose herself through a patient-controlled analgesia (PCA) pump, while in other units this is managed by the midwife who will 'top-up' the drug via the epidural catheter, which remains in situ.

The anaesthetic agent that is usually given for maintenance is a low concentration of local anaesthetic and opioid solution. In the UK, 0.0625–0.1% bupivacaine with 1–2.0 micrograms/mL fentanyl is recommended. This combination allows some limited sensation and mobility during labour, enabling the woman to feel the urge to push during the second stage. Even though the anaesthetist administers the test dose, it is the midwife's responsibility to check that this mixture of medication has been correctly labelled and has not passed its expiry date.

Before the procedure

The midwife's role begins antenatally. During follow-up meetings or parent preparation, time should be available to discuss the benefits and risks of this pain relief and this should be reviewed at the onset of labour to ensure informed consent to the procedure. Whilst regional anaesthesia is effective in relieving pain, it is not without risk (Box 78.1).

With this information the woman should be armed with a clear understanding of the choice she is making. The anaesthetist should further explain the procedure, which should better empower her to make a well-informed choice.

Immediately before the procedure the midwife will have made an assessment of the mother and fetus to include her pulse, blood pressure and the fetal heart rate; all of which can be affected by the anaesthetic agents.

In most cases as intravenous access is required prior to initiating the procedure to allow rapid administration of fluid to prevent the risk of hypotension. The midwife may need to cannulate to expedite the whole process.

Due to a limited sensation to urinate and possible urinary retention, once the epidural is established, an indwelling urinary catheter may need to be inserted.

There should be clear documentation of all observations and the stage of labour with an indication of cervical dilation, fetal position and descent. This will all help with monitoring the progress of labour and alert the midwife to any deviation from normal, which may affect the outcome of the labour.

During the procedure

At the insertion of the epidural catheter, it is imperative that the midwife supports the woman and her partner, while assisting the anaesthetist. This would involve:
- Communicating with the woman to ensure that she understands the information from the anaesthetist
- Preparing the equipment and establishing the sterile field with the anaesthetist to enable the sterile technique
- Supporting the woman to maintain an adequate position, which allows maximum curvature of her spine to enable access through the skin and tissues into the epidural space (Figure 78.1)
- Monitoring the fetal wellbeing during the procedure.

After the procedure

The woman's blood pressure must be recorded every 5 minutes for 15 minutes after the first dose and subsequent bolus doses of anaesthesia for any indication of acute hypotension. This is not uncommon and may be corrected by increasing the rate of the intravenous fluids.

In addition, a change of position to ensure that she is not supine will prevent compression of the inferior vena cava by the uterus. If there is no improvement, guidelines should stipulate that the anaesthetist be urgently summoned to administer a vasopressor.

The analgesic effect of the epidural is monitored, which necessitates observing the woman's behaviour whilst checking her experience of any existing pain. Furthermore, the midwife is required to monitor the height of sensory block hourly, often by using an approved cold spray or ice on the skin of the abdomen. As the spray or ice is gradually moved upwards the woman's reaction is observed to ascertain if she can feel the coldness on the skin. The block should be kept at a height between thoracic vertebrae 8 (T8) and thoracic vertebrae 10 (T10).

The impact of the epidural on the woman's ability to move her legs must also be monitored hourly and according to local policy. The midwife will need to observe the epidural catheter site and record urine output, fetal wellbeing and be vigilant about the possible development of decubitus ulcers.

The aim is provision of adequate comfort and analgesia for the woman who chooses to have regional anaesthesia in labour and provide the care that enables her to safely birth her baby.

Service user's view

'I had made up my mind that I was going to have an epidural this time. Even though I knew it could be a faster labour, I did not care! I was able to sleep for most of the labour. The midwife kept topping it up and made sure that the pains did not come back. I started to feel the contractions in my back passage a little bit towards the end but my midwife made me channel that into pushing. I guess I could have done it without the epidural again but I am pleased I chose to have the epidural.'

Verbal feedback from a second time mother 15 hours after a normal delivery, West London

79 Non-pharmacological methods of pain relief

Figure 79.1 Benefits of water immersion in labour.

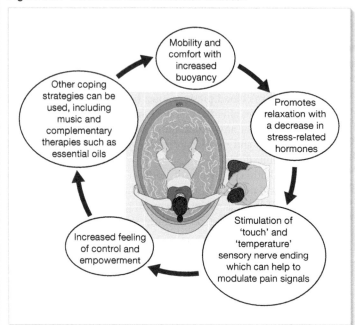

Figure 79.2 Areas on the back where the TENS electrodes are placed between T10 and L1 (just under the bra line) and between S1 and S4.

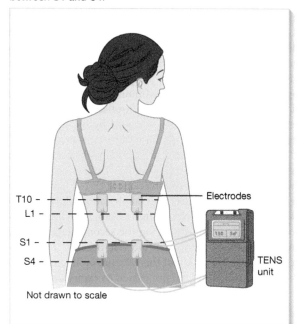

Figure 79.3 A variety of complementary, alternative therapies and coping techniques the woman may choose from to use for pain relief in labour.

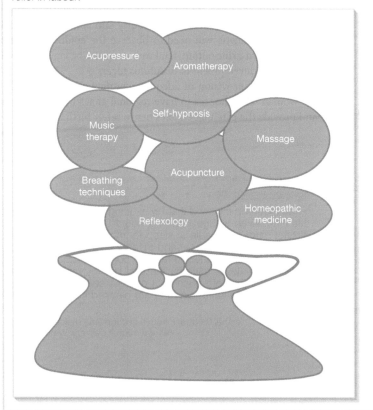

Key point

It is not uncommon for women to consult a trained practitioner in the antenatal period and be been shown how to use the various methods. When a woman presents in labour and has expressed her desire to utilise these methods, the attending midwife should facilitate this; beginning with a discussion with the woman ensuring that what occurs is underpinned by existing policies and guidelines. Thereby as stipulated by the Nursing and Midwifery Council (2015) the midwife remains accountable at all times and work within her professional remit.

Midwifery Skills at a Glance, First Edition. Edited by Patricia Lindsay, Carmel Bagness and Ian Peate.
© 2018 John Wiley & Sons, Ltd. Published 2018 by John Wiley & Sons, Ltd.

There are a number of non-pharmacological forms of pain relief and coping strategies that can be used during labour. Those that are supported by the evidence would usually have been discussed or taught in antenatal sessions by midwives or independent practitioners.

The physiology related to methods such as hydrotherapy, transcutaneous electrical nerve stimulation and massage is based on stimulating sensory nerve endings in the skin and muscles, which affects the transmission of nerve impulses from nociceptors (pain receptors) in the contracting uterus at the spinal cord before they activate the higher centres of the brain for interpretation. The experience, particularly in the early stages of labour, can be relaxing as production of naturally occurring pain relieving endogenous opioids (e.g. beta-endorphins) increases to a level that modulates pain impulses, providing relief and a sense of euphoria.

Hydrotherapy

Women may underestimate the effect of immersion or use of warm water during labour; however, it is beneficial and decreases the use of pharmacological methods for alleviating pain (Figure 79.1). While immersion in a warm bath or a birthing pool are common methods, there is also the option of using a warm shower. Birthing pools are available in midwifery-led birthing units and can be hired for use in the home. If the woman wants to use the pool to cope with her pain, there will need to be an initial discussion on her eligibility to do so. The option is usually only available for the woman who meets the criterion of low risk, that is an uncomplicated pregnancy, after 37 weeks' gestation, and where spontaneous rupture of the membranes have occurred less than 24 hours before using the pool.

The midwife will also need to discuss and advise the woman on other safety issues, such as how to appropriately clean the bath or pool, keeping the water around 37.5°C and how to avoid slipping while using the shower or bath at home. The woman should be informed about what may happen if there is a deviation from the norm during labour, as any divergence from normality may mean that immersion has to be abandoned. She should also be sufficiently agile and able to rapidly exit the pool in case of any unexpected change in her condition or that of the fetus.

If the woman chooses to remain in water for her labour, maternal temperature should be checked hourly for possible pyrexia. The fetal heart should be intermittently auscultated with a water-proof Doppler ultrasound, as per the frequency and duration for any labour and according to the intrapartum guidelines.

As birth can often be sudden and rapid when water is used, the midwife should be skilled (or supported by a colleague who is competent) in facilitating birth in water, whether it is planned or unexpected.

Transcutaneous electrical nerve stimulation

Transcutaneous electrical nerve stimulation (TENS) involves applying electrode pads to the skin on either side of the spine between thoracic vertebrae 10 (T10) and lumbar vertebrae 1 (L1) and between the sacral vertebrae 1 (S1) and sacral vertebrae 4 (S4) (Figure 79.2).

The National Collaborating Centre for Women's and Children's Health (NCC-WCH) outline that TENS is ineffective in established labour therefore most women who choose to use TENS usually need to buy or hire them for home use in early labour. The midwife will need to advise women on how to obtain a device and demonstrate how and where to position the pads so she can apply it at home and use it effectively in the latent phase of labour. TENS must not be used if the woman is labouring in water.

Complementary, alternative therapies and coping strategies

An array of complementary and alternative therapies, as well as coping strategies exist with some being shown to improve perception of pain and positively impact on overall satisfaction with the experience of childbirth (Figure 79.3). There is evidence to suggest that acupuncture, acupressure, aromatherapy and hypnosis do work for some women but there is not enough research-based support to suggest that they should be offered as standard forms of pain relief or coping strategies within the NHS maternity service. Midwives should be familiar with methods used.

Women may consult a trained practitioner antenatally and be shown various methods. When a woman presents in labour and expresses a desire to utilise particular methods, the midwife should try and facilitate this; beginning with discussion ensuring that request are underpinned by policies and guidelines.

Mind–body interventions such as relaxation and focused breathing techniques to enable conscious awareness of muscular tension, together with music therapy for distraction are supported for use in national guidelines. Massage, particularly on the lower back area, also works to stimulate nerve impulses, which modulate pain signals from the uterus and should be encouraged if the woman wishes and can tolerate being touched in labour.

Each midwife needs to understand the evidence underpinning non-pharmacological methods of pain relief and be able to facilitate the recommended coping strategies in labour according to the woman's requests. Birthing companions can also become involved in supporting the woman to utilise some of the techniques in labour.

Service user's view

'I really wanted to have a natural labour and to use as little drugs as possible. I knew some of it could pass to my baby, and I wanted to avoid that from happening. I was keen to try labouring in water but I did not want a water birth. We had seen the birthing unit on our tour when I was about 28 weeks pregnant and was fortunate enough to get a room with a pool. It was so good! I am so pleased!

We had downloaded a set of those types of instrumental relaxing music before coming in, as the midwife at our antenatal classes recommended. The music took my mind off the pain for a bit. We also had sounds of the seaside and some others things my friends recommended. It was good. No regrets.'

First time mother, 7 hours after a normal delivery, West London

80 Transfusion of blood and blood products

Box 80.1 Pretransfusion cross checks.

Before the blood component is collected the midwife must:
- Check blood product has been prescribed and the woman has given consent.
- Ensure patent venous access.
- Perform a baseline set of observations including blood pressure (BP), temperature (T), respiration rate (RR) and pulse (P). These should be taken and recorded no more than 60 minutes before starting the transfusion.
- Gather all necessary equipment to take to the bedside. This includes a blood administration set with an integral mesh filter (170-200 micron), non-sterile gloves, alcohol wipes, and a drip stand.
- Once the blood is received, visually inspect it for any discolouration, leaking and date and time of expiration.

Box 80.2 Setting up a transfusion.

- Wash hands
- Don non-sterile gloves
- Clean the cannula port with the alcohol wipe
- Open the blood giving set and ensure the roller clamp is closed
- Break the seal on the blood component bag, insert the spike end of administration set and hang on drip stand
- Squeeze the drip chamber to allow the blood enter
- Open roller clamp slowly and prime the the giving set
- Attach the port of giving set to the cannula and commence the infusion at the prescribed rate

---

Table 80.1 Signs and symptoms of potential reactions to transfusion.

Mild Reaction	Severe Reaction
Pyrexia – a rise of more than 2 degrees Centigrade Urticaria Rash	Pyrexia, rigors Hypotension Loin/back pain Pain at the transfusion site Tachycardia Dark urine Bleeding (DIC)

Key points

- Always ensure you have the right blood for the right patient at the right time.
- The majority of inappropriate or unnecessary transfusions were due to knowledge gaps and/or lack of training and education. It is an individual's professional responsibility to ensure that they have adequate knowledge, skills and understanding before performing any task in the transfusion process. Midwives must familiarise themselves with the hospital major haemorrhage protocol as these may vary from unit to unit.

Blood transfusion involves giving blood or components of blood from one (the donor) to another person (the recipient). Examples of blood products include red cell concentrate, platelet concentrate and fresh frozen plasma.

For the majority of women during childbirth, a blood transfusion is never necessary. There are, however, a small number who may require it either due to severe anaemia or where there has been a significant loss of blood due to medical or obstetrical complications.

It can be a life-saving procedure but is not without its risks. Recipients rarely develop transfusion-transmitted infection or immunological sequelae such as red cell alloimmunisation. The major risk is of receiving an incorrect blood component. It is therefore paramount that local transfusion policy and procedures are strictly adhered to at all times, even in an emergency.

The decision to transfuse is made by an obstetrician and/or anaesthetist based on the situation and haematological

Midwifery Skills at a Glance, First Edition. Edited by Patricia Lindsay, Carmel Bagness and Ian Peate.
© 2018 John Wiley & Sons, Ltd. Published 2018 by John Wiley & Sons, Ltd.

blood values. Once that decision has been made, a number of subsequent considerations should follow.

Positive patient identification: This is essential at all stages of the blood transfusion process.

Patient core identifiers are: last name, first name, date of birth, unique identification number.

Whenever possible ask the woman to state their full name, date of birth and confirm the Unique Patient Identification number in full on their ID wristband.

Where possible, women should have the risks, benefits and alternatives to transfusion explained in a timely and understandable manner.

Pretransfusion documentation: The minimum dataset to be recorded in clinical records should contain the reason for transfusion (clinical and laboratory data), details of the information provided to the woman (risks, benefits and alternatives to transfusion) and consent to proceed.

The prescription: This must contain the woman's core identifiers and must, as a minimum, specify what components are to be transfused, date of transfusion, the volume/number of units to be transfused, the rate of transfusion and any other special instructions or requirements, such as irradiated.

Transfusion request: This must include core identifiers, gender, current diagnosis and any relevant significant comorbidities, a clear unambiguous reason for the request, type of component and volume/ number of units required, any special requirements, time needed, the location of the woman (and location where transfusion will occur if known to be different), name and contact number of the requester.

Pretransfusion testing: Where a recent blood group and screen result for transfusion is unavailable, a blood test will required prior to transfusion.

Pre-transfusion cross checks are outlined in Box 80.1.

Administration

Step 1: Identifying the **right patient**. The final administration check must be conducted next to the woman by the midwife.

Remember, 61% of the cases in the wrong blood transfused category reported by SHOT (Serious Hazards of Transfusion) in 2014 would have been prevented had the final bedside check been performed correctly.

The woman must be positively identified again – ask her to tell you her **full name** and her **date of birth** and check this against the **identification band** for accuracy. Many NHS Trusts now use electronic bar coding to assist with identification. All core identifiers on the identification wristband must match the details on the blood component label.

Step 2: Ensure the **right blood** product has been received.

Before commencing the transfusion, the midwife must check the laboratory produced label attached to the blood component against the blood component. Check:
- The component numbers are the same
- The blood groups are the same
- The RhD types are the same
- If there are any special requirements, e.g. cytomegalovirus-negative blood components.

Step 3: Once satisfied that the right woman has been identified and all the required checks have been undertaken, transfusion can proceed.

See Box 80.2 for setting up a transfusion.

Observations

Women receiving a blood transfusion should be in an environment where they can be observed throughout the transfusion. They should be advised of possible adverse effects and ensure they have access to the call bell so they can alert staff in the event of experiencing any symptoms of a reaction.

The early check is the most important observation. The majority of major adverse reactions occur within the first 15 minutes, thereafter observation should be conducted according to agreed local policy. The minimum observations recommended for each unit are:
- Temperature, pulse, respiratory rate and blood pressure 15 minutes after start of each unit
- Temperature, pulse, respiratory rate and blood pressure on completion of each unit.
- More frequent observations may be required in certain circumstances, e.g. rapid transfusion.

Transfusion completion: Transfusion of each blood component must be completed within 4 hours of removal from a clinical fridge. If a further blood component unit is prescribed, repeat the administration and identity check with each unit. If no further units are prescribed, disconnect and discard of the blood bag as per hospital policy.

Management of a transfusion reaction

If a transfusion reaction is suspected, **stop** the transfusion and seek medical advice immediately. A mild reaction (Table 80.1) may be the early stages of a severe reaction, which should not be ignored.

Check that the component is compatible with the woman, continue to observe and assess any signs/ symptoms of a reaction appropriately. In the case of a severe reaction ensure airway is maintained and anticipate the need to resuscitate. Any adverse event must be explained to the woman, documented in notes and recorded on the hospital's clinical risk incident form.

A record of the transfusion should be kept in the woman's case notes. The prescription chart should also be completed in full to confirm administration.

The midwife must sign the transfusion documentation to say the component has been checked against the woman's ID band. Record the blood component number on the transfusion documentation and complete traceability documentation and return to laboratory as per local policy.

81 Anti-D: preventing rhesus isoimmunisation

Figure 81.1 Rhesus positive, Rh D antigen present or rhesus negative, Rh D antigen not present.

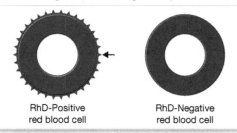

RhD-Positive red blood cell

RhD-Negative red blood cell

Box 81.1 Potentially sensitising events.

- Birth of a rhesus-positive baby (most common time for FMH)
- Following medical intervention
  - Chorionic villus sampling
  - Amniocentesis
  - External cephalic version
  - Termination of pregnancy
- Ectopic pregnancy
- Miscarriage or threatened miscarriage
- Antepartum haemorrhage
- Abdominal trauma
- Intrauterine death or stillbirth

Figure 81.2 Isoimmunisation.

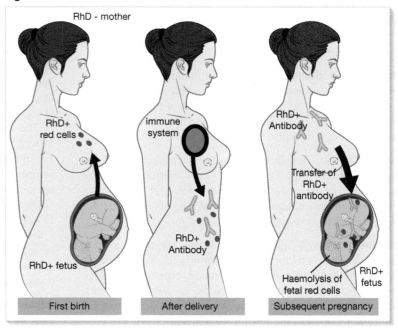

RhD - mother

RhD+ red cells

RhD+ fetus

First birth

immune system

RhD+ Antibody

After delivery

RhD+ Antibody

Transfer of RhD+ antibody

Haemolysis of fetal red cells

RhD+ fetus

Subsequent pregnancy

Box 81.2 Maternal and cord blood tests.

Booking: Mother's blood group ABO and Rh type is identified. Women who are Rh negative are screened for antibodies (*indirect Coombs test*)

16–26 weeks: New maternal blood test using cell-free fetal DNA (cff DNA) that identifies whether the fetus is rhesus positive or rhesus negative. This test will reduce number of anti-D injections needed but anti-D will still be needed for fetus/newborn known to be rhesus positive or when the rhesus status of the fetus is unknown.

28 weeks: Blood is retested for antibodies and RAADP is given (one dose schedule). For mothers where the cff DNA test has identified the fetus as Rh D negative, RAADP is not required.

Birth: Cord blood taken to check baby's blood group, rhesus type (anti-D only required if found to be rhesus positive) and presence of maternal antibodies on fetal red blood cells (*direct Coombs test*).

Kleihauer test on maternal blood taken after birth or any potentially sensitising event to assess extent of feto-maternal haemorrhage.

Box 81.3 Factors that may contribute to a larger fetal maternal haemorrhage (FMH).

- Traumatic deliveries including caesarean section
- Manual removal of the placenta
- Stillbirths and intrauterine deaths
- Abdominal trauma during the third trimester
- Twin pregnancies (at delivery)

Figure 81.3 The deltoid muscle.

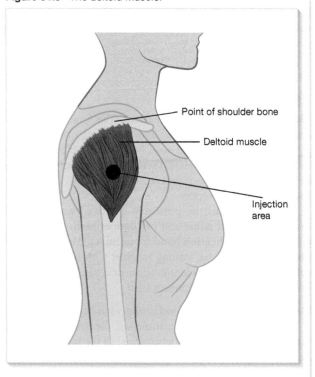

Point of shoulder bone

Deltoid muscle

Injection area

Key point

Timely administration of the correct dose of anti-D to women at risk of developing rhesus antibodies is crucial in preventing haemolytic disease of fetus or newborn.

Midwifery Skills at a Glance, First Edition. Edited by Patricia Lindsay, Carmel Bagness and Ian Peate.
© 2018 John Wiley & Sons, Ltd. Published 2018 by John Wiley & Sons, Ltd.

Midwives have a key role in preventing rhesus isoimmunisation. This occurs when a rhesus-negative mother develops antibodies, which may subsequently cause destruction of the red blood cells of a rhesus-positive fetus. Timely use of anti-D has been very successful in reducing perinatal death and morbidity associated with isoimmunisation. A maternal blood test can identify the fetal blood type during pregnancy and this will allow a more targeted approach for anti-D administration.

Rhesus factor (Rh D) is one of the substances used to classify human blood with regard to its compatibility for transfusion. Individuals are classified as either rhesus positive (Rh D antigen present) or rhesus negative (Rh D antigen not present) (Figure 81.1). Rhesus isoimmunisation occurs when a mother's blood type is rhesus negative and her fetus's blood type is Rh D positive (inherited from the father).

The placenta normally acts as a barrier to fetal blood cells entering the maternal circulation. However, during late pregnancy, following a potentially sensitising event (PSE) (Box 81.1) but particularly at birth with the separation of the placenta, small amounts of fetal blood can enter the maternal circulation. This is known as a fetal maternal haemorrhage (FMH). The Rh D-negative mother's immune system mounts an immune response to the fetal Rh D-positive cells in her system and produces Rh D antibodies. This process is called isoimmunisation, also known as sensitisation, and once sensitisation occurs it cannot be reversed (Figure 81.2).

The antibodies do not normally affect the current pregnancy but subsequent pregnancies, where the mother is carrying a rhesus-positive baby, then the antibodies will cross the placenta and attack the fetal red blood cells. This can cause haemolytic disease of fetus or newborn (HDFN). Features of HDFN include anaemia and jaundice, which may result in significant perinatal morbidity or mortality.

Preventing rhesus isoimmunisation through administration of anti-D

The exact mechanism of how anti-D works is unclear but it appears the passive anti-D binds to any fetal Rh D-positive cells and removes them from the maternal circulation before the mother's immune system can trigger antibody production. There are two strategies to prevent rhesus isoimmunisation with administration of anti-D:

1 Anti-D administration of a rhesus-negative mother following a sensitising event, predominantly the birth of a rhesus-positive infant but also following a known PSE in pregnancy (Box 81.1)
2 Routine antenatal anti-D prophylaxis (RAADP) most commonly given as a one-dose injection of anti-D (1500 i.u. IM) at 28–30 weeks of pregnancy. The anti-D is given as a preventative measure to cover the possibility of an unknown FMH during the last trimester of pregnancy.

Administration of anti-D

Anti-D is a prescription drug, included under the midwives exemptions allowing midwives to administer it without a prescription. The correct timing of administration, the correct dose and giving it to the correct woman is essential. The **correct dose** depends on the stage of the pregnancy and the size of the FMH and the **correct time** requires that anti-D be administered as soon as possible, but within 72 hours, of birth or any other PSE. Intramuscular anti-D should be given into the deltoid muscle (Figure 81.3) as injections into the gluteal region often only reach the subcutaneous tissues and absorption may be delayed. Anti-D is a blood product and as such there is a small risk of the transmission of blood-borne infections. There is also a risk of an allergic reaction although these are rare. The midwife should therefore provide the woman with both written and verbal information prior to obtaining consent for administration. Some women may choose to decline anti-D for religious reasons, if they anticipate only having children with a partner known to be rhesus negative, or if she is not intending any further children. The woman's reason for declining should be discussed and documented.

A clear audit trail of anti-D administration is required with details of the prescriber/midwife, the batch number, the dose, route, date and time of administration recorded. Local protocols for administration should be followed as product and dose may vary, although national guidelines from Serious Hazards of Transfusion (SHOT) and the British Committee for Standards in Haematology (BCSH) are recommended.

Box 81.2 outlines maternal and cord blood tests.

The **Kleihauer test** on maternal blood is done after birth and after any PSE to determine the extent of fetal–maternal haemorrhage. A standard dose of anti-D (500 i.u. IM) is usually enough to cover a bleed of up to 4 mL and anti-D should be given as soon as possible after birth or any PSE, and within 72 hours, without waiting for the test result.

Box 81.3 list situations that have been associated with a larger FMH. In very large FMH (greater than 100 mL) intravenous anti-D should be considered.

Errors in administration of anti-D

SHOT (Serious Hazards of Transfusion) reports a rise in errors relating to the use of anti-D, mostly due to omission or late administration of anti-D. Reports suggest:
- Lack of knowledge of when and how anti-D should be administered, although factors such as understaffing and the rapid turnover of women, probably play a part
- Misuse and misinterpretation of Kleihauer test, (performed solely to determine if more than the standard dose is required)
- Confusion between the administration of RAADP and in response to a sensitising event.

Anti-D must still be administered in response to a PSE, even if the woman has received or is due to receive her RAADP and vice versa.

Service user's view

'I was told it was an awful injection to have, so I was worried about it. I don't like injections. But it wasn't that bad – stings a bit. I have heard that women refuse it but I wouldn't be able to forgive myself if I didn't have it and something happened to the baby.'

Sally, service user, London

Figure 2.3 Five moments of hand washing.
Source: *Nursing Practice: Knowledge and Care*, First Edition. Edited by Ian Peate, Karen Wild and Muralitharan Nair. © 2014 John Wiley & Sons, Ltd. Reproduced with permission of John Wiley & Sons.

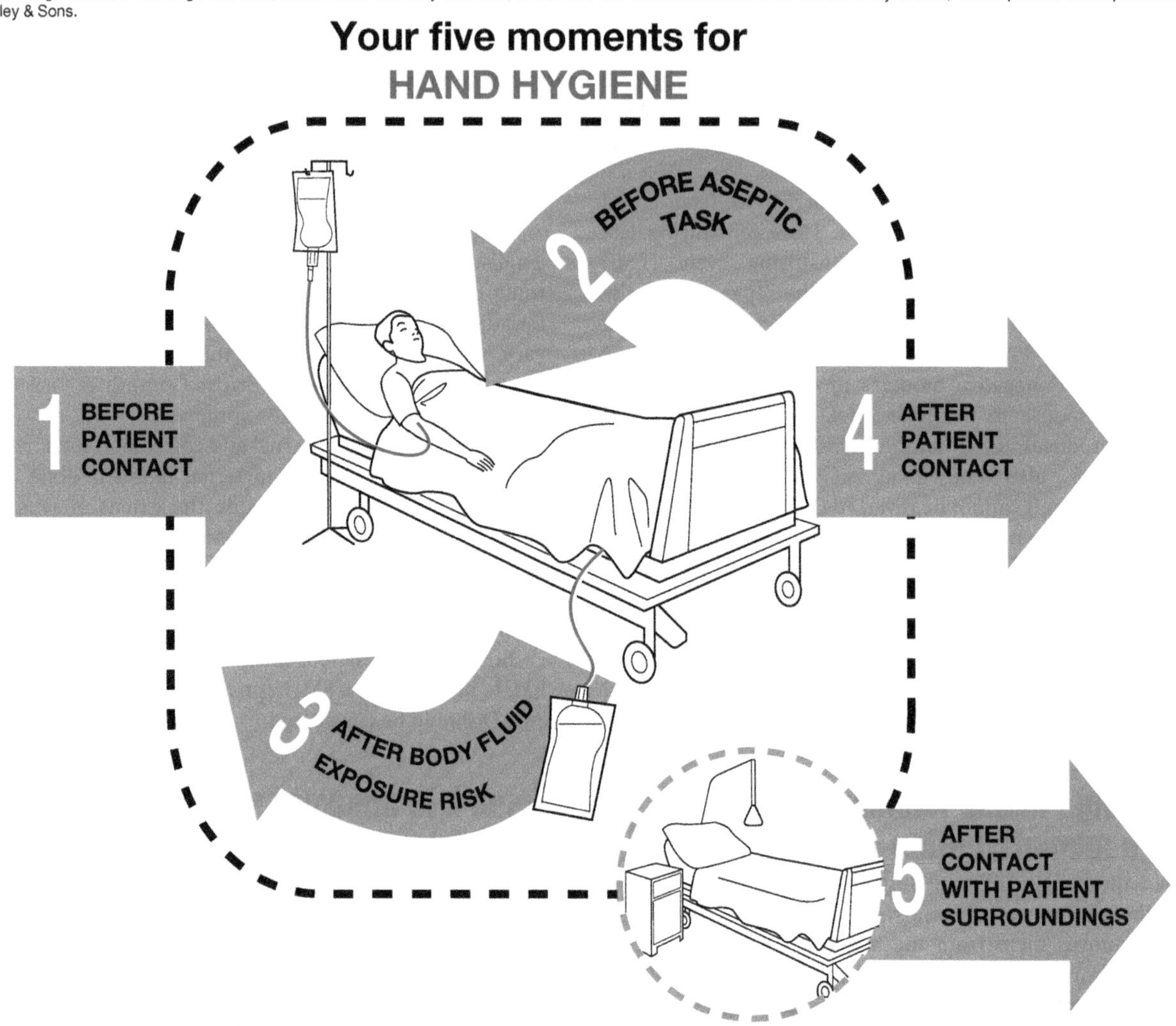

Your five moments for
HAND HYGIENE

1 **BEFORE PATIENT CONTACT**	WHEN? Clean your hands before touching a patient when approaching him or her	
	WHY? To protect the patient against harmful germs carried on your hands	
2 **BEFORE AN ASEPTIC TASK**	WHEN? Clean your hands immediately before any aseptic task	
	WHY? To protect the patient against harmful germs, including the patient's own germs, entering his or her body	
3 **AFTER BODY FLUID EXPOSURE RISK**	WHEN? Clean your hands immediately after an exposure risk to body fluids (and after glove removal)	
	WHY? To protect yourself and the healthcare environment from harmful patient germs	
4 **AFTER PATIENT CONTACT**	WHEN? Clean your hands after touching a patient and his or her immediate surroundings when leaving	
	WHY? To protect yourself and the healthcare environment from harmful patient germs	
5 **AFTER CONTACT WITH PATIENT SURROUNDINGS**	WHEN? Clean your hands after touching any object or furniture in the patient's immediate surroundings, when leaving - even without touching the patient	
	WHY? To protect yourself and the healthcare environment from harmful patient germs	

Figure 33.1 Customised growth chart. Note: FH or EFW measurements may also have been recorded electronically.
Source: Gestation Network - www.gestation.net. Accessed May 2017. Reproduced with permission of Perinatal Institute, Birmingham, UK.

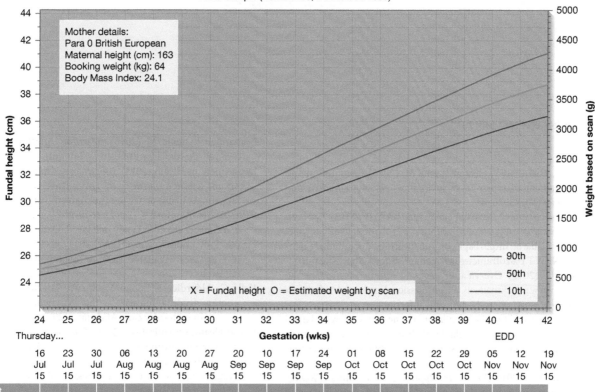

Antenatal GROW Chart
Anna Sample (Ref:123456, DOB:01/01/1990)

Mother details:
Para 0 British European
Maternal height (cm): 163
Booking weight (kg): 64
Body Mass Index: 24.1

X = Fundal height   O = Estimated weight by scan

— 90th
— 50th
— 10th

Fundal height (cm) — left axis: 24, 26, 28, 30, 32, 34, 36, 38, 40, 42, 44
Weight based on scan (g) — right axis: 0, 500, 1000, 1500, 2000, 2500, 3000, 3500, 4000, 4500, 5000

Gestation (wks): 24 25 26 27 28 29 30 31 32 33 34 35 36 37 38 39 40 41 42

Thursday...   EDD

| 16 Jul 15 | 23 Jul 15 | 30 Jul 15 | 06 Aug 15 | 13 Aug 15 | 20 Aug 15 | 27 Aug 15 | 20 Sep 15 | 10 Sep 15 | 17 Sep 15 | 24 Sep 15 | 01 Oct 15 | 08 Oct 15 | 15 Oct 15 | 22 Oct 15 | 29 Oct 15 | 05 Nov 15 | 12 Nov 15 | 19 Nov 15 |

Date of visit
Fundal height (cm)
For growth scan?
Scan EFW result (g)
Signature

The GROW chart (Gestation Related Optimal Weight) is customised for the characteristics of each pregnancy.

The centile lines provide the reference curves (not absolute values) for the expected growth velocity of fundal height and fetal weight.

Fundal height measurements to monitor growth: Should be done every 2-3 weeks, from 26 or 28 weeks gestation onwards; preferably by same care provider; mother semi-recumbent, bladder empty.

Hold end of non-elastic tape at top of uterine fundus.

Lead the tape down to top of symphysis pubis.

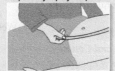

Measure along longitudinal uterine axis and plot on chart.

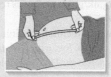

Referrals for growth scan* should be arranged if:
- the first fundal height measurement plots below 10th centile line on the customised chart
- consecutive measurements suggest NO growth (static or flat curve), or
- SLOW growth (curve not following slope of any curve on the chart); or
- EXCESSIVE growth (curve steeper than any curve on the chart) **.

* Ultrasound biometry for estimated fetal weight (EFW) and amniotic fluid assessment (plus Doppler flow if scan suggests growth problems).

** A first measurement above the 90th centile is NOT an indication for a growth scan. A scan would however be indicated if there was clinical suspicion of polyhydramnios or there was excessive growth on subsequent measurements. Please refer to your local guideline.

If result of ultrasound assessment is: Normal >> revert to serial fundal height measurement.
Abnormal >> refer for urgent obstetric review.

GROW (UK) Chart ID:15669867   © Gestation Network - www.gestation.net

Key references and further reading

All websites accessed July 2017.

Chapter 1

Barnden J, Diamond V, Heaton P, Paul SP (2016) Recognition and management of sepsis in early infancy. *Nursing Children and Young People*, 28, 36–45.

British Association of Perinatal Medicine (BAPM) (2015) *Newborn early warning trigger and track (NEWTT) A framework for practice*. Available at: http://bapm.org/publications/documents/guidelines/NEWTT%20framework%20final%20for%20website.pdf

Caserta MT (2015) *Overview of neonatal infections*. Available at: https://www.merckmanuals.com/professional/pediatrics/infections-in-neonates/overview-of-neonatal-infections

Gibson E, Nawab U (2015) *Hypothermia in neonates*. Merck Manual Professional Version. Available at: https://www.merckmanuals.com/professional/pediatrics/perinatal-problems/hypothermia-in-neonates

Moldenhauer JS (2016) *Premature Rupture of Membranes (PROM)*. Available at: https://www.merckmanuals.com/professional/gynecology-and-obstetrics/abnormalities-and-complications-of-labor-and-delivery/premature-rupture-of-membranes-prom

National Childbirth Trust (NCT) (2016) *Group B Streptococcus (GBS)*. Available at: https://www.nct.org.uk/pregnancy/group-b-streptococcus-gbs

National Institute for Health and Care Excellence (NICE) (2014a) *Intrapartum care for healthy women and babies*. CG 190. Available at: https://www.nice.org.uk/guidance/cg190/chapter/1-recommendations

National Institute for Health and Care Excellence (NICE) (2014b) Neonatal Infection: Quality Standard. Available at https://www.nice.org.uk/guidance/qs75/resources/neonatal-infection-pdf-2098849787845

National Perinatal Epidemiology Unit (NPEU). *MBRRACE – UK: Mothers and Babies: Reducing Risk through Audits and Confidential Enquiries across the UK*. Available at: https://www.npeu.ox.ac.uk/mbrrace-uk

Robinson D, Kumar P, Cadichan S (2008) Neonatal sepsis in the emergency department. *Clinical Paediatric Emergency Medicine*, 9, 160–168.

Chapter 2

Dougherty L, Lister S (2015) *The Royal Marsden Manual of Clinical Nursing Procedures: Professional Edition*, 9th edn. John Wiley & Sons, Ltd., Oxford.

Loveday H, Wilson JA, Pratt RJ, *et al.* (2014) epic3: National Evidence-Based Guidelines for Preventing Healthcare-Associated Infections in NHS Hospitals in England. *Journal of Hospital Infection*, 86, S1–S70.

National Institute for Health and Care Excellence (NICE) *Quality Statement 3: Hand Decontamination* (QS61). Available at: https://www.nice.org.uk/guidance/qs61/chapter/quality-statement-3-hand-decontamination

Chapter 3

Bothamley J, Boyle M (2015) *Infections Affecting Pregnancy and Child Birth*. Radcliffe Publishing, London.

Department of Health (2011) *Tuberculosis, Chapter 32. Immunisation Against Infections Diseases; the Green Book*. Department of Health, London. Available at: www.gov.uk/government/publications

Gillespie SH, Bamford K (2012) *Medical Microbiology and Infection at a Glance*, 4th edn. Wiley Blackwell, Oxford.

Health Protection Agency(HPA) (2011) *Guidance on Viral rashes in Pregnancy*. Available at: www.hpa.org.uk/webc/HPAwebFile/HPAweb

Kelly C, Alderdice F, Lohan M, Spence D (2013) Every pregnant woman needs a midwife – the experiences of HIV affected women in maternity care. *Midwifery*, 29, 132–138.

World Health Organisation (2016) *Zika Virus Fact Sheet*. Available at: www.who.int/mediacentre/factsheets/zika/en/

World Health Organisation (2017) *Zika Virus and Complications*. Available at: www.who.int/features/qa/zika/en/

Chapter 4

Dougherty L, Lister S (2015) *The Royal Marsden Manual of Clinical Nursing Procedures: Professional Edition*, 9th edn. John Wiley & Sons, Ltd., Oxford.

Loveday H, Wilson JA, Pratt RJ, *et al.* (2014) epic3: National Evidence-Based Guidelines for Preventing Healthcare-Associated Infections in NHS Hospitals in England. *Journal of Hospital Infection*, 86, S1–S70.

National Institute for Health and Care Excellence (NICE) (2014) *Infection Prevention and Control* (QS61). Available at: https://www.nice.org.uk/guidance/qs61/resources/infection-prevention-and-control-2098782603205

Weston D (2013) *Fundamentals of Infection Prevention and Control: Theory and Practice*, 2nd edn. John Wiley & Sons, Ltd., Oxford.

Chapter 5

Gallagher R (2015) Aseptic technique and specimen collection. In: Delves-Yates C (ed.) *Essentials of Nursing Practice*. Sage, London, 403–422.

National Institute for Health and Care Excellence (NICE) (2016) *Sepsis: Recognition, Diagnosis and Early Management* (NG51). Available at: https://www.nice.org.uk/guidance/ng51?unlid=280104107201611917351

National Institute for Health and Care Excellence (NICE) (2017) *Healthcare-Associated Infections: Prevention and Control in Primary and Community Care* (CG 139). Available at: https://www.nice.org.uk/Guidance/CG139

National Perinatal Epidemiology Unit (NPEU) (2016) *MBRRACE-UK Mothers and Babies: Reducing Risk through Audits and Confidential Enquiries across the UK. Saving Lives2016*.

NHS Choices (2016) *Sepsis*. Available at: http://www.nhs.uk/Conditions/Blood-poisoning/Pages/Introduction.aspx

Royal College of Obstetricians and Gynaecologists (2012) *Sepsis following Pregnancy, Bacterial* (Green-top Guideline No.64b).

Royal College of Obstetricians and Gynaecologists (2012) *Sepsis in Pregnancy, Bacterial* (Green-top Guideline No.64a).

Chapter 6

Health and Safety Executive (HSE) (2004) *Manual Handling Operations Regulations1992; Guidance on Regulations*, 3rd edn.

Health and Safety Executive (HSE) (2012) *Moving and Handling: A Brief Guide*.

Health and Safety Executive (HSE) *What you Need to do – Moving and Handling*. Available at: http://www.hse.gov.uk/healthservices/moving-handling-do.htm

Johnson R, Taylor W (2016) *Skills for Midwifery Practice*. Elsevier, London.

Chapter 7

Health and Safety Executive (HSE) *Control of Substances Hazardous to Health (COSHH)*. Available at: www.hse.gov.uk/coshh

Health and Safety Executive (HSE) *Latex Allergies*. Available at: http://www.hse.gov.uk/skin/employ/latex.htm

Robertson A (2006) No laughing matter. *Midwifery Matters*, 109, 13–18.

Royal College of Nursing (2012) *Tools of the Trade – guidance for Healthcare Staff on Glove Use and the Prevention of Contact Dermatitis*.

Chapter 8

Department of Health (2013) *Safe Management of Healthcare Waste*. Available at https://www.gov.uk/government/publications/guidance-on-the-safe-management-of-healthcare-waste.

Health and Safety Executive (2014) *Preventing Slips and Trips at Work*. Available at: http://www.hse.gov.uk

Health and Safety Executive (2016) *Equipment Safety*. Available at: http://www.hse.gov.uk/healthservices/equipment-safety.htm

Health and Safety Executive. *Health and Social Care Services*. Available at: http://www.hse.gov.uk/healthservices/index.htm

Royal College of Nursing (2014) *The Management of Waste from Health, Social and Personal Care*. Available at: http://www.rcn.org.uk

Chapter 9

Health and Safety Executive (HSE) *Management of Risk when Planning Work: The Right Priorities*. Available at: http://www.hse.gov.uk/construction/lwit/assets/downloads/hierarchy-risk-controls.pdf

Health and Safety Executive (HSE) *Sharps Injuries*. Available at: http://www.hse.gov.uk/healthservices/needlesticks/

Jeong J, Son H, Jeong I, *et al.* (2016) Qualitative content analysis of psychologic discomfort and coping process after needlestick injuries among health care workers. *American Journal of Infection Control*, 44,183–188.

Public Health England (2014) *Eye of the Needle. United Kingdom Significant Occupational Exposure to Bloodborne Viruses in Healthcare Workers*. PHE, London.

Royal College of Nursing (RCN) (2015) *Sharps safety. RCN Guidance to Support the Implementation of the Health and Safety (Sharp Instruments in Healthcare Regulations) 2013*.

Chapter 10

NHS Business Services Authority (NHSBSA) Lone Worker Protection Service. Available at: https://www.nhsbsa.nhs.uk/nhs-protect

NHS Employers (2013) *Improving Safety for Lone Workers*. Available at: http://www.nhsemployers.org/case-studies-and-resources/2013/10/improving-safety-for-lone-workers-a-guide-for-lone-workers

NHS Protect (2017) *A Guide for the Better Protection of Lone Workers in the NHS*. Available at: https://www.nhsbsa.nhs.uk/sites/default/files/2017-04/Lone%20worker%20guidance_Final%20March%202017.pdf

Royal College of Nursing (RCN) (2012) *RCN Lone Working Survey 2011*. Available at: https://my.rcn.org.uk/__data/assets/pdf_file/0007/424096/RCN_lone_working_survey_2011.pd

Chapter 11

Bailey L (2009) Patient dignity in an acute hospital setting: a case study. *International Journal of Nursing Studies*, 46, 23–36.

Department of Health (2010) *Essence of Care: Benchmarks for Personal Hygiene*. Available at: Department of Health, London. https://www.gov.uk/government/uploads/system/uploads/attachment_data/file/216697/dh_119976.pdf

Knight M, Kenyon S, Brocklehurst P, *et al.* (2014) *Saving Lives, Improving Mothers' Care*. MBRRACE-UK. Available at: https://www.npeu.ox.ac.uk/downloads/files/mbrrace-uk/reports/Saving%20Lives%20Improving%20Mothers%20Care%20report%202014%20Full.pdf

Chapter 12

Bick D, Bassett S (2013) *How to Provide Postnatal Perineal Care*. Royal College of Midwives. Available at: https://www.rcm.org.uk/news-views-and-analysis/analysis/how-to-provide-postnatal-perineal-care

Cohen S. (2009) Orthopaedic patients perceptions of using a bedpan *Journal of Orthopaedic Nursing*, 13, 78–84.

Johnson R, Taylor W (2016) *Skills for Midwifery Practice*. Elsevier, London.

Chapter 13

Baharestani M, Ratliff C (2007) Pressure ulcers in neonates and children: a NPUAP white paper *Advances in Skin and Wound Care*, 20, 208–220.

Hopkins A, Dealey C, Bale S, *et al.* (2006) Patient stories of living with pressure ulcer. *Journal of Advanced Nursing*, 56, 345–353.

Morison B, Baker C (2001) How to raise awareness of pressure sore prevention. *British Journal of Midwifery*, 9, 147–150.

National Institute for Health and Care Excellence (NICE) (2014) *Pressure Ulcers: Prevention and Management*, CG179. Available at: https://www.nice.org.uk/guidance/cg179/resources/pressure-ulcers-prevention-and-management-35109760631749

NHS *Stop the Pressure*. Available at: http://nhs.stopthepressure.co.uk/

Wicks G (2007) A guide to the treatment of pressure ulcers from grade 1 to grade 4. *Wound Essentials*, 2, 106–113.

Chapter 14

Fox R, Yelland A, Draycott T (2013) Analysis of legal claims – informing litigation systems and quality improvement. *BJOG*, 121, 6–10.

National Health Service Litigation Authority (NHSLA). Available at: http://www.nhsla.com/Pages/Home.aspx

NHS England (2016) *Safer Maternity Care: Next Steps Towards the National Maternity Ambition*. Available at: https://www.gov.uk/government/publications/safer-maternity-care

O'Connor D (2016) *Saving Babies Lives A Care Bundle for Reducing Stillbirth*. NHS England. Available at: https://www.england.nhs.uk/wp-content/uploads/2016/03/saving-babies-lives-car-bundl.pdf

Smith A, Dixon A, Page L (2009) Health-care professionals' views about safety in maternity services: a qualitative study. *Midwifery*, 25, 29–31.

Chapter 15

National Patient Safety Agency (NPSA) National Reporting and Learning Service. *Root Cause Analysis Investigation Tools*. Available at: http://www.nrls.npsa.nhs.uk/EasySiteWeb/getresource.axd?AssetID=60180

National Patient Safety Agency. Available at: http://www.npsa.nhs.uk/

NHS Litigation Authority (NHSLA) (2010) *Maternity Claims – Information Sheet 11 Midwifery Care*. Available at: http://www.nhsla.com/safety/Documents/Midwifery%20Care%20-%2011.pdf

Wu A, Steckelberg R (2012) Medical error, incident investigation and the second victim: doing better but feeling worse? *BMJ Quality and Safety*, 21, 267–270.

Chapter 16

NHS National Maternity Review Team (2016) *Better Births*. NHS England. Available at: https://www.england.nhs.uk/wp-content/uploads/2016/02/national-maternity-review-report.pdf

NHS Litigation Authority (2012) *CNST Maternity Clinical Risk Management Standards – Clinical Audit Report Template*. Available at: http://www.nhsla.com/safety/Documents/Maternity%20Clinical%20Audit%20Template.doc

Royal College of Obstetricians and Gynaecologists (RCOG) (2008) *Standards for Maternity Care: Maternity Audit Indicators*. Available at: https://www.rcog.org.uk/globalassets/documents/guidelines/maternityauditindicators0608.pdf

Chapter 17

British Medical Association (BMA) *Safeguarding Vulnerable Adults – A Toolkit for General Practitioners*. Available at: https://www.bma.org.uk/-/media/files/pdfs/.../safeguardingvulnerableadults.pdf

Hutchinson S, Page A, Sample E (2015) *Rebuilding Shattered Lives*. St Mungo's. Available at: http://rebuildingshatteredlives.org/wp-content/uploads/2014/03/Rebuilding-Shattered-Lives-Final-Report.pdf

National Institute for Health and Care Excellence (NICE) (2010) *Pregnancy and Complex Social Factors: a Model for Service Provision for Pregnant Women with Complex Social Factors* (CG110). Available at: https://www.nice.org.uk/Guidance/CG110

Royal College of Nursing (RCN). *Safeguarding*. Available at: https://www.rcn.org.uk/clinical-topics/safeguarding

Safelives (2106) *Getting it Right First Time for Victims of Domestic Violence*. Available at: http://www.safelives.org.uk/policy-evidence/getting-it-right-first-time

Chapter 18

Dumbrill GC (2006) Parental experience of child protection intervention: A qualitative study. *Child Abuse and Neglect*, 30, 27–37.

HM Government (2015) *What to do if you are Worried a Child is being Abused: Advice for Practitioners*. Department for Education, London. Available at https://www.gov.uk/government/uploads/system/uploads/attachment_data/file/419604/What_to_do_if_you_re_worried_a_child_is_being_abused.pdf

HM Government (2015) *Working Together to Safeguard Children: A Guide to Inter-agency Working to Safeguard and Promote the Welfare of Children*. Department for Education, London. Available at https://www.gov.uk/government/uploads/system/uploads/attachment_data/file/419595/Working_Together_to_Safeguard_Children.pdf

National Society for the Prevention of Cruelty to Children. Available at: www.nspcc.org.uk

Powell C (2016) *Safeguarding and Child Protection for Nurses, Midwives and Health Visitors*, 2nd edn. Open University Press, Maidenhead.

Chapter 19

Health Education England (2015). *e-FGM Educational Programme*. Available at: http://www.e-lfh.org.uk/programmes/female-genital-mutilation/

HM Government (2016) *Multi-agency Statutory Guidance on Female Genital Mutilation*.

Royal College of Nursing (RCN) (2016) *Female Genital Mutilation: An RCN Resource for Nursing and Midwifery Practice*, 3rd edn.

Royal College of Obstetricians and Gynaecologists (RCOG) (2015) *Female Genital Mutilation and its Management*, Green-top Guideline No.53.

Chapter 20

National Institute for Health and Care Excellence (NICE) (2016a) *Antenatal Care for Uncomplicated Pregnancies* (CG62). Available at: https://www.nice.org.uk/Guidance/CG62

National Institute for Health and Care Excellence (NICE) (2016b) *Antenatal and Postnatal Mental Health*. Available at: https://pathways.nice.org.uk/pathways/antenatal-and-postnatal-mental-health

NHS Antenatal and Newborn Screening Programme (2016) *NHS Antenatal and Newborn Screening Programme*. Available at: https://www.gov.uk/topic/population-screening-programmes

Which. *Helping you Decide Where to Give Birth*. Available at: http://www.which.co.uk/birth-choice

Chapter 21

Bagness C, Shakespeare J (2016) Perinatal mental health and practice nursing. *Journal of Practice Nursing*, 2, 56–60.

Department of Health (2010) *Midwifery 2020: Delivering Expectations*. Available at: https://www.gov.uk/government/publications/midwifery-2020-delivering-expectations

National Institute for Health and Care Excellence (NICE) (2016) *Antenatal Care for Uncomplicated Pregnancies* (CG62). Available at: https://www.nice.org.uk/guidance/cg62/chapter/Woman-centred-care

National Institute for Health and Care Excellence (NICE) (2016) *Antenatal and Postnatal Mental Health*. Available at: https://pathways.nice.org.uk/pathways/antenatal-and-postnatal-mental-health

National Maternity Review (2016) *Better Births. Improving Outcomes of Maternity Services in England. A Five Year Forward View for Maternity Care*. Available at: https://www.england.nhs.uk/wp-content/uploads/2016/02/national-maternity-review-report.pdf

Chapter 22

Baston H (2014) Antenatal care. In: Marshall J, Raynor M (eds) *Myles' Textbook for Midwives*. Elsevier.

healthtalk.org. *Maternity Care and Antenatal Visits*. Available at: http://www.healthtalk.org/peoples-experiences/pregnancy-children/pregnancy/maternity-care-and-antenatal-visits

Johnson R, Taylor W (2016) *Skills for Midwifery Practice*. Elsevier, London.

National Institute for Health and Care Excellence (NICE) (2016) *Antenatal Care for Uncomplicated Pregnancies*, CG62. Available at: https://www.nice.org.uk/guidance/cg62/chapter/Woman-centred-care

Royal College of Obstetricians and Gynaecologists (RCOG) (2013). *The Investigation and Management of Small-for-Gestational-Age Fetus*. Green Top Guideline No. 31.

Chapter 23

Centre for Maternal and Child Enquiries (CMACE) (2011). Saving Mothers' Lives: reviewing maternal deaths to make motherhood safer: 2006-08. The Eighth Report on Confidential Enquiries into Maternal Deaths in the United Kingdom. *BJOG*, 118 (Suppl.1),1–203.

Knight M, Kenyon S, Brocklehurst P, *et al.* (eds) on behalf of MBRRACEUK (2014) *Saving Lives, Improving Mothers' Care – Lessons Learned to Inform Future Maternity Care from the UK and Ireland Confidential Enquiries into Maternal Deaths and Morbidity 2009–12*. Oxford: National Perinatal Epidemiology Unit, University of Oxford.

Knight M, Tuffnell D, Kenyon S, *et al.* (eds) on behalf of MBRRACE-UK (2015) *Saving Lives, Improving Mothers' Care – Surveillance of Maternal Deaths in the UK 2011–13 and Lessons Learned to Inform Maternity Care from the UK and Ireland Confidential Enquiries into Maternal Deaths and Morbidity 2009–13*. Oxford: National Perinatal Epidemiology Unit, University of Oxford.

National Institute for Health and Care Excellence (NICE) (2006) *Postnatal Care up to 8 Weeks After Birth (updated 2015)*, CG37. Available at: https://www.nice.org.uk/guidance/cg37/resources/postnatal-care-up-to-8-weeks-after-birth-pdf-975391596997

Chapter 24

Marshall JE, Raynor MD (2014) *Myles Textbook for Midwives*, 16th edn. Churchill Livingstone.

National Collaborating Centre for Women's and Children's Health (2014) *Intrapartum Care – Care of Healthy Women and their Babies During Childbirth*. Clinical Guideline. Draft Guidelines. RCOG Press, London.

National Institute for Health and Care Excellence (NICE) (2014) *Intrapartum Care for Healthy Women and Babies (updated 2017)*, CG190. Available at: https://www.nice.org.uk/guidance/cg190/resources/intrapartum-care-for-healthy-women-and-babies-pdf-35109866447557

Chapter 25

Chalmers B, Kaczorowski J, Levitt C, *et al.* (2009) Use of routine interventions in vaginal labor and birth: findings from the maternity experience survey. *Birth*, 36, 22.

Johnstone R, Taylor W (2016) *Skills for Midwifery Practice*, 4th edn. Churchill Livingstone Elsevier, Edinburgh.

Murray ML, Huelsmann GM (2009) *Labor and Delivery Nursing: A Guide to Evidence-Based Practice*. Springer, New York.

National Institute for Health and Care Excellence (NICE) (2014) *Intrapartum Care for Healthy Women and Babies*, CG190. Available at: https://www.nice.org.uk/guidance/cg190

Chapter 26

Dixon l, Foureur M (2010) The vaginal examination during labour: is it benefit or harm? *New Zealand College of Midwives Journal*, 42, 21–26.

Downe S, Gyte ML, Dahlen HG, *et al.* (2013) Routine vaginal examinations for assessing progress of labour to improve outcomes for women and babies at term. *Cochrane Database of Systematic Reviews*, (7), CD010088.

Jackson K, Marshall JE, Brydon S (2014) Physiology and care during the first stage of labour. In: Marshall J, Raynor M (eds) *Myles Textbook for Midwives*, 16th edn. Churchill Livingstone, Edinburgh.

National Institute for Health and Care Excellence (NICE) (2014) *Intrapartum Care for Health Women and Babies* (CG190) Available at: https://www.nice.org.uk/guidance/cg190?UNLID=6240145162015781406

Chapter 27

Johnson R, Taylor W (2016) *Skills for Midwifery Practice*. Elsevier, London.

Leap N, Hunter B (2016) *Supporting Women for Labour and Birth*. Routledge, London.

Royal College of Midwives (2012) *Evidence Based Guidelines for Midwifery-Led Care in Labour. Positions for Labour and Birth*. RCM, London.

Royal College of Midwives (RCM) *Better Births*. Available at: http://betterbirths.rcm.org.uk/normal-births/

Royal College of Midwives (RCM) *Positions Used in Birth and Labour*. Available at: https://www.rcm.org.uk/clinical-practice-and-guidance/better-births/positions-used-in-birth-and-labour

Walsh D (2011) *Evidence and Skills for Normal Labour and Birth: A Guide for Midwives*, 2nd edn. Routledge, Oxfordshire.

Chapter 28

Hodnett ED, Gates S, Hofmeyr GJ, *et al.* (2013) Continuous support for women during childbirth. *Cochrane Database of Systematic Reviews*, (7), CD003766.

National Childbirth Trust (NCT) *Birth*. Available at: https://www.nct.org.uk/Birth

National Institute for Health and Care Excellence (NICE) (2014) *Intrapartum Care for Healthy Women and Babies*, CG190. Available at: https://www.nice.org.uk/guidance/cg190

Chapter 29

Dahl B, Malterud K (2015) Neither father nor biological mother: a qualitative study about lesbian co-mothers' maternity care experiences. *Sexual and Reproductive Healthcare*, 6, 169–173.

healthtalk.org. *Conditions that Threaten Women's Lives in Childbirth and Pregnancy*. Available at: http://www.healthtalk.org/peoples-experiences/pregnancy-children/conditions-threaten-womens-lives-childbirth-pregnancy/fathers-partners-experiences-hospital#ixzz4kTNAq9T5

Ledenfors A, Berterö C (2016) First time fathers' experiences of normal childbirth. *Midwifery*, 40, 26–31.

Snowdon C, Elbourne D, Forsey M, *et al.* (2012) Information-hungry and disempowered: a qualitative study of women and their partners' experiences of postpartum haemorrhage. *Midwifery*, 28, 791–799.

Steen M, Downe S, Bamford N, *et al.* (2012) Not-patient and not-visitor: a metasynthesis fathers' encounters with pregnancy, birth and maternity care. *Midwifery*, 28, 422–431.

Chapter 30

Lodge F, Haith-Cooper M (2016) The effect of maternal position at birth on perineal trauma. *British Journal of Midwifery*, 24, 172–180.

Priddis H, Schmied V, Dahlen H (2014) Women's experiences following severe perineal trauma: a qualitative study. *BMC Women's Health*, 14, 32.

Royal College of Midwives (2012) *Evidence Based Guidelines for Midwifery-led Care in Labour – Suturing the Perineum*. RCM, London.

Royal College of Midwives (2013) *How to Suture Correctly.* Available at: https://www.rcm.org.uk

Royal College of Obstetricians and Gynaecologists (2015) *The Management of Third- and Fourth-Degree Perineal Tears.* Green-top Guideline No. 29 RCOG, London. Available at: https://www.rcog.org.uk/globalassets/documents/guidelines/gtg-29.pdf

Chapter 31

Baergen RN (2011) *Manual of Pathology of the Human Placenta*, 2nd edn. Springer, New York.

Ceallaigh ME, Lotus Fertility. *Common Questions about Neonatal Umbilical Integrity(Lotus Birth): A Resource.* Available at: www.lotusfertility.com/Lotus_Birth_Q/Lotus_Birth_QA.html

Johnson R, Taylor W (2016) *Skills for Midwifery Practice.* Elsevier, London

Rankin W (2017) *Physiology in Childbearing.* Bailliere Tindall.

Chapter 32

Baston H (2011) Female bladder catheterisation: step by step. *Practising Midwife*, 14, 26–28.

Johnson R, Taylor W (2016) *Skills for Midwifery Practice*, 4th edn. Elsevier, Edinburgh.

National Institute for Health and Care Excellence (NICE) (2014) *Intrapartum Care for Healthy Women and Babies*, CG190. Available at: https://www.nice.org.uk/guidance/cg190

National Institute for Health and Care Excellence (NICE) (2014) *Quality Statement 4: Urinary Catheters*, QS61. Available at: www.nice.org.uk/guidance/qs61/chapter/Quality-statement-4-Urinary-catheters

Chapter 33

National Institute for Health and Care Excellence (NICE) (2008) *Antenatal Care for Uncomplicated Pregnancies*, CG62. Available at: https://www.nice.org.uk/guidance/cg62/chapter/1-guidance

National Institute for Health and Care Excellence (NICE) (2014) *Intrapartum Care for Healthy Women and Babies*, CG190. Available at https://www.nice.org.uk/guidance/cg190?unlid=624025600201579

Perinatal Institute. Available at: https://www.perinatal.org.uk/

Royal College of Midwives (RCM) (2012) *Evidence Based Guidelines for Midwifery-Led Care in Labour: Intermittent Auscultation (IA).* Available at: https://www.rcm.org.uk/sites/default/files/Intermittent%20Auscultation%20(IA)_0.pdf

Chapter 34

Ayres-De-Campos D, Spong CY, Chandraharan E (2015) FIGO consensus guidelines on intrapartum fetal monitoring: cardiotocography. *International Journal of Gynecology and Obstetrics*, 131, 13–24.

International Confederation of Midwives (ICM) (2011) *International Definition of the Midwife.* ICM, The Hague.

National Institute of Health and Care Excellence (NICE) (2014) *Intrapartum care for Healthy Women and Babies.* Available at: https://www.nice.org.uk/guidance/cg190/resources/intrapartum-care-for-healthy-women-and-babies-35109866447557

Chapter 35

Committee on Fetus and Newborn, American Academy of Pediatrics, and Committee on Obstetric Practice, American College of Obstetricians and Gynecologists (2015) *The Apgar Score. Committee Opinion no. 644.*

Li F, Wu T, Lei X, *et al.* (2013) The Apgar score and infant mortality. *PLOS One*, 8, e69072.

Chapter 36

England C (2014) Recognizing the healthy baby at term through examination of the newborn screening. In: Marshall JEM, Raynor MD (eds) *Myles Textbook for Midwives*, 16th edn. Churchill Livingstone, Edinburgh.

Lomax A (ed.) (2015) *Examination of the Newborn. An Evidence-Based Guide*, 2nd edn. Wiley Blackwell, Chichester.

National Patient Agency (2008) *Identification of Neonates: Antenatal.* NRLS-0798-ID-neonates-antenatal-2008-10-v1.pdf. Available at: http://www.nrls.npsa.nhs.uk

NHS England (2016) *National Maternity Review Better Births: Improving Outcomes of Maternity Services in England: A Five Year Forward View for Maternity Care.* Available at: https://www.england.nhs.uk/2016/02/maternity-review-2

UK National Screening Committee. Available at: www.gov.uk/government/groups/uk-national-screening-committee-uk-nsc

Chapter 37

Healthtalk (2016) *Comments for Health Professionals.* Available at: http://www.healthtalk.org/peoples-experiences/pregnancy-children/breastfeeding/comments-health-professionals

Lissauer T, Fanaroff A, Miall L, *et al.* (2016) *Neonatology at a Glance*, 3rd edn. John Wiley & Sons, Ltd., Oxford.

Michaelides S, Johnson G (2017) Physiology, assessment and care of the newborn. In: Macdonald S (ed.), *Mayes' Midwifery: a Textbook for Midwives*, 15th edn. Bailliere Tindall, London, 705–740.

Stanford Medicine. *Newborn Nursery at Lucile Packard Children's Hospital.* Available at: http://newborns.stanford.edu/PhotoGallery/AGA1.html

Chapter 38

Guerra L, Leonard M, Castagnetti M (2014) Best practice in the assessment of bladder function in infants. *Therapeutic Advances in Urology*, 6, 148–164.

Johnson R, Taylor W (2016) Assessment of the baby: daily examination. In: *Skills for Midwifery Practice*, 4th edn. Elsevier, Edinburgh, 301–306.

McNally S, Napier K, Welford H (2010) *What's in a Nappy?* A joint NCT/Simpson Centre for Reproductive Health Publication. Available at: https://www.nct.org.uk/sites/default/files/related_documents/What's%20in%20a%20nappy%20(ENGLISH%20VERSION)%20FINAL%20WITHOUT%20BLEED.pdf

National Institute for Health and Care Excellence (NICE) (2006) *Postnatal Care up to 8 Weeks after Birth*, CG37. Available at: https://www.nice.org.uk/guidance/cg37

Chapter 39

UK National Screening Committee (2016). *Newborn and Infant Physical Examination: Screening Programme Standards 2016/17.* Available at: https://www.gov.uk/government/uploads/system/uploads/attachment_data/file/524424/NIPE_Programme_Standards_2016_to_2017.pdf

Chapter 40

Healthtalk. *Looking Back – Preterm Birth and Special Care.* Available at: http://www.healthtalk.org/peoples-experiences/pregnancy-children/pregnancy/looking-back-preterm-birth-and-special-care

Lissauer T, Fanaroff A, Miall L, *et al.* (2016) *Neonatology at a Glance.* John Wiley & Sons, Ltd., Oxford.

Office for National Statistics (ONS) (2015) *Birth Characteristics in England and Wales 2014.* Available at: http://www.ons.gov.uk/ons/dcp171778_419005.pdf

Royal College of Obstetricians and Gynaecologists (RCOG) (2013) *The Investigation and Management of the Small-for-Gestational-Age Fetus*. Available at: https://www.rcog.org.uk/globalassets/documents/guidelines/gtg_31.pdf

Chapter 41

Barnes C, Adamson-Macedo E (2007) Perceived maternal parenting self-efficacy (PMP S-E) tool: development and validation with mothers of hospitalized preterm neonates. *Journal of Advanced Nursing*, 60, 550–560.

Brazelton Centre UK. Available at: http://brazelton.co.uk/

Imdad A, Bautista M, Senen K, *et al.* (2013) Umbilical cord antiseptics for preventing sepsis and death among newborns. *Cochrane Database of Systematic Reviews*, (5), CD008635.

Mumsnet. *Podcast*. Available at: http://www.mumsnet.com/babies/podcast

National Institute for Health and Care Excellence (NICE) (2006) *Postnatal Care up to 8 weeks After Birth*, CG37. Available at: https://www.nice.org.uk/guidance/cg37

National Institute for Health and Care Excellence (NICE) (2013) *Nappy Rash*. Available at: http://cks.nice.org.uk/nappy-rash#!scenario

NHS Choices (2015) *How to Change your Baby's Nappy*. Available at: http://www.nhs.uk/conditions/pregnancy-and-baby/pages/nappies.aspx

Nugent J, Keefer C, Minear S, *et al.* (2007) *Understanding Newborn Behavior and Early Relationships: The Newborn Behavioral Observations (NBO) System Handbook*. Paul Brooks Publishing Co, Maryland.

Public Health Agency (2016) *Birth to Five*. Available at: http://www.publichealth.hscni.net/publications/birth-five

Chapter 42

Alergy UK. *Childhood Food Allergy*. Available at: https://www.allergyuk.org/information-and-advice/conditions-and-symptoms/42-childhood-food-allergy

Baby Centre. *Bathing Equipment*. Available at: http://www.babycentre.co.uk/c559959/bathing-equipment

Baby Centre. *Bathing your Baby*. Available at: http://www.babycentre.co.uk/a37/bathing-your-baby#ixzz490vlpOAl

Blume-Peytavi U, Hauser M, Stamatas GN, *et al.* (2012) Skin care practices for newborns and infants: review of the clinical evidence for best practices. *Pediatric Dermatology*, 29, 1–14.

Care Quality Commission (CQC) (2015) *Maternity Services Survey*. Available at: http://www.cqc.org.uk/content/maternity-services-survey-2015

McCall E, Alderdice F, Halliday H, *et al.* (2010) Interventions to prevent hypothermia at birth in preterm and/or low birth-weight infants. *Cochrane Database of Systematic Reviews*, (3), CD004210.

Moore E, Anderson G, Bergman N, *et al.* (2012) Early skin-to-skin contact for mothers and their healthy newborn infants. *Cochrane Database of Systematic Reviews*, (5), CD003519.

Mums net. *Newborn Baby Bath Time*. Available at: http://www.mumsnet.com/Talk/parenting/479543-newborn-baby-bath-time

NHS Choices. *Washing and Bathing your Baby*. Available at: http://www.nhs.uk/conditions/pregnancy-and-baby/pages/washing-your-baby.aspx

Visscher MO, Adam R, Brink S, *et al.* (2015) Newborn infant skin: physiology, development and care. *Clinics in Dermatology*, 33, 271–280.

World Health Organisation (WHO) (2013) *Recommendations on Postnatal care of the Mother and Newborn*. Available at: http://apps.who.int/iris/bitstream/10665/97603/1/9789241506649_eng.pdf

Chapter 43

Colson S, Meeks J, Hawdon J (2008) Optimal positions for the release of primitive neonatal reflexes stimulating breastfeeding. *Early Human Development*, 84, 441–449.

Entwistle F (2013) *The Evidence and Rationale for the UNICEF UK Baby Friendly Initiative Standards*. UNICEF UK. Available at: http://www.unicef.org.uk/Documents/Baby_Friendly/Research/baby_friendly_evidence_rationale.pdf

UNICEF UK. *The Baby Friendly Initiative*. Available at: http://www.unicef.org.uk/BabyFriendly/

Widström A, Lilja G, Aaltomaa-Michalias P, *et al.* (2010) Newborn behaviour to locate the breast when skin-to-skin: A possible method for enabling early self-regulation. *Acta Pædiatrica*, 100, 79–85.

Chapter 44

Earle S (2000) Why some women do not breast feed: bottle feeding and fathers' role. *Midwifery*,16, 323–330.

Health and Social Care Information Centre (HSCIC) (2012) *Infant Feeding Survey 2010*. HSCIC, London.

National Institute for Health and Care Excellence (NICE) (2015) *Postnatal Care up to 8 Weeks after Birth*, CG37. Available at: https://www.nice.org.uk/guidance/cg37

UNICEF (2015) *A Guide to Bottle Feeding: How to Prepare Infant Formula and Sterilise Equipment to Minimise the Risks to your Baby*. Available at: http://www.unicef.org.uk/Documents/Baby_Friendly/Leaflets/start4life_guide_to_bottle_%20feeding.pdf

World Health Organisation (WHO) (1981) *The International Code of Marketing of Breastmilk Substitutes*. WHO Geneva.

Chapter 45

Cleft Lip and Palate Society (CLAPA). Available at: https://www.clapa.com/

Flint A, New K, Davis M (2016) Cup feeding versus other forms of supplemental enteral feeding for newborn infants unable to fully breastfeed. *Cochrane Database of Systematic Reviews*, (8), CD005092.

Johnson R, Taylor W (2016) *Skills for Midwifery Practice*, 4th edn. Elsevier, London.

National Patient Safety Agency (NPSA) (2005) *Reducing the Harm Caused by Misplaced Naso and Orogastric Feeding Tubes in Babies under the Care of Neonatal Units*. Available at: http://www.nrls.npsa.nhs.uk/resources/?entryid45=59798

Stevens E, Gazza E, Pickler R (2014) Parental experience learning to feed their preterm infant. *Advances in Neonatal Care*, 14, 354–361.

Chapter 46

Population Screening Programmes. *NHS Newborn Blood Spot (NBS) screening Programme*. Available at: https://www.gov.uk/topic/population-screening-programmes/newborn-blood-spot

Public Health England (PHE) (2016) *Guidelines for Newborn Blood Spot Sampling*. PHE Publications (Crown Copyright), London.

Public Health England (PHE) (2016) *Screening Tests for You and Your Baby*. PHE Publications (Crown Copyright), London.

Chapter 47

Brooks N (2014) *Venepuncture and Canulation*. M&K Publishing, Cumbria.

Johnson R, Taylor W (2016) *Skills for Midwifery Practice*. Elsevier, London.

National Institute of Health and Care Excellence (NICE) (2015) *Diabetes in Pregnancy: Management from Preconception to the Postnatal Period*, NG3. Available at: https://www.nice.org.uk/guidance/ng3

Royal College of Obstetricians and Gynaecologists (RCOG) (2013) *Gestational Diabetes*. Available at: https://www.rcog.org.uk/globalassets/documents/patients/patient-information-leaflets/pregnancy/pi-gestational-diabetes.pdf

Chapter 48

National Institute of Health and Care Excellence (NICE) (2014) *Intrapartum Care for Healthy Women and Babies*, CG190. Available at: https://www.nice.org.uk/guidance/cg190

Public Health England (2016) *Guidelines for Newborn Blood Spot Sampling*. Available at: https://www.gov.uk/government/uploads/system/uploads/attachment_data/file/511688/Guidelines_for_Newborn_Blood_Spot_Sampling_January_2016.pdf

Uga E, Candriella M, Perino A, *et al.* (2008) Heel lance in newborn during breastfeeding: an evaluation of the analgesic effect of this procedure. *Italian Journal of Paediatrics*, 34, 3.

Chapter 49

Jackson A. *Andrew Jackson's VIP Video*. Available at: https://ipsuk.wordpress.com/2008/01/23/andrew-jacksons-vip-video-2/

Keedle H, Schmied V, Burns E, *et al.* (2015) Women's reasons for, and experiences of, choosing a homebirth following a caesarean section. *BMC Pregnancy and Childbirth*, 15, 206.

McCallum L, Higgins D (2012) Care of peripheral venous cannula sites. *Nursing Times*, 108, 12–15.

National Health Service (NHS) (2007) *High Impact Intervention No. 2 Peripheral Intravenous Cannula Care Bundle*. Available at: http://webarchive.nationalarchives.gov.uk/20130107105354/http://www.dh.gov.uk/prod_consum_dh/groups/dh_digitalassets/@dh/@en/documents/digitalasset/dh_078121.pdf

Thomas R (2015) *Practical Medical Procedures at a Glance*. John Wiley & Sons Ltd., Oxford.

Chapter 50

Beetz R (2012) Evaluation and management of urinary tract infections in the neonate. *Current Opinion in Pediatrics*, 24, 205–211.

Graham H (2002) Urine analysis in the neonate: an important diagnostic aid. *Journal of Neonatal Nursing*, 8, 151–154.

National Institute for Health and Care Excellence (NICE) (2008) *Diabetes in Pregnancy: Management of Diabetes and its Complications from Pre-conception to the Postnatal Period*, CG63. Available at: https://www.nice.org.uk/guidance/cg63

Waugh J, Bell S, Kilby M, *et al.* (2005) Optimal bedside urinalysis for the detection of proteinuria in hypertensive pregnancy: a study of diagnostic accuracy. *BJOG*, 112, 412–417.

Chapter 51

Dougherty L, Lister S (eds) (2015) *The Royal Marsden Manual of Clinical Nursing Procedures: Professional Edition*, 9th edn. John Wiley & Sons, Ltd., Oxford.

Lecky D, Hawking M, McNulty C (2014) Patients' perspectives on providing a stool sample to their GP: a qualitative study. *British Journal of General Practice*, 64, 684–693.

NHS Choices (2016) *How Should I Collect and Store a Stool (Faeces) Sample?* Available at: http://www.nhs.uk/chq/Pages/how-should-i-collect-and-store-a-stool-faeces-sample.aspx?CategoryID=69

Public Health England (2014) *UK Standards for Microbiology Investigations. Investigation of Faecal Specimens for Enteric Pathogens*. Available at: https://www.gov.uk/government/uploads/system/uploads/attachment_data/file/343955/B_30i8.1.pdf

Royal College of Nursing (RCN) (2014) *The Management of Waste Arising from Health, Social and Personal Care*. RCN, London.

Chapter 52

Public Health England (2016) *UK Standards for Microbiology Investigations B11: Investigation of Swabs from Skin and Superficial Soft Tissue Infections*. Available at: https://www.gov.uk/government/uploads/system/uploads/attachment_data/file/544453/B_11i6.1.pdf

Patient. *Wound Infection*. Available at http://patient.info/health/wound-infection

Chapter 53

Evans A, Morgan M (2012) The high vaginal swab in general practice. *Practice Nursing*, 23, 330–337.

Johnson R, Taylor W (2016) *Skills for Midwifery Practice*, 4th edn. Elsevier.

Royal College of Obstetricians and Gynaecologists (RCOG) (2010) *Preterm Prelabour Rupture of Membranes*, Green Top Guideline No. 44. RCOG, London.

Chapter 54

Boulvain M, Stan C, Irion O (2005) Membrane sweeping for induction of labour. *Cochrane Database of Systematic Reviews*, (1), CD000451.

De Miranda E, van der Bom J, Bonsel G, *et al.* (2006) Membrane sweeping and prevention of post-term pregnancy in low-risk pregnancies: a randomised controlled trial. *BJOG*, 113, 402–408.

McCarthy F, Kenny L (2014) Induction of labour. *Obstetrics, Gynaecology and Reproductive Medicine*, 24, 9–15.

Rogers H (2010) Does a cervical membrane sweep in a term healthy pregnancy reduce the length of gestation? *MIDIRS Midwifery Digest*, 20, 315–319.

Royal College of Midwives (RCM) Available at: www.rcm.org.uk

Chapter 55

Goonewardene M, Rameez MFM, Kaluarachchi A, *et al.* (2011) WHO recommendations for induction of labour: RHL commentary. *WHO Reproductive Health Library*. World Health Organization, Geneva.

National Institute for Health and Care Excellence (NICE) (2008) *Inducing Labour*, CG70. Available at: https://www.nice.org.uk/guidance/cg70

National Institute for Health and Care Excellence (NICE) (2014) *Inducing Labour*, QS60. Available at: https://www.nice.org.uk/guidance/qs60

Chapter 56

National Institute for Health and Care Excellence (NICE) (2008) *Inducing Labour*, CG70. Available at: https://www.nice.org.uk/guidance/cg70

National Institute for Health and Care Excellence (NICE) (2014) *Intrapartum Care for Healthy Women and Babies*, CG190. Available at: https://www.nice.org.uk/guidance/cg190

Nursing and Midwifery Council (NCM) (2015) *The Code*. Available at: https://www.nmc.org.uk/standards/code/

Royal College of Midwives (2012) *Evidence Based Guidelines for Midwifery Led Care in Labour. Rupturing Membranes*. Available at: https://www.rcm.org.uk/sites/default/files/Rupturing%20Membranes.pdf

Smyth RMD, Markham C, Dowsell T (2013) Amniotomy for shortening spontaneous labour. *Cochrane Database of Systematic Reviews*, (6), CD006167.

Chapter 57

Hinton L, Locock L, Knight M (2015) Maternal critical care: what can we learn from patient experience? *BMJ Open*, 5, e006676.

KnightM,KenyonS,BrocklehurstP,*etal.*(eds)onbehalfofMBRRACE-UK. *Saving Lives, Improving Mothers' Care – Lessons learned to inform future maternity care from the UK and Ireland Confidential Enquiries into Maternal Deaths and Morbidity 2009–12.* National Perinatal Epidemiology Unit, University of Oxford. Available at: https://www.npeu.ox.ac.uk/downloads/files/mbrrace-uk/reports/Saving%20Lives%20Improving%20Mothers%20Care%20report%202014%20Full.pdf

Resuscitation Council (UK) Available at: https://www.resus.org.uk/

Royal College of Obstetricians and Gynaecologists (RCOG) (2011) *Maternal Collapse in Pregnancy and the Puerperium.* Green-top Guideline No. 56. Available at: https://www.rcog.org.uk/globalassets/documents/guidelines/gtg_56.pdf

Chapter 58

Schroeder R, Barbeito A, Bar-Yosef S, *et al.* (2015) Cardiovascular monitoring. In: Miller RD (ed.) *Miller's Anesthesia*, 8th edn. Churchill Livingstone, 2009.

Taylor RW, Palagiri AV (2007) Central venous catheterization: concise definitive review. *Critical Care Medicine*, 35, 1390–1396.

Veille JC, Kitzman DW, Bacevice AE (1996) Effects of pregnancy on the electrocardiogram in healthy subjects during strenuous exercise. *American Journal of Obstetrics and Gynecology*, 175, 1360–1364.

World Health Organisation. *Pulse OximetryTraining Manual.* Available at: http://www.who.int/patientsafety/safesurgery/pulse_oximetry/who_ps_pulse_oxymetry_training_manual_en.pdf

Chapter 59

Dougherty L, Lister S (2015) Fluid balance. In: *The Royal Marsden Manual of Clinical Nursing Procedures: Professional Edition*, 9th edn. John Wiley & Sons, Ltd., Oxford, pp. 254–265.

Mothers and Babies Reducing Risk through Audit and Confidential Enquiries (MBRRACE) (2014) *Saving Lives, Improving Mothers' Care. Lessons Learned to Inform Future Maternity Care from the UK and Ireland Confidential Enquiries into Maternal Deaths and Morbidity 2009-2012.* Available at: https://www.npeu.ox.ac.uk/downloads/files/mbrrace-uk/reports/Saving%20Lives%20Improving%20Mothers%20Care%20report%202014%20Full.pdf

Shepherd A (2011) Measuring and managing fluid balance. *Nursing Times*, 107, 12–16.

Welch K (2010) Fluid balance. *Learning Disability Practice*, 13, 33–38.

Chapter 60

Asthma UK. Available at: https://www.asthma.org.uk

De Swiet M, Williamson C, Lewis G (2011) Other indirect deaths in CMACE (Centre for Maternal and Child Enquiries) saving mother's lives: reviewing maternal deaths to make motherhood safer 2006-2008. The eighth report on confidential enquires into maternal deaths in the United Kingdom. *International Journal of Obstetrics and Gynaecology*, 118 (Suppl. 1), 119–131

Durrani S, Busse W (2014) Management of asthma in adolescents and adults. In: Adkinson N, Bochner B, Burks A, *et al.* (eds), *Middleton's Allergy Principles and Practice*, 8th edn. Elsevier Saunders, Philadelphia, PA, 902–922.

Jensen D, Webb, K, Davies G, *et al.* (2009) Mechanisms of activity-related breathlessness in healthy human pregnancy. *European Journal of Applied Physiology*, 106, 253–265.

Jones A, Pill R, Adams S (2000) Qualitative study of views of health professionals and patients on guided self management plans for asthma. *British Medical Journal*, 321, 1507.

National Institute for Health and Care Excellence (NICE) (2013) *Asthma*, QS25. Available at: www.nice.org.uk/guidance/QS25

National Institutes of Health, US National Library of Medicine. Available at: https://www.nlm.nih.gov

NHS Choices. *Asthma.* Available at: http://www.nhs.uk/conditions/asthma/pages/introduction.aspx

Chapter 61

Knight M, Tuffnell D, Kenyon S, *et al.* (eds) on behalf of MBRRACE-UK (2015) *Saving Lives, Improving Mothers' Care - Surveillance of Maternal Deaths in the UK 2011-13 and Lessons Learned to Inform Maternity Care from the UK and Ireland Confidential Enquiries into Maternal Deaths and Morbidity 2009-13.* National Perinatal Epidemiology Unit, University of Oxford.

Lewis G (2007) *The Confidential Enquiry into Maternal and Child Health (CEMACH) Saving Mother's Lives: Reviewing Maternal Deaths to Make Motherhood Safer.* The Seventh Report on Confidential Enquiries into Maternal Deaths in the United Kingdom. CEMACH, London. Available at: http://www.publichealth.hscni.net/sites/default/files/Saving%20Mothers%27%20Lives%202003-05%20.pdf

Resuscitation Council (UK). Available at: https://www.resus.org.uk/

Resuscitation Council UK (2016) *Immediate Life Support*, 4th edn. Resuscitation Council (UK), London.

Teasdale G (2014) *Glasgow Coma Scale.* Available at: http://www.glasgowcomascale.org/

Teasdale G, Jennett B (1974) Assessment of coma and impaired consciousness. A practical scale. *Lancet*, 2, 81–84.

Chapter 62

Hospice UK (2015) *Updated Guidance for Professionals who Provide Care after Death.* Hospice UK, London. Available at: https://www.hospiceuk.org/media-centre/press-releases/details/2015/04/22/updated-guidance-for-professionals-who-provide-care-after-death

Jessica's Trust (2008) Available at: http://www.jessicastrust.org.uk/

Stillbirth and Neonatal Death Society (SANDS) (2007) *Pregnancy Loss and the Death of a Baby.* Bosun Press, Shepperton.

Chapter 63

Bedford Russell A (2015) Neonatal sepsis. *Paediatrics and Child Health*, 25, 271–275.

National Institute for Health and Clinical Excellence (NICE) (2012) *Neonatal Infection (Early Onset): Antibiotics for Prevention and Treatment*, CG149. Available at: http://www.nice.org.uk/guidance/cg149

Royal College of Obstetricians and Gynaecologists (RCOG) (2012) *The Prevention of Early-onset Neonatal Group β Streptococcal Disease.* Green-top Guideline No.36. RCOG, London.

Watson G, Caldwell C, Kennea N (2016) *Neonatal early onset sepsis: a reflection on the NICE guidance. Infant*, 12, 133–135.

Chapter 64

Ives NK (2015) Management of neonatal jaundice. *Paediatrics and Child Health*, 25, 276–281.

National Institute for Health and Care Excellence (NICE) (2016) *Jaundice in Newborn Babies under 28 Days*, CG98. Available at: https://www.nice.org.uk/guidance/cg98

Stowkowski L (2011) Fundamentals of phototherapy for neonatal jaundice. *Advances in Neonatal Care*, 11 (5 Suppl.), S10–S21.

Wentworth S (2005) Neonatal phototherapy – today's lights, lamps and devices. *Infant*, 1, 14–19.

Chapter 65

British Association of Perinatal Medicine (2017) *Identification and Management of Neonatal Hypoglycaemia in the Full Term Infant*

– *A Framework for Practice.* Available at: http://www.bapm.org/publications/Hypoglycaemia%20F4P%20May%202017.pdf

Deshpande S, Ward Platt M (2005) The investigation and management of neonatal hypoglycaemia. *Seminars in Fetal and Neonatal Medicine*, 10, 351–361.

National Institute for Health and Care Excellence (NICE) (2015) *Diabetes in Pregnancy: Management from Preconception to the Postnatal Period*, NG3. Available at: https://www.nice.org.uk/guidance/ng3/chapter/1-recommendations?unlid=87047696620 1671419458ations?unlid=87047696620167141945 8#/postnatal-care-2

World Health Organisation (WHO) (1997) *Hypoglycaemia of the Newborn. Review of the Literature.* WHO, Geneva.

Chapter 66

Knobel R (2014) Fetal and neonatal thermal physiology. *Newborn and Infant Nursing Reviews*, 14, 45–49.

Laptook A, Watkinson M (2008) Temperature management in the delivery room. *Seminars in Fetal and Neonatal Medicine*, 13, 383–391.

Thomas K (1994) Thermoregulation in neonates. *Neonatal Network*, 13, 15–22.

World Health Organisation (WHO) (1997) *Thermal Protection of the Newborn: a Practical Guide.* Available at: http://apps.who.int/iris/bitstream/10665/63986/1/WHO_RHT_MSM_97.2.pdf

Chapter 67

Peate I, Glencross W (2015) *Wound Care at a Glance.* John Wiley & Sons, Ltd., Oxford.

Kettle C (2015) Perineal pain: a neglected area. *13th National Conference on Current Issues in Midwifery. The Changing Landscape of Maternity Care.* London.

Wound Care Alliance UK. *Achieving Effective Outcomes in Patients with Over Granulation.* Available at: www.wcauk.org

Chapter 68

Abdelrahman T, Newton H (2011) Wound dressings: principles and practice. *Surgery*, 29, 491–495.

Hatfield A, Tronson M (2008) *The Complete Recovery Room Book*, 4th edn. Oxford University Press.

Jones V, Grey JE, Harding KG (2006) ABC of wound healing: wound dressings. *British Medical Journal*, 332, 777–780.

Kirk RM (2010) *Basic Surgical Techniques*, 6th edn. Churchill Livingstone, Edinburgh.

Chapter 69

Johnson R, Taylor W (2016) *Skills for Midwifery Practice*, 4th edn. Elsevier, Edinburgh.

Mainstone A (2004) Sutures, surgical needles and perineal trauma. *British Journal of Midwifery*, 12, 771–776.

Pudner R (2010) *Nursing the Surgical Patient*, 3rd edn. Bailliere Tindall, Edinburgh.

Royal College of Obstetricians and Gynaecologists (RCOG) (2015) *The Management of Third- and Fourth- Degree Perineal Tears*, Green-top Guideline No. 29. Available at: https://www.rcog.org.uk/globalassets/documents/guidelines/gtg-29.pdf

Chapter 70

Knight M, Kenyon S, Brocklehurst P, *et al.* (eds) on behalf of MBRRACE-UK (2014) *Saving Lives, Improving Mothers' Care. Lessons Learned to Inform Future Maternity Care from the UK and Ireland Confidential Enquiries into Maternal Deaths and Morbidity 2009-2012.* National Perinatal Epidemiology Unit, University of Oxford.

National Institute for Health and Care Excellence (NICE) (2015) *Venous Thromboembolism: Reducing the Risk for Patients in Hospital*, CG92. Available at: https://www.nice.org.uk/guidance/cg92.

Royal College of Obstetricians and Gynaecologists (RCOG) (2015) *Reducing the Risk of Venous Thromboembolism during Pregnancy and the Puerperium*, Green Top Guideline No 37a. RCOG, London.

Scottish Intercollegiate Guideline Network (SIGN) (2010) *Prevention and Management of Venous Thromboembolism*, No 122. SIGN, Edinburgh.

Chapter 71

Bates SM, Greer IA, Pabinger I, *et al.* (2008) Venous thromboembolism, thrombophilia, antithrombotic therapy and pregnancy: American College of Chest Physicians Evidence-Based Clinical Practice Guidelines, 8th edition. *Chest*, 6 (Suppl), 844S–846S.

National Institute for Health and Care Excellence (NICE) (2015) *Venous Thromboembolism: Reducing the Risk for Patients in Hospital*, CG92. Available at: https://www.nice.org.uk/guidance/cg92

Royal College of Obstetricians and Gynaecologists (RCOG) (2015) *Reducing the Risk of Venous Thromboembolism during Pregnancy and the Puerperium*, Green Top Guideline No. 37a. RCOG, London.

Sajid MS, Tai NRM, Goli G, *et al.* (2006) Knee versus thigh length graduated compression stockings for prevention of deep vein thrombosis: a systematic review. *European Journal of Vascular and Endovascular Surgery*, 32, 730–736.

Chapter 72

British National Formulary (BNF) (2016) Available at: https://www.bnf.org/

Medicines and Healthcare Products Regulatory Agency (MHRA) (2014) *Patient Group Directions: Who Can Use Them.* Available at: www.gov.uk/government/publications/patient-group-directions-pgds/patient-group-directions-who-can-use-them

Nursing Midwifery Council (NMC) (2010) *Standards for Medicines Management.* Available at: www.nmc.org.uk/standards/additional-standards/standards-for-medicines-management/

Nursing Midwifery Council (NMC) (2011) *Annexe 1 to NMC 07/2011 Changes to Midwives Exemptions.* Available at: https://www.nmc.org.uk/globalassets/siteDocuments/Circulars/2011Circulars/nmcCircular07-2011_Midwives-Exemptions-Annexes.pdf

Chapter 73

Chadwick A, Withnell N (2015) How to administer intramuscular injections. *Nursing Standard*, 30, 36–39.

Clinical Skills.net. Available at: https://www.clinicalskills.net/

Johnson R, Taylor W (2016) *Skills for Midwifery Practice*, 4th edn. Elsevier, Edinburgh.

Nursing and Midwifery Council (2010) *Standards for Medicines Management.* Available at: www.nmc.org.uk

Chapter 74

Dougherty L, Lister S (eds) (2015) *The Royal Marsden Manual of Clinical Nursing Procedures: Professional Edition*, 9th edn. John Wiley & Sons, Ltd., Oxford.

Institute for Safe Medication Practice (ISMP) (2015) *ISMP Safe Practice Guidelines for Adult IV Push Medications.* Available at: http://www.ismp.org/Tools/guidelines/ivsummitpush/ivpushmedguidelines.pdf

Lavery I, Ingram P (2008) Safe practice in intravenous medicines administration. *Nursing Standard*, 22, 44–47.

Medicines and Healthcare products Regulatory Agency (MHRA) (2014). *Patient Safety Alert, Stage Three: Directive. Improving*

Medication Error Incident Reporting and Learning. NHS England. Available at: https://www.england.nhs.uk/wp-content/uploads/2014/03/psa-sup-info-med-error.pdf

Chapter 75

British National Formulary. Available at: https://www.bnf.org/products/bnf-online/

Johnson R, Taylor W (2016) *Skills for Midwifery Practice.* Elsevier, London.

Nursing and Midwifery Council (NMC) (2007) *Standards for Medicine Management.* NMC, London.

Royal College of Midwives (RCM) *RCM Entonox Guidance.* Available at: https://www.rcm.org.uk/content/entonox

Twigg M, Lupattelli A, Nordeng H (2016) Women's beliefs about medication use during their pregnancy: a UK perspective. *International Journal of Clinical Pharmacology,* 38, 968–976.

Chapter 76

National Institute for Health and Care Excellence (NICE) *BNF for Children.* Available at: https://bnfc.nice.org.uk/

Nursing and Midwifery Council (NMC) (2010) *Standards for Medicines Management.* Available at: https://www.nmc.org.uk/standards/additional-standards/standards-for-medicines-management/

Pape TM (2003) Applying airline safety practices to medication administration. *Medsurg Nursing,* 12, 77–93.

Shah V, Taddio A, Rieder M (2009) Effectiveness and tolerability of pharmacologic and combined interventions for reducing injection pain during routine childhood immunizations: Systematic review and meta-analyses. *Clinical Therapeutics,* 31 (Suppl. 2), S104–151.

Chapter 77

Oxford Vaccine Group (2016) *Vaccines in Development: Respiratory Syncytial Virus (RSV) and Group B Streptococcus.* Available at: https://www.ovg.ox.ac.uk/research

Public Health England (PHE) (2016) *Immunisation Against Infectious Disease: the Green Book.* Available at: https://www.gov.uk/government/collections/immunisation-against-infectious-disease-the-green-book

Public Health England (PHE/NHS) (2016) *Screening Programmes. Continuing Professional Development for Screening, Resource Cards.* Available at: http://cpd.screening.nhs.uk/resource-cards

World Health Organization, Global Advisory Committee for Vaccine Safety (WHO GAVS) (2014) *Safety of Immunization during Pregnancy: A Review of the Evidence.* Available at: http://www.who.int/vaccine_safety/publications/safety_pregnancy_nov2014.pdf

Chapter 78

Anaesthesia UK. Available at: http://www.anaesthesiauk.com

Anim-Somuah M, Smyth RMD, Jones L (2011) Epidural versus non-epidural or no analgesia in labour. *Cochrane Database of Systematic Reviews,* (12), CD000331.

Jones L, Othman M, Dowswell T, *et al.* (2013) Pain management for women in labour: an overview of systematic reviews. *Cochrane Database of Systematic Reviews,* (3), CD009234.

National Collaborating Centre for Women's and Children's Health (NCC-WCH) (2014) *Intrapartum Care: Care of Healthy Women and their Babies during Childbirth.* NCC-WCH, London.

Chapter 79

Expectancy. *Natural Therapies for Natural Births.* Available at: http://www.expectancy.co.uk

Jones L, Othman M, Dowswell T, *et al.* (2013) Pain management for women in labour: an overview of systematic reviews. *Cochrane Database of Systematic Reviews,* (3), CD009234.

National Collaborating Centre for Women's and Children's Health (NCC-WCH) (2014) *Intrapartum Care: Care of Healthy Women and their Babies during Childbirth.* NCC-WCH, London.

Chapter 80

British Society for Haematology (BSH) (2009) Guideline on the Administration of Blood Components. Available at: http://www.bcshguidelines.com/documents/Admin_blood_components_bcsh_05012010.pdf

Learn Blood Transfusion. Available at: http://www.learnbloodtransfusion.org.uk

Royal College of Obstetrics and Gynaecology (RCOG) (2015) Blood Transfusion in Obstetrics, Green-top Guideline No. 47. Available at: https://www.rcog.org.uk/globalassets/documents/guidelines/gtg-47.pdf

Serious Hazards of Transfusion Report (SHOT) (2014) Annual SHOT Report 2014. Available at: https://www.shotuk.org/wp-content/uploads/report-2014.pdf

Chapter 81

Bolton-Maggs PHB, Davies T, Poles D, *et al.* (2013) Errors in anti-D immunoglobulin administration: retrospective analysis of 15 years' reports to the UK confidential haemovigilance scheme. *British Journal of Obstetrics and Gynaecology,* 120, 873–878.

National Institute for Health and Care Excellence (NICE) (2008) *Routine Antenatal anti-D Prophylaxis for Women who are Rhesus D Negative,* TA 156. Available at: https://www.nice.org.uk/guidance/ta156/resources/routine-antenatal-antid-prophylaxis-for-women-who-are-rhesus-d-negative-82598318102725

Serious Hazards of Transfusion (SHOT) *Anti-D Administration Checklist.* Available at: http://www.shotuk.org/wp-content/uploads/2010/03/SHOT-Anti-D-Administration-Checklist-v12-Oct-2012.pdf

Serious Hazards of Transfusion (SHOT) *SHOT Resources.* Available at: http://www.shotuk.org/wp-content/uploads/Resource-List.pdf

Soothill PW, Finning K, Latham T, et al. (2015) Use of cffDNA to avoid administration of anti-D to pregnant women when the fetus is RhD-negative: implementation in the NHS. *British Journal of Obstetrics and Gynaecology,* 122, 1682–1686.

Glossary

Ankyloglossia Ubiquitously referred to as 'tongue-tie'. It is apparent in some babies where a tight piece of skin between the underside of the tongue and the lingual frenulum (floor of the mouth) is visible.

Apgar score A crude measure of the neonate's condition in the first minute at birth based on five criteria on a scale of 0 to 2. The Apgar score is repeated at 5 minutes and again at 10 minutes if necessary. It accounts for: appearance (of skin colour); pulse; grimace (reflex irritability); activity (muscle tone) and respiration.

Asepsis Absence or avoidance of contamination by micro-organisms.

Aseptic technique A process (technique) used to achieve asepsis.

Asynclitism Situation in a cephalic presentation where a parietal bone of the fetal head is tilted towards one or other shoulder.

Bilirubin encephalopathy (kernicterus) A condition that arises when unconjugated bilirubin is high and deposits in the fatty tissues of the brain and results in brain injury. Damage can result in hearing loss, visual problems, cerebral palsy and intellectual disability.

Bolus A substance, usually a medicine, given as a single large dose.

Brown adipose tissue (BAT) (brown fat) The main source of energy used to generate heat in the newborn, a process called non-shivering thermogenesis. It is heavily innervated by the sympathetic nervous system and has a rich blood supply (giving it a dark appearance). It develops late in the second trimester and can be found down the scapulae, neck, sternum and the adrenal glands.

Cannula A thin tube inserted into a vein to deliver fluids or drugs.

Capillary refill time (CRT) A measure of peripheral perfusion to the tissues. It is defined as the time it takes in seconds for colour to return to the capillaries under the skin after pressure or blanching is applied. A normal CRT in a neonate is less than 3 seconds.

Caput succedaneum An oedematous swelling under the scalp but above the periosteum.

Circulatory system The organ system that allows blood to travel round the body. Also known as the cardiovascular system.

Competent person A competent person is someone who has sufficient training and experience or knowledge and other qualities that allow them to carry out the role. The level of competence required will depend on the complexity of the situation.

Conduction (heat loss) Occurs when a warm infant loses or transfers heat to a cooler object in direct contact. For example, using weighing scales not covered with a paper towel or blanket.

Conjugation The process that takes place in the liver whereby unconjugated or fat-soluble bilirubin is converted to conjugated or water-soluble bilirubin by the enzyme uridine diphosphate (UDP) glucuronyl transferase so that it can be excreted by the gut.

Convection (heat loss) Occurs when heat is lost or transferred from the warmer infant to the cooler surrounding air. For example, as a result of a fan on in the delivery room after the infant is born.

Counter-regulation The process by which the body makes glucose available in the fasted state.

Controlled drugs These are classified by law based on their benefit when used in medical treatment and their harm if misused. Controlled drugs should be administered in line with relevant legislation and local standard operating procedures.

C-reactive protein (CRP) A non-specific inflammatory product produced by the liver in response to infection or tissue injury.

Dipsticks Reagent strips coated with chemicals.

Evaporation (heat loss) Occurs when a liquid is converted to a vapour. Energy is required and therefore lost when this change in state occurs. For example, the evaporation of amniotic fluid from the newborn's skin at delivery results in heat loss and cools the baby.

Exudate Produced as a result of inflammation. It consists of cells and fluid that has moved out of the circulatory system.

Female genital mutilation (FGM) Deliberate cutting of a female's genitals, a practice that has cultural and societal roots and is believed to protect young women from promiscuity.

Gluconeogenesis The formation of glucose from non-carbohydrate substances such as lactate, pyruvate, glycerol (from the breakdown of fat) and alanine. Takes place in the liver.

Glycogenolysis The breaking down of glycogen. It is the initial counter-regulatory process in the newborn.

Grunting An expiratory sound made by infants in respiratory distress. In an effort to retain air in the lungs at end expiration, the infant close the glottis and the sound is made by air forced past the closed glottis.

Hypoglycaemia Occurs when the blood glucose is below 2.6 mmol/L.

Hypothermia Occurs when the infant's body temperature is less than 36.5°C.

Infusion The introduction of a fluid into a vein.

Intravenous Into a vein.

Irritant contact dermatitis An irritant directly damages cells if in contact with the skin in sufficient concentration and for sufficient time The signs and symptoms of irritant contact dermatitis can include redness, soreness, dryness or cracking of the skin.

Jitteriness Defined by UNICEF as 'excessive repetitive movements of one or more limbs, which are unprovoked and usually relatively fast. It is important to be sure that this movement is not simply a response to stimuli' (UNICEF (2013) Guidance on the development of policies and guidelines for the prevention and management of Hypoglycaemia of the Newborn, p. 6).

Ketone bodies Formed from the metabolism of fatty acids and can be used by the neonatal brain as an alternative fuel to glucose.

Lanugo Fine, downy hair that is usually found on the body of the fetus/some newborn babies, especially if preterm.

M, C & S Microscopy, culture and sensitivity.

Midwives exemptions (ME) Medicinal products that midwives can supply and administer on their own initiative provided it is appropriate and within the course of their professional midwifery practice.

Neutral thermal environment The temperature of the infant's environment that allows the infant to use the least amount of oxygen to maintain a normal body temperature. This temperature will vary from baby to baby and will be determined by gestation, postnatal age and wellbeing.

Non-accidental injury Physical injury to a child (under the age of 18) deliberately carried out.

Occupational exposure incident An incident whereby a healthcare worker is exposed to blood or other high-risk body fluids. The highest risk to the healthcare worker is the transmission of blood-borne infections.

Patient group direction (PGD) A written instruction for the sale, supply and administration of medicines to patients, usually in planned circumstances or an identified clinical situation.

Patient specific direction A written instruction from a qualified and registered prescriber for a medicine including the dose, route

Midwifery Skills at a Glance, First Edition. Edited by Patricia Lindsay, Carmel Bagness and Ian Peate.
© 2018 John Wiley & Sons, Ltd. Published 2018 by John Wiley & Sons, Ltd.

and frequency or appliance to be supplied or administered to a named patient.

Percutaneous injury An injury that occurs when the skin of the healthcare worker is broken by a human bite, needle, scratch or other sharp item.

Personal protective equipment (PPE) Equipment that is intended to be worn or held by a person at work and that protects them against one or more risks to health or safety.

Pharmacovigilance The science and activities relating to ensuring the detection, assessment, understanding and prevention of adverse effects or any other drug-related problem.

Phototherapy A common neonatal treatment that uses light to reduce unconjugated bilirubin levels by converting it into a water soluble and excretable product without passing through the conjugation step.

Postexposure prophylaxis (PEP) Antiretroviral medication used to reduce the risk of seroconversion to HIV following a significant exposure incident. Its use should only follow a risk assessment and should be started within 72 hours.

Pyuria Pus cells in urine.

Pus A liquid produced in the presence of infection, often yellow in colour. It is made up of debris, white blood cells and bacteria.

Radiation (heat loss) Occurs when the infant loses heat to a cooler object that is not in direct contact with the infant. For example, the infant placed near a cool window will lose heat to that window. Radiant losses can be reduced by dressing the infant in clothing.

Reasonably practicable Balancing the level of risk against the measures needed to control the real risk in terms of money, time or trouble.

SBAR (situation background assessment recommendation) A tool used in healthcare to logically and effectively communicate to key team members information and concerns about a patient to ensure assessment and safe management.

Scavenger system A medical device used in hospitals to collect and remove gas after it is exhaled from the patient.

Sensorineural hearing loss (SNHL) Results from damage to the hair cells in the cochlea (inner ear) and/or 8th cranial nerve.

Sharp An item used in the delivery of healthcare that can cut or pierce the skin.

Skin surveillance A type of health surveillance required under health and safety law where employers have a system in place to ensure that exposures to hazardous substances are controlled and not causing skin conditions such as dermatitis.

Standard operating procedures (SOP) Step by step instructions that should specify in writing what should be done, when, where and by whom.

Sterile An item free from micro-organisms.

Transepidermal water loss (TEWL) A measure of water in $g/m^2/h$ that passes through the skin by means of diffusion. Evaporation of this water can lead to heat loss and dehydration as it evaporates from the neonate's skin. The more immature the skin is, the greater the TEWL.

Type I allergy Type l allergic reaction is an immediate allergic reaction to natural rubber latex (NRL) proteins. In rare cases can result in anaphylactic shock. Clinical reactions can involve the skin, eyes, mucous membranes and respiratory system, including localised or generalised rash (urticaria), inflammation of the mucous membranes in the nose (rhinitis), red and swollen eyes with discharge (conjunctivitis) and asthma.

Type IV allergy Type lV allergic reactions or allergic contact dermatitis. This is an allergic response to the chemical additives, known as accelerators, used in the manufacture of natural rubber latex (NRL) gloves. The signs and symptoms may be indistinguishable from those of irritant contact dermatitis, and diagnosis will require clinical assessment. Sensitisation can take months or years but, once sensitised, a type IV allergic response occurs between 10 and 24 hours after exposure and can get worse over the subsequent 72 hours.

Vernix (caseosa) A creamy white substance that covers and protects the fetus's skin from the effects of the amniotic fluid, and is commonly present at birth.

Vulnerable site A body site that if contaminated by micro-organisms can result in infection, e.g. open wound, vascular access device, epidural catheter site.

Index

Page numbers in **bold** refer to tables; those in *italics* refer to illustrations

Printed and bound by CPI Group (UK) Ltd, Croydon, CR0 4YY